The People's Hospital
1903-2003

By David Lowe and Paul Swift

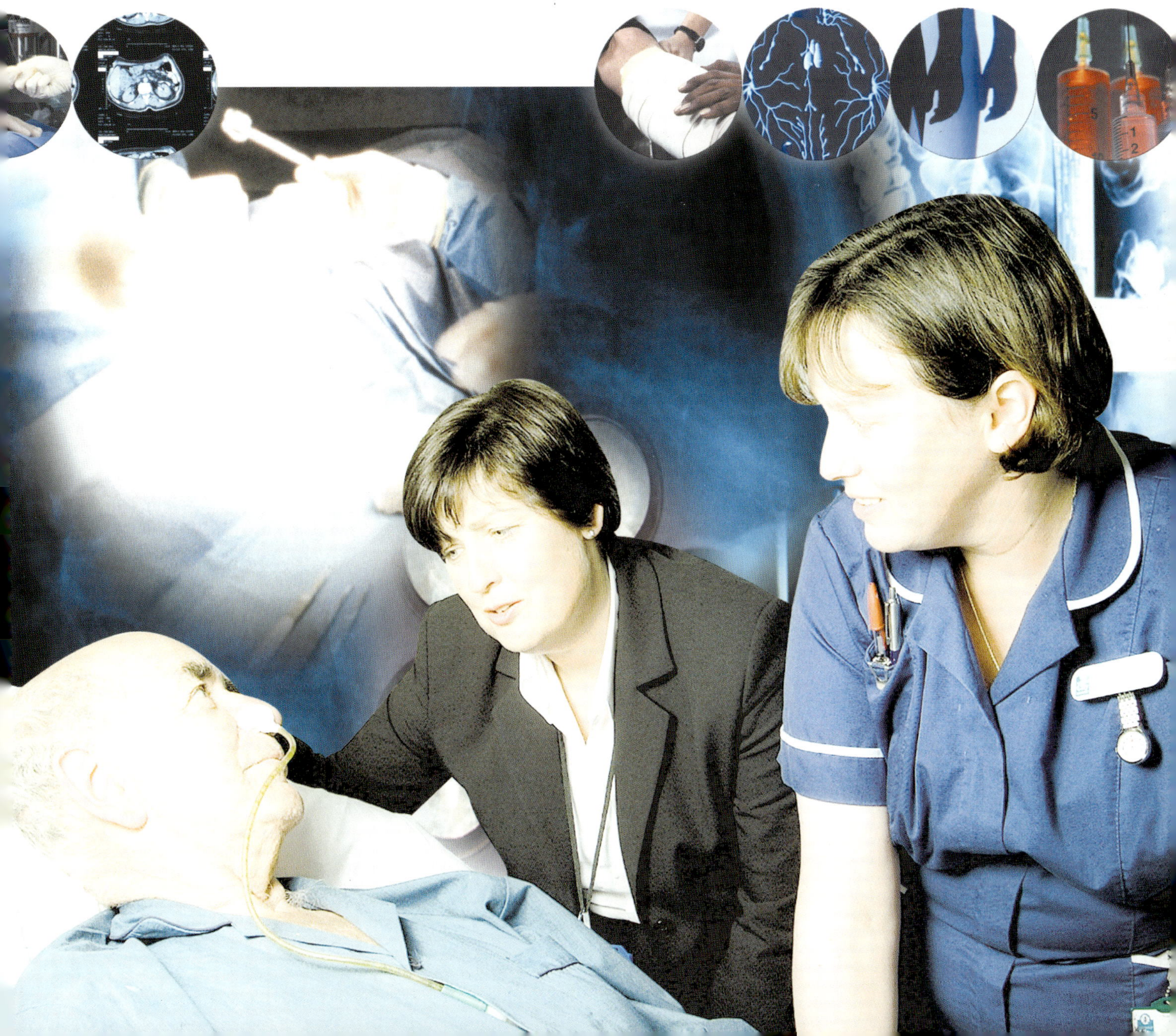

The People's Hospital

Published by Nottingham City Hospital NHS Trust,
Hucknall Road,
Nottingham
NG5 1PB
First published March 2003

© Paul Swift and David Lowe

All rights reserved. No part of this work may be reproduced or used in any form without permission

ISBN 0-9544506-0-4

Designed by Tony Rose and Beckie Best

Printed in Great Britain by Piggott Printers Limited, Cambridge

The People's Hospital

Foreword

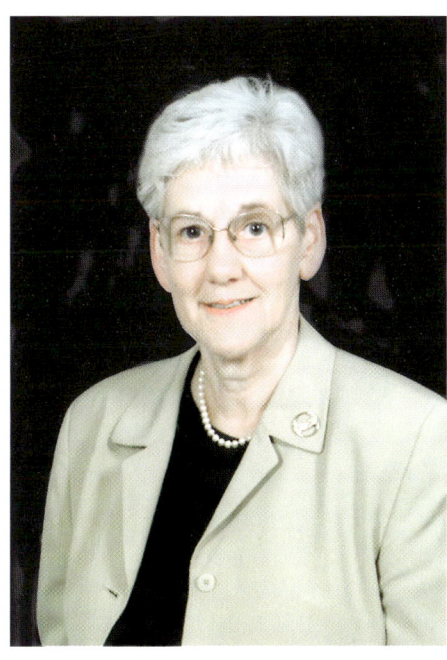

Christine Bowering is the Chairman of the Board of Directors of Nottingham City Hospital. She was a former headmistress of Nottingham High School for Girls and Non-Executive Director of Queen's Medical Centre from 1994 to 1998

WHEN I first came to this hospital as Chairman in 1998, two things became immediately obvious: first of all the warmth and friendliness of all I met who worked here, and secondly the size of the site and the quantity of old buildings. Since then my feelings concerning the staff have been strengthened and reinforced and I have grown to appreciate the history of those buildings and the changing uses to which they have been put over the years.

I am therefore delighted to have been asked to write the foreword for this history of Nottingham City Hospital, which has been produced to celebrate our centenary.

Over recent years Paul Swift, one of our porters, has developed an interest in our history and, by delving into the archives and meeting many interested staff and people associated with us, he has built up an extensive knowledge of what has led to the hospital being as it is today. His enthusiasm has been infectious and many people have given him pictures, articles and artefacts which have enabled him to assemble a wide range of material which has been put to good use.

We are grateful to David Lowe from the *Nottingham Evening Post* for joining with Paul to write this very accessible and lively history, which traces our development from the early days of the workhouse through to the centre of excellence which the hospital is today. Methods and attitudes have certainly changed over the years, but this site has always been a place of care for the people of Nottingham and this is clearly demonstrated by the many accounts which fill the pages of this book. It outlines a past of which all those who work in the hospital can feel justly proud as it has become an acute teaching hospital with a national, and in some areas international, reputation, and one which cares for hundreds of thousands of patients each year from an increasingly wide area.

In the final chapter our Chief Executive Gerry McSorley brings us up-to-date and outlines his vision for the future.

I hope you will enjoy this book as I have done, and will also share with us in Nottingham City Hospital's centenary celebrations.

Christine Bowering
Chairman

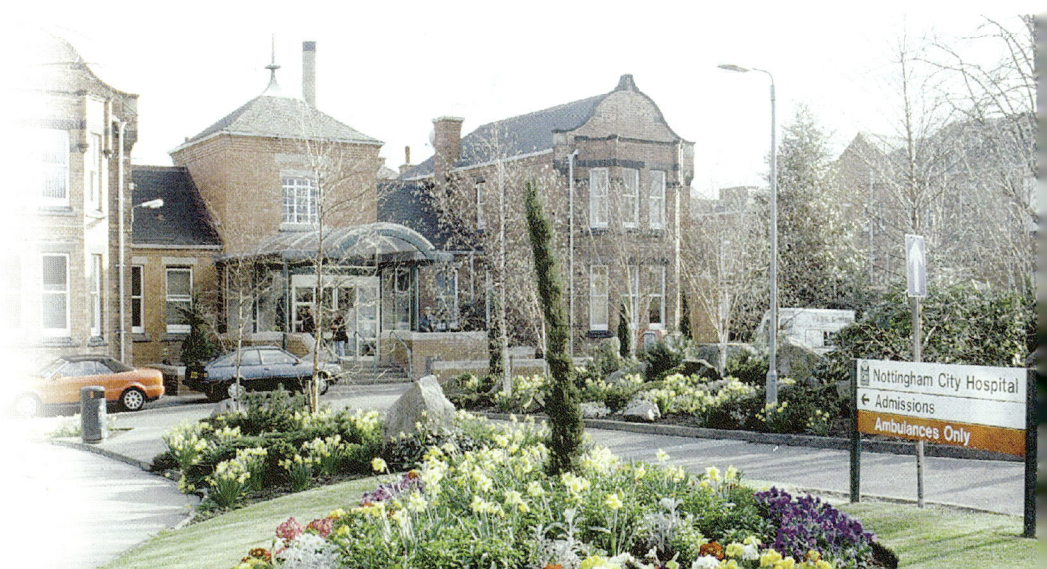

THE PEOPLE'S HOSPITAL PRINCIPAL SPONSORS

Nottingham City Hospital would like to thank the following for their generous support of its centenary publication *The People's Hospital*:

Royal Bank of Scotland Group plc, Nottingham Corporate Office

The League of Friends of the City Hospital, Nottingham

The hospital also acknowledges the support of other individuals and organisations who have helped to contribute to the success of this project:

Cedric Ford

HSBC Bank plc, Nottingham

Nottingham City Council Social Services Department

Sherwood Sunrisers Rotary Club

The University of Nottingham

The White Foundation

ACKNOWLEDGEMENTS

They say you cannot produce a book by a committee. But this publication, marking the centenary of Nottingham City Hospital, is truly a team effort.

Charting 100 years of change in words and pictures was a challenge we, as joint authors, were honoured to accept. Paul Swift, a porter in the radiotherapy department and the hospital's honorary archivist, is a dedicated local historian. Since starting his research six years ago, he's motivated many others to recognise the importance of preserving hospital records. David Lowe, who has reported on Nottingham's health and community scene for more than 30 years as an *Evening Post* journalist, also has a personal interest in the hospital. His sister Iris died in April, 2002, having benefited, like thousands of others, from marvellous care in the hospital and as a day care patient at Hayward House.

This book is a tribute to Nottingham City Hospital and the many staff, volunteers and community organisations who have contributed to its development.

We are indebted to the Chairman of the Centenary Project Steering Group Dr David Banks and Nottingham City Hospital Public Relations Manager Elisabeth Reeson for their enormous help in guiding, editing and bringing the book to its publication stage.

We are particularly grateful to the *Nottingham Evening Post* for their help throughout the publication. Senior Editorial Designer Tony Rose and Editorial Designer Beckie Best supplied the expertise on style, design and content of the book. We also wish to acknowledge the help given by the Imaging Department staff.

We appreciate the advice of medical writer Stephen Morris, who read the proofs, Marian Anderson, who compiled the index, and Piggott Printers Limited in Cambridge.

We extend our thanks to the many people who loaned photographs. They came from a wide range of sources and we are particularly grateful to Sasha Andrews, of Nottingham City Hospital Medical Illustration Department, John Birdsall, of John Birdsall Social Issues Photo Library, the *Nottingham Evening Post* and its library staff, especially Phil Meakin, as well as Dorothy Ritchie and staff of the Local Studies Library in Angel Row, Nottingham.

Finally, it is no exaggeration to say that this book would not have been possible without the many contributors, who gave generously of their time in providing personal recollections. We received letters, illustrations and memoirs literally from all over the world. This response shows why Nottingham City Hospital has come to be loved and respected as *The People's Hospital* . . .

DAVID LOWE and PAUL SWIFT, January, 2003

The People's Hospital

Contents

	INTRODUCTION By David Lowe	**1**
	CITY HOSPITAL MILESTONES Notable events that shaped the history of Nottingham City Hospital	**2**
1	**TURNING THE CLOCK BACK** From workhouse to the birth of the NHS	**5**
	WHAT'S IN A NAME? Great figures behind the ward names	**14**
2	**EXCITING TIMES — AND REAL PROGRESS** The growth years (1948-1982)	**17**
3	**THE SPIRIT OF NURSING** A century of memories from the front line	**33**
4	**THE EMERGENCE OF SPECIALIST SERVICES** A thriving centre of excellence	**47**
5	**TWO DECADES OF DEVELOPMENT** Looking ahead with optimism	**69**
6	**SUPPORT SERVICES: A WINNING TEAM** Working together to keep the wheels turning	**81**
7	**MEDICAL TRAINING: MAJOR BENEFITS FOR EVERYONE** Integrated approach to education brings real gains to patients, students and services	**89**
8	**COMMUNITY INVOLVEMENT** Tremendous team effort boosts hospital	**95**
	THE FUTURE VISION By Chief Executive Gerry McSorley	**103**
	GLOSSARY Medical terminology explained	**104**
	PICTURE CREDITS AND BIBLIOGRAPHY	**105**
	INDEX	**106**

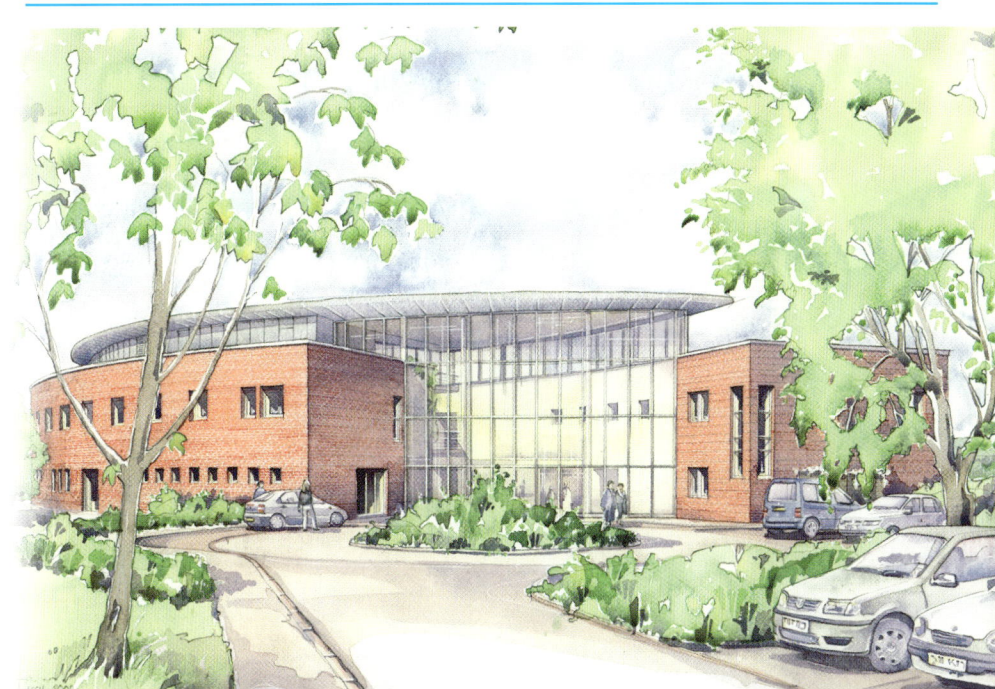

The Nottingham Breast Institute, scheduled to open at Nottingham City Hospital in the autumn of its centenary year

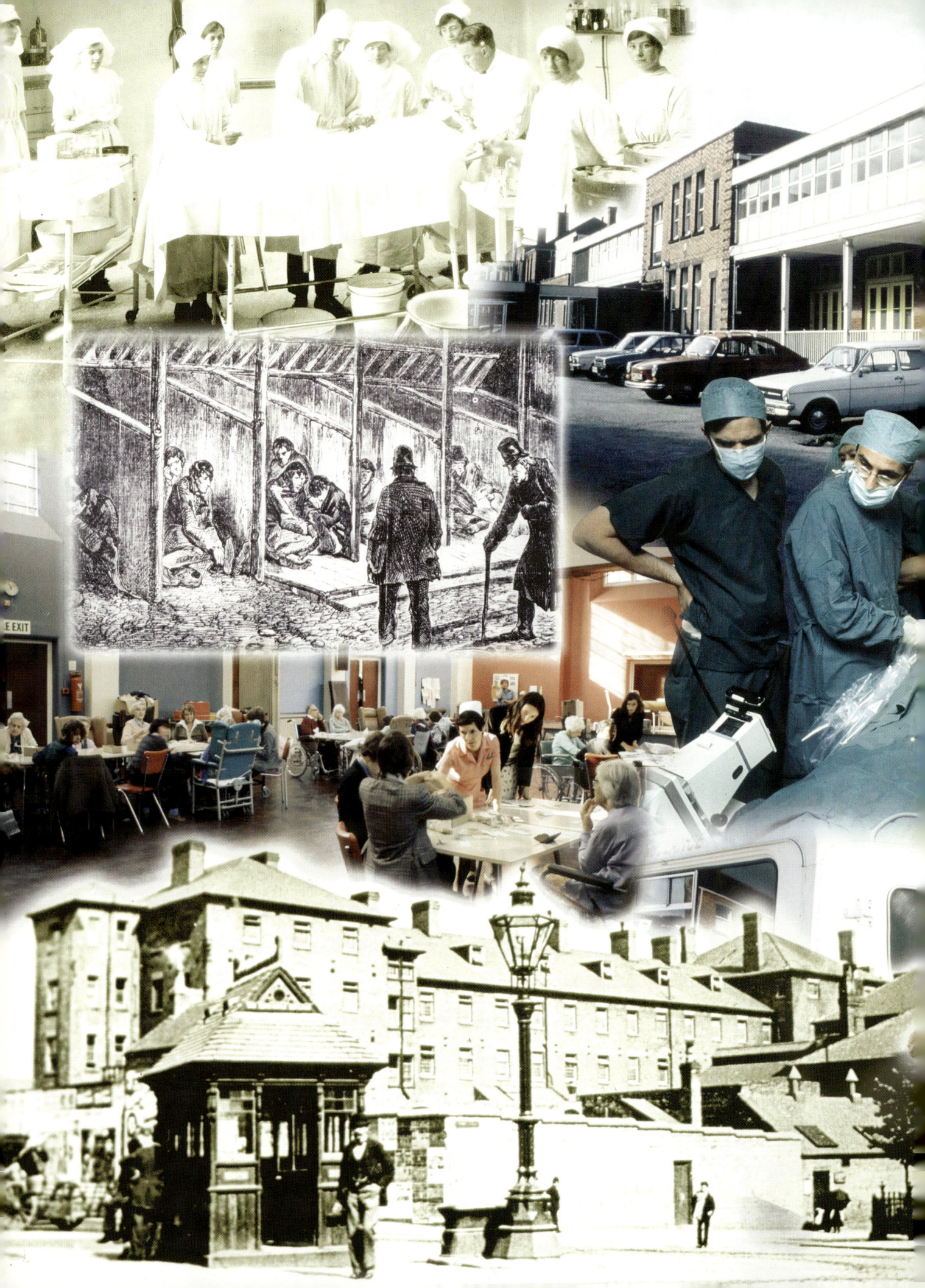

Introduction

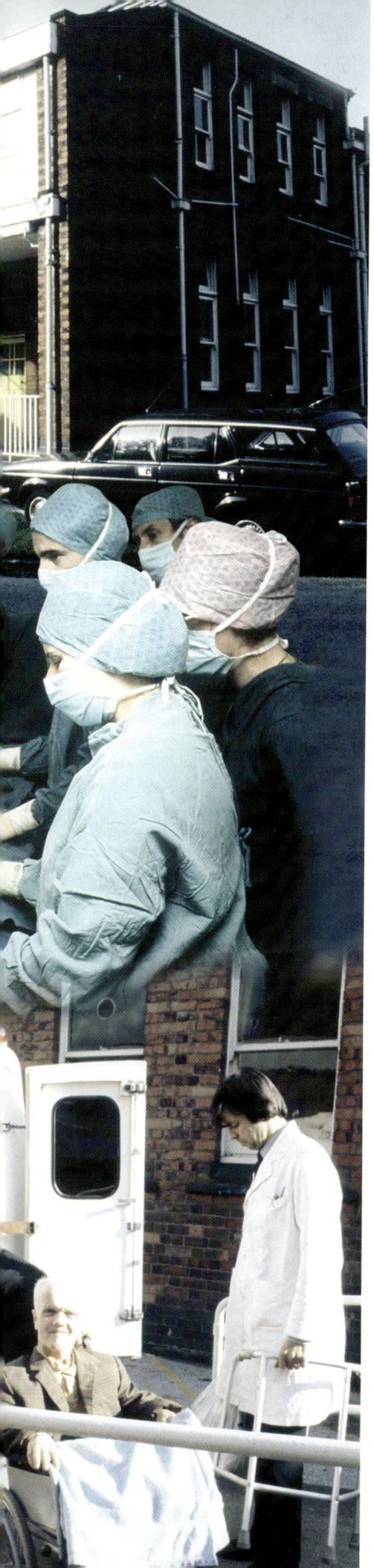

NOTTINGHAM City Hospital has served the community with great distinction for 10 decades. It started life as a humble workhouse for the poor. It cared for thousands of wounded soldiers during the First and Second World Wars and was already a major municipal hospital when the National Health Service was born in 1948. The 1970s - a key decade for development - saw the City Hospital gain teaching status and the campus expand rapidly to meet new demands. The pace of change has been equally swift and significant since Dr James Macfie wrote a history of the City Hospital in 1983. In the intervening two decades, major new departments have appeared on the site and dramatic developments in medical science have forged ahead for the benefit of patients.

So 2003 - the hospital's centenary year - is an ideal and auspicious time to update the records. This publication, celebrating the hospital's momentous achievements over the past century, also incorporates its vision for the future.

Rather than produce a measured sequential history, hospital archivist Paul Swift and myself both felt the remarkable story of progress from a Victorian workhouse and infirmary to a major teaching hospital was best told through photographs, drawings and illustrations.

We were equally interested in the human aspirations that lay behind the century of care. For the spirit and work of a hospital is more important than the bricks and mortar.

With the generous help of former and current members of staff, as well as members of the public, we have attempted to record key milestones and mention some of the influential personalities who shaped the hospital's history. We have also sought expert contributions to reflect the City Hospital's important educational, training and research roles and its strong links with the local community.

Inevitably in exploring the past and taking a glimpse into the future, there will be gaps, omissions and oversights for which the authors take full responsibility.

Our objective was a centenary book that can be dipped into at leisure, taking readers on a journey into Nottingham City Hospital's memorable past and looking ahead to an exciting future.

David Lowe

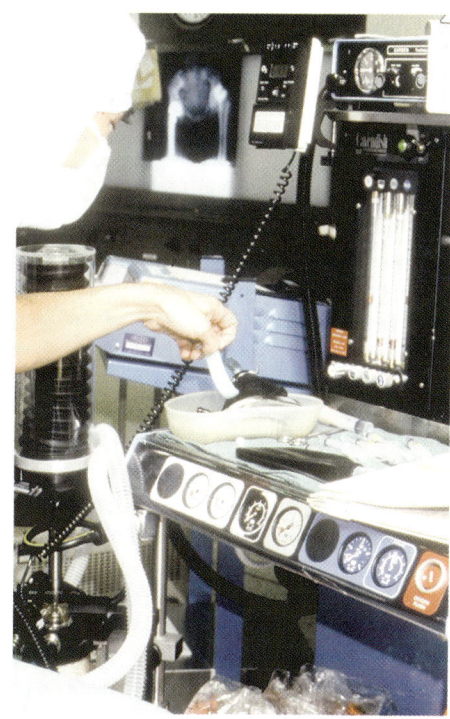

City Hospital Milestones

These notable events shaped the history of Nottingham City Hospital

1888 Nottingham Corporation Health Committee recommends building a permanent isolation hospital to cope with outbreaks of smallpox and scarlet fever.

Ceremonial trowel used at the laying of the foundation stone in April 1899

1892 The new isolation hospital and sanitorium is opened at Bagthorpe.

1899 Foundation stone is laid for the new workhouse and infirmary on a 64-acre site off Hucknall Road. The Board of Guardians, responsible for running the institution, purchase the land for £12,900 from the Nottingham Corporation.

March 18, 1903 Official opening of the Bagthorpe Workhouse and Infirmary. The workhouse houses 624 people, plus married couples, and the infirmary accommodates 750 patients. Its other facilities include the Bagthorpe Infirmary School of Nursing, later to become the Nottingham City Hospital School of Nursing.

1909 The word workhouse is dropped following a Royal Commission into the Poor Law. So the Bagthorpe Workhouse and Infirmary becomes the Institute and Infirmary.

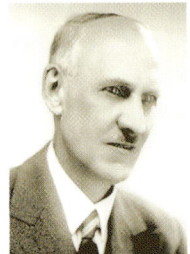
Geoffrey Gould MBE, Workhouse Master, 1920-1947

1914-18 During the First World War the infirmary becomes known as Bagthorpe Military Hospital and receives many casualties from the Western Front.

1929 The City Hospital School of Nursing opens in one large classroom in Nurses' Home One.

1930 Purpose-built children's wards and an additional operating theatre is opened. Nottingham Board of Guardians is abolished and replaced by the Local Assistance Committee. The old workhouse building known as the Institute is re-named Valebrook Lodge and the Infirmary is renamed the City Infirmary.

1934 A plaque is unveiled in memory of long-serving Medical Superintendent Dr Herbert George Ashwell. The first of two new nurses' homes is opened.

1935 The City Infirmary assumes the full functions of a municipal general hospital and is renamed the City Hospital.

1938 Mr John Barr Cochrane is appointed the first full-time Obstetrician and Gynaecological Officer.

1939 Nurses' Homes Two is opened.

1939-45 During the Second World War the hospital receives its share of military patients as well as wounded German prisoners-of-war.

1942 Sir William Beveridge publishes a report outlining the creation of a modern Welfare State and the National Health Service.

1943 The 'Forces Sweetheart' Vera Lynn visits the hospital to give an impromptu concert on Lister Two ward.

1946 Dr William Morton is appointed resident Medical Officer.

1948 Birth of the National Health Service. Under the new administrative system, the City Hospital becomes part of the Nottingham No. 2 Hospital Management Committee.

1950 Introduction of a compulsory pre-registration year for newly qualified doctors greatly eases the problem of finding suitable house physicians and house surgeons.

1951 The hospital's occupational therapy department is opened.

1954 The Duchess of Gloucester opens the new twin operating theatre suite. The City Hospital League of Friends is formed.

1955 The hospital's first plastic surgeon Mr David Wynn-Williams is appointed.

1957 A major scheme begins to modernise the hospital's main wards.

1958 The new outpatients department is opened.

1959 The new X-ray department is opened.

1963 The pathology department is reorganised and the microbiology service is taken over by Dr E R Mitchell,

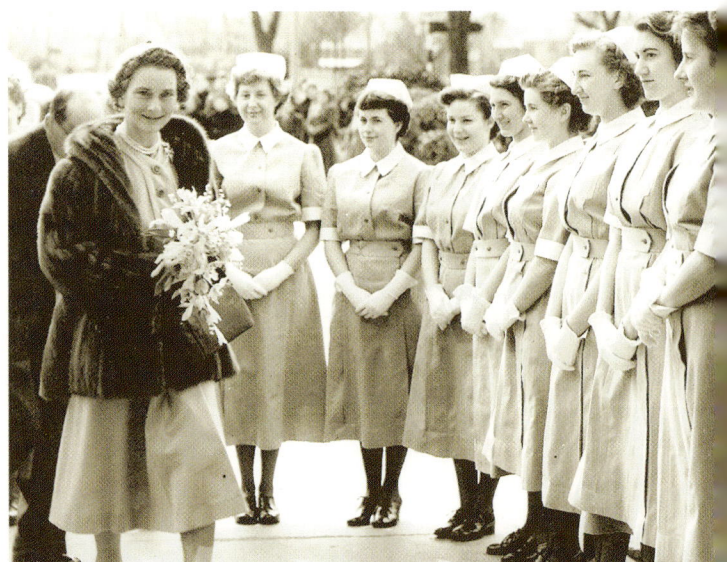
The Duchess of Gloucester opens the new twin operating theatre suite

The People's Hospital

Director of the Public Health Laboratory Service.

1965 Group Captain Douglas Bader opens the Nottingham School of Physiotherapy. A new hospital roadway leading to Edwards Lane is constructed.

1967 The first kidney dialysis machine is presented to the hospital.

1969 Sherwood Day Hospital and the artificial limb appliance centre - now known as the Mobility Centre - opened.

1970 The City Hospital is awarded teaching hospital status. Lady Hamilton opens the new physiotherapy department and the local authority begins to vacate the former 'workhouse' wards in the old Sherwood Hospital.

1972 The Post Graduate Medical Centre is opened. The coronary care unit opens and the Hospital Management Committee votes in favour of dropping the name Sherwood from the City Hospital title.

1973 Six more operating theatres open and the central sterile supplies department is established. Three more outpatient clinics open to add to the three already in existence.

1974 A new 168-bed maternity hospital is officially opened. Its facilities include a 46-cot special care baby unit. The first kidney transplant operation is performed at the City Hospital; the urology department is strengthened by the appointment of two consultants and the staff Leisure Centre opens. As part of a major reorganisation of the NHS, the City Hospital comes under the North Nottingham (Teaching) District.

1975 The hospital's first renal unit is established in the former maternity unit.

1976 The Sandfield children's unit is opened.

1977 A £50,000 bequest - the largest gift in the hospital's history - gives a flying start to the £1m CARE Appeal to fund a medical research centre.

1979 The Helen Garrod breast screening unit is opened.

1980 The new H Block is opened. It incorporates children's services, a dedicated burns unit, plastic surgery, renal dialysis and the department of clinical genetics. In the same year, Hayward House, a specialist palliative care unit, is opened.

1981 Linden Lodge, a 26-bed unit for younger chronically ill patients, is opened.

1986 The Duchess of Gloucester opens the Medical Research Centre.

Patients and staff are reaping the rewards of changes which have taken place in our radiography department — changes which other hospitals are now being encouraged to follow. Pictured here is Senior Radiographer Mark Smith

1988 Princess Margaret visits the new occupational therapy department and officially opens a CT body scanner. A new outpatient reception area is opened and a portable breast screening unit is installed.

1989 Phase four of the new health care of the elderly wards is opened.

1990 A purpose-built genito-urinary medicine unit is opened, following the transfer of the special clinic from the Nottingham General Hospital. The refurbished children's outpatients department is opened - thanks to generous backing from the City Hospital League of Friends.

1991 After an extensive refurbishment, Nightingale Two ward is re-opened to treat patients with infectious diseases.

1992 The hospital becomes an NHS Trust. A lithotriptor machine for shattering kidney stones without the need for an operation is installed - thanks to a successful £500,000 public appeal. The Duke of Kent officially opens the department of clinical radiology and medical physics.

1993 The renal/oncology building is commissioned. The project - one of the largest joint capital developments ever commissioned by the Regional Health Authority - enables cancer services to be transferred from the Nottingham General Hospital and the acute renal wards to be relocated alongside the dialysis unit in the H Block.

1994 The new £10m maternity unit is opened to replace the asbestos-clad unit built in the early 1970s. The new unit includes a Patient Hotel - the first in the UK. The women's endoscopy unit and the new day surgery unit is opened.

1995 The upper limb unit - named the Charnley Suite - is opened at the City Hospital following the closure of Harlow Wood Orthopaedic Hospital, near Mansfield. The cardiac intensive care unit is opened.

1996 The last of the old Sherwood wards are demolished to make way for a new endoscopy unit.

1999 Chief Medical Officer Professor Sir Liam Donaldson opens the University of Nottingham's Clinical Sciences Building on the hospital site.

2000 The cardiac surgery unit is opened.

2001 The new endoscopy centre is opened.

March 18, 2003 Nottingham City Hospital celebrates its 100th anniversary.

2003 Opening of the Nottingham Breast Institute.

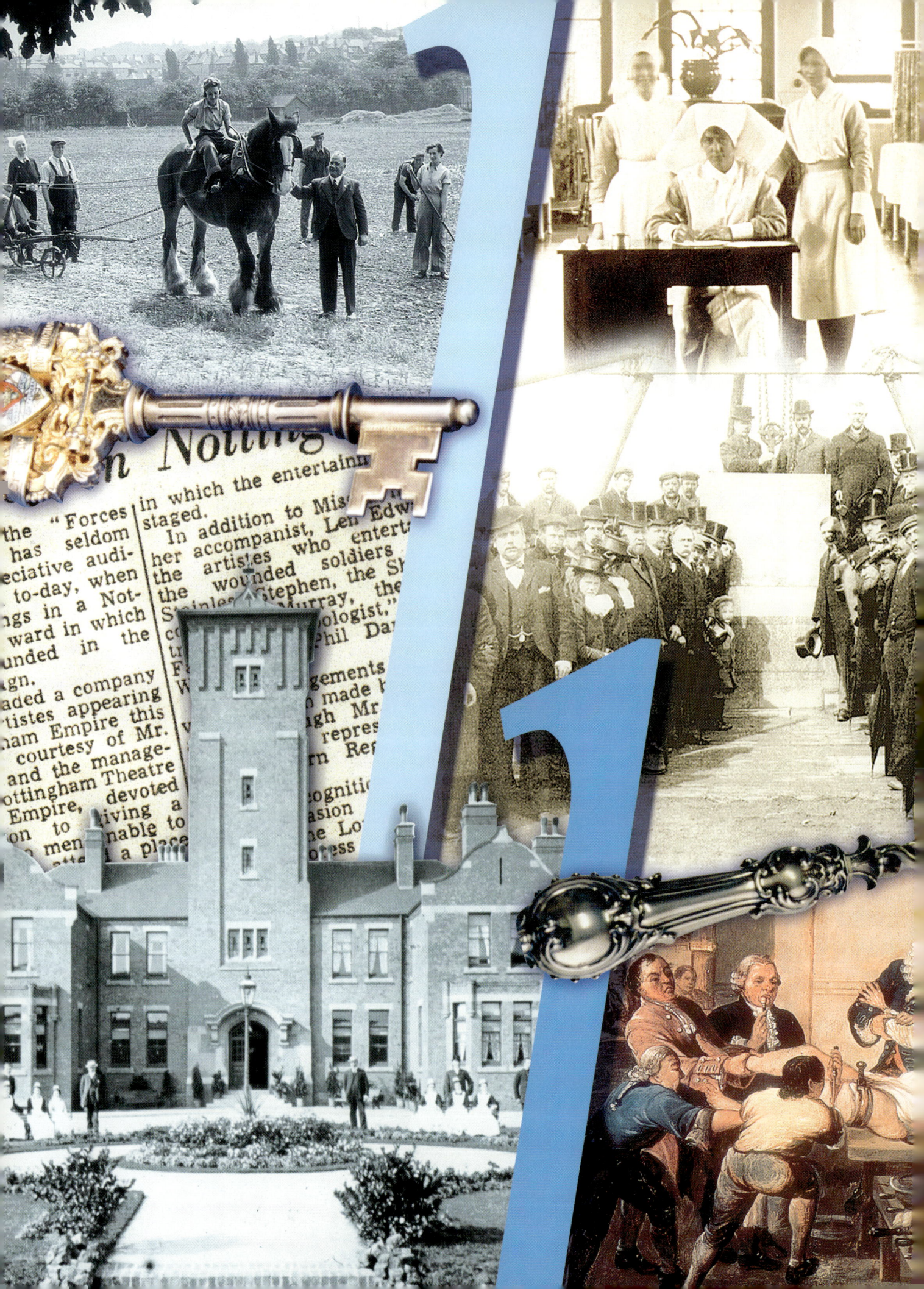

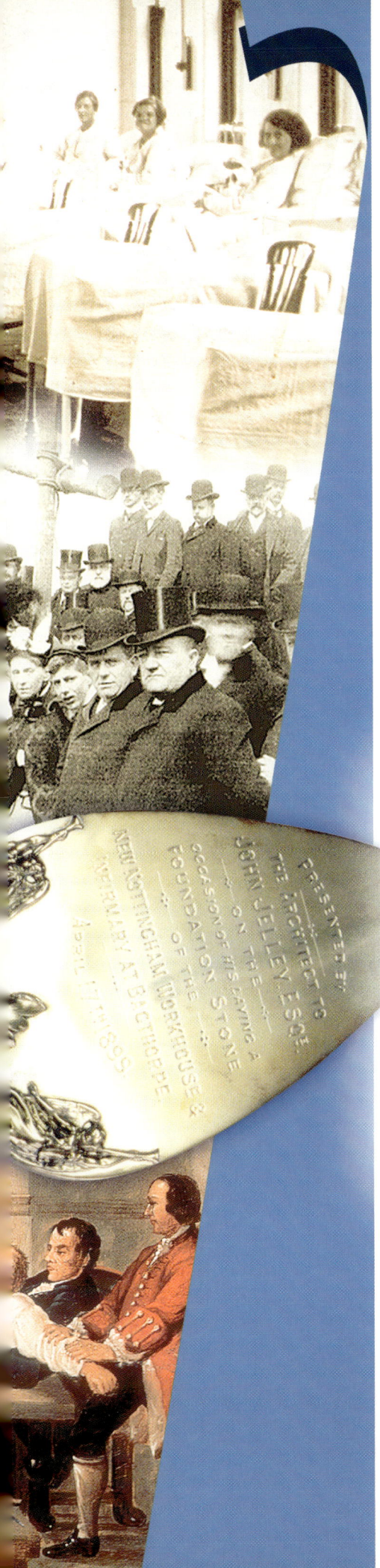

Turning the clock back

From workhouse to the birth of the NHS

HISTORY is important because delving into the past can sometimes give us an insight into the future. So let's step aboard an imaginary time machine and embark on a journey of discovery aimed at uncovering the history of the Nottingham City Hospital. Certainly the founding fathers who established a workhouse at Bagthorpe a century ago would be amazed to find their vision had led to the development of one of Britain's leading hospitals.

Today the entire City Hospital staff, all 5,700 of them, are dedicated to meeting 21st century challenges and providing premier care for hundreds of thousands of patients every year.

So how did the hospital grow to its present stature? To answer that question we must turn the medical clock back to Victorian times.

For more than a decade before Bagthorpe Workhouse and Infirmary was opened on March 18, 1903, staff in the neighbouring isolation hospital were already hard at work tackling a formidable array of diseases such as diphtheria, enteric fever (typhoid), smallpox, scarlet fever and TB.

It's worth noting that Nottingham was in the grip of a smallpox epidemic. So in the interests of public health the actual opening and official opening of the new workhouse were performed on the same day. To reduce the risk of the disease spreading, two temporary workhouses on Great Freeman Street, Nottingham and Leslie Road in Forest Fields were kept open. Of course the staff in the adjoining isolation hospital, opened in 1892, lacked today's powerful antibiotics; X-rays had still to be discovered and although the first microscope had arrived in Nottingham in 1852, diagnosis remained an inexact science. The introduction of anaesthesia brought the biggest breakthrough with the development of chloroform, followed by the acceptance of Lister's antiseptic techniques, paving the way for modern surgery. Until then, wound infection was almost universal.

Surprising as it sounds, the Nottingham City Hospital owes its origins as much to transport as medical science. By 1893 the railways were growing rapidly and Parliament had given approval for a Nottingham to London extension to the Manchester, Sheffield and Lincolnshire Railway. This was later renamed the Great Central Railway, founded by Victorian magnate Sir Edward Watkin. The line, completed in 1899, linked Sheffield, Nottingham, Loughborough and Leicester with the new Marylebone terminus in London. More than half a million cubic yards of sandstone were excavated for the new Nottingham Victoria Station and the tunnels at either end. Buildings on a 13-acre site had to be demolished, including 1,300 homes, 20 pubs and the Nottingham Union Workhouse in York Street.

And this is where the City Hospital story really begins.

With the construction of Victoria Station under way, the Nottingham Board of Guardians, who ran the workhouse, decided in 1896 to seek a suitable location for a new institution. They eventually bought from

The People's Hospital

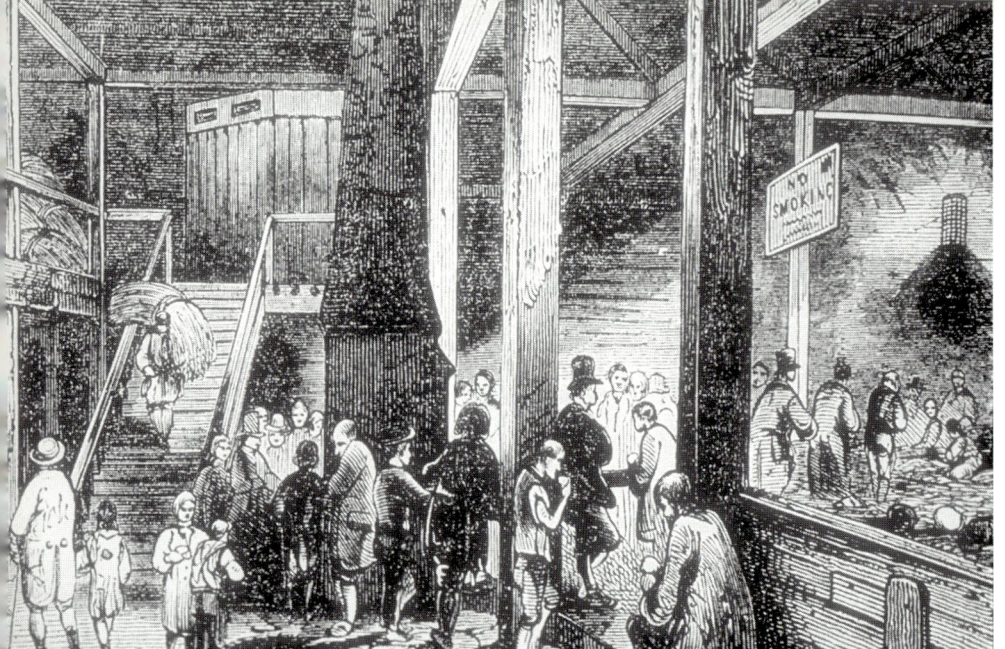

Nottingham Corporation a 64-acre plot of land off Hucknall Road for £12,900. The land had been originally purchased by the Corporation's health department from the Vicar of Basford. Although only 26 acres was required, the health department had to buy the whole site because the vicar felt that if only part of the land was sold it would reduce the value of the remaining church land. Acquiring a larger site than was needed was to prove invaluable to the hospital in later years.

This massive project was also tackled without assembling umpteen committees. The building specifications were simply sent out to five competing architects. Arthur Marshall, of Marshall and Turner, on Angel Row, won the prize for the best design - and he quickly got to work on his new commission.

The foundation stone for Bagthorpe Workhouse - laid by Councillor Charles Smith, Chairman of the Board of Guardians, on April 17, 1899 - can still be seen on an outside wall of the main headquarters entrance to the Nottingham City Hospital.

The foundation stone for the infirmary was laid by Alderman John Jelley, Chairman of the Building Committee, on what is now the

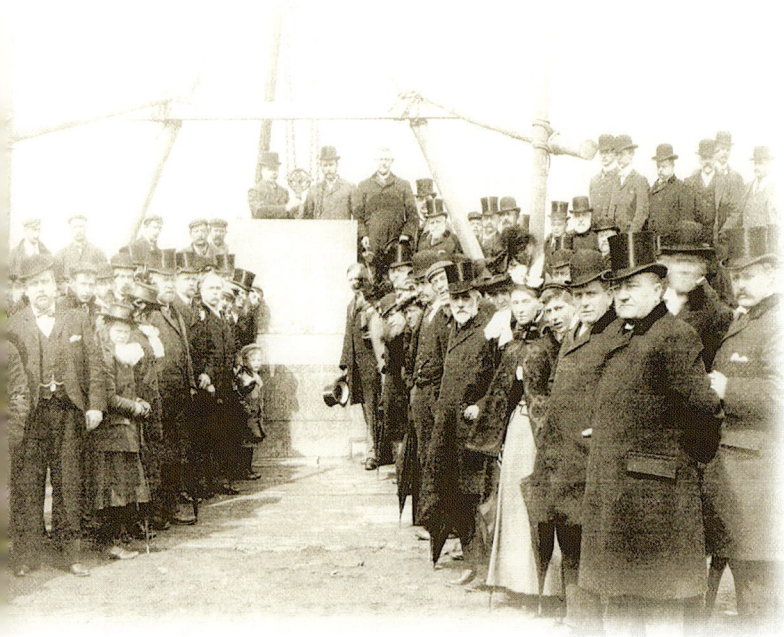

Above: Illustration shows what life was like in a workhouse

Left: The foundation stone for Bagthorpe Workhouse was laid by Councillor Charles Smith, Chairman of the Board of Guardians, on April 17, 1899. Four years later the hospital opened its doors to its patients

Below: The hospital as it looked in 1903. Picture taken from a footpath that is now Valley Road

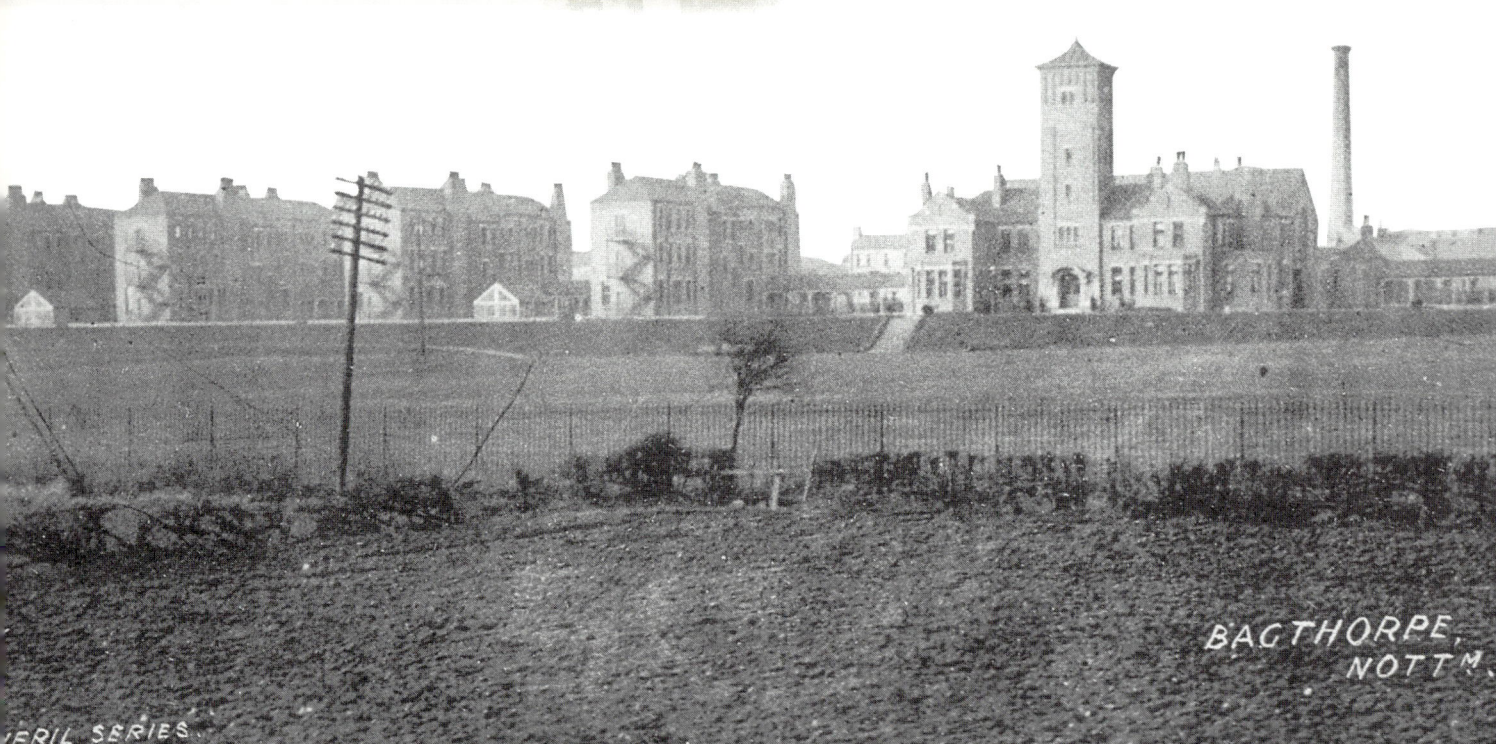

The People's Hospital

hospital's main north corridor entrance. Of the two foundation stones laid that day, he regarded the hospital stone of greater importance because he foresaw a time when workhouses would no longer be needed. But the hospital, he declared, would stand for ever to answer a useful purpose. He argued that old age pensions might mean the end of workhouses but he added sagely: "You can't do away with illness."

While the workhouse was publicly described as 'a palace for paupers', the Board of Guardians carefully avoided any outlay deemed extravagant. Total cost of the workhouse and infirmary buildings was £163,240 - and, until recently, some of the original red brick buildings were still in use.

A report in the *Nottingham Guardian* described the workhouse as one of the most extensive and completely equipped in the country. From start to finish the project took six years to complete. More than 100,000 tons of goods and materials were brought on to the site; workmen installed seven miles of drains and bricklayers laid 13.5 million bricks. If placed end to end they would have stretched from London to Constantinople. The Board of Guardians were particularly pleased with the 10 miles of piping used in the heating and water supply, making its circulation the longest in the British Isles.

The Chairman of the Board of Guardians Councillor Thomas Palmer performed the opening ceremony after the architect presented him with a massive gold key, banded with pearls and suitably inscribed.

The workhouse housed 624 people, plus accommodation for married couples, while the infirmary comprised 16 wards, each with 28 beds. Another 250 beds were set aside on wards for the mentally ill and those with learning disabilities. Other buildings housed children and people suffering from consumption. There were also receiving wards, an isolation ward, a workshop, mortuary, bakery, laundry, boiler and engine houses and a chapel to seat a congregation of 600. There was a stable block for 10 horses and even a coffin-making shed. The infirmary had 55 nurses, a matron, a medical officer and 72 other staff. When the new complex opened, the yearly salary of Mrs Burrows, Matron of the training institution, increased from £50 to £60.

Public visiting to the workhouse and infirmary was prohibited because of the smallpox epidemic in Nottingham. Fortunately Dr Philip Boobbyer, Medical Superintendent to the Bagthorpe Isolation Hospital for 40 years until he retired in 1929, was an authority on smallpox. At times during a remarkable career he was regarded as an 'open air' crank because of his belief in pure air as a healing agent. In an account for the *British Medical Journal* he described the practice of nursing all serious smallpox cases in individual bell tents with open sides. He also reported just one death among 128 vaccinated patients.

Dr Boobbyer battled long and hard

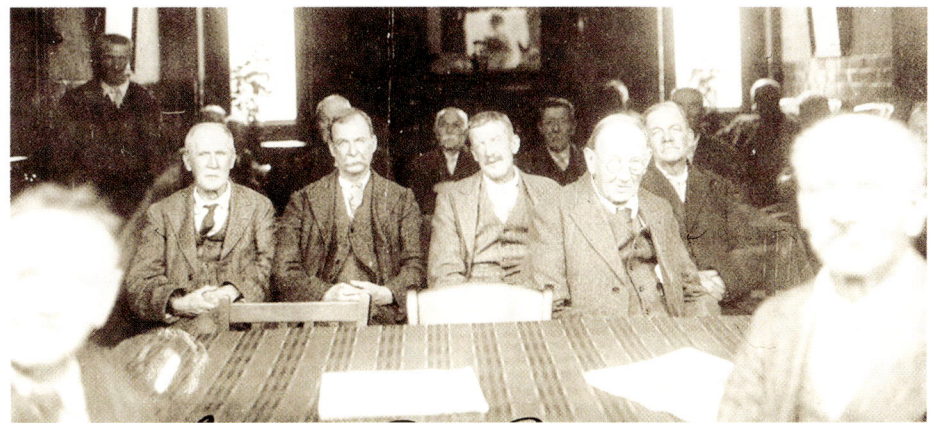

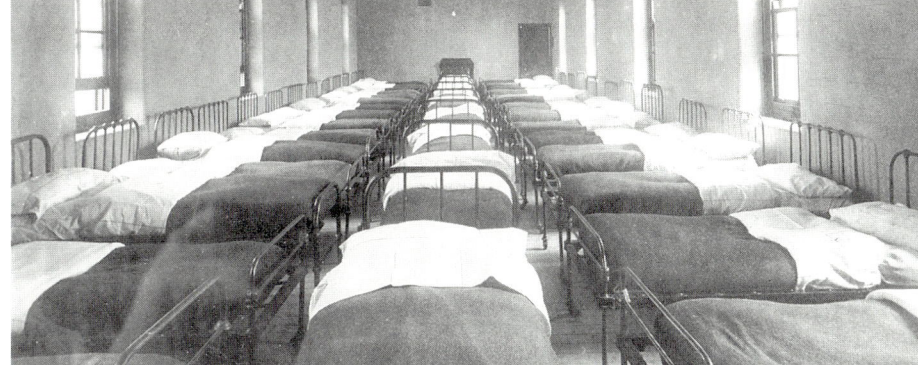

Above: *The dayroom and inmates' dormitory at Bagthorpe Institute (workhouse) in 1925*

Right: *Together in a Moses basket are babies James Mulray, Elizabeth Woodford and Elizabeth Coulton who were born at the City Hospital on the day of the Queen's Coronation in 1953*

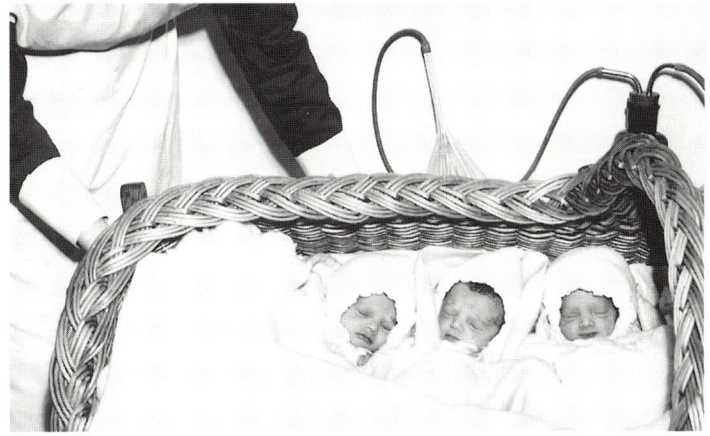

The People's Hospital

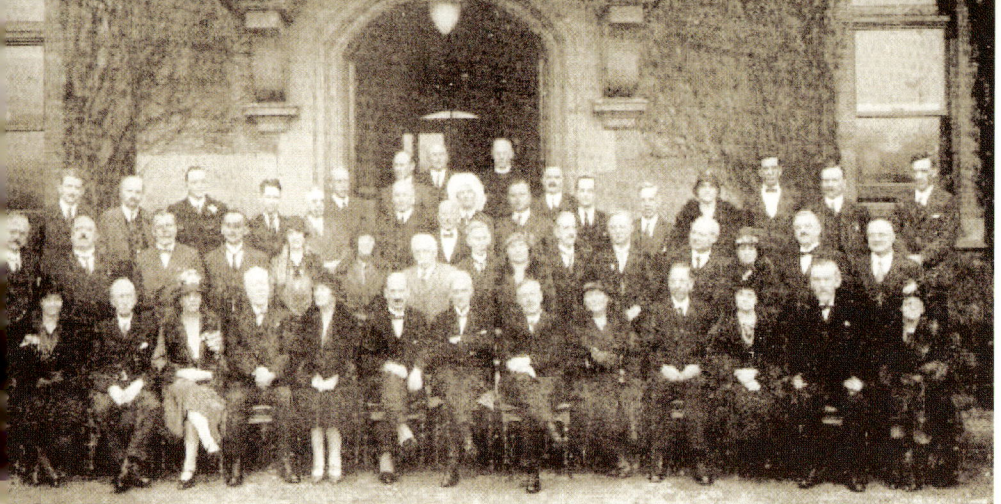

to convince the health and civic authorities that outbreaks of typhoid and other diseases were largely due to the insanitary conditions arising from the 'pail closet' system in Nottingham's overcrowded streets. He was also instrumental in the introduction of child health and tuberculosis services.

His 'open air' methods undoubtedly saved many lives. But, perhaps ironically, Dr Boobbyer died, aged 72, after taking his daily cold bath before breakfast.

During the First World War, Bagthorpe Military Hospital, as it became known, received many casualties from the Western Front. Wounded soldiers arrived via a special railway siding on the site of the present Post Graduate Education Centre.

The first annual report of the Ministry of Health in 1919/20 praised the part played by the Board of Guardians during the war and described Bagthorpe as one of the finest military hospitals in the country.

"The Guardians of the Parish of Nottingham at once placed their separate infirmary at the disposal of the War Office. This large infirmary, built some 24 years ago, had accommodation for 750 patients, and could be described as thoroughly up-to-date with every appliance which could be required, an excellent operating theatre and X-ray apparatus, and generally a model hospital in every respect.

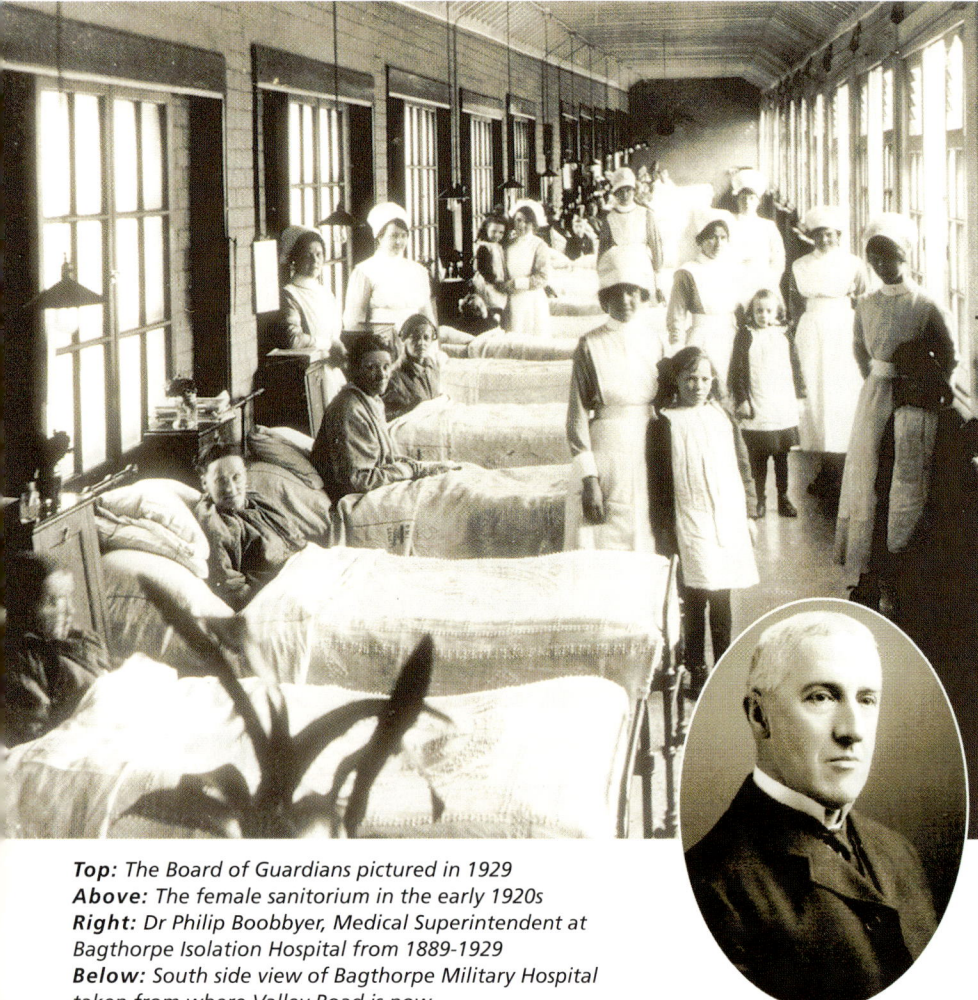

Top: The Board of Guardians pictured in 1929
Above: The female sanitorium in the early 1920s
Right: Dr Philip Boobbyer, Medical Superintendent at Bagthorpe Isolation Hospital from 1889-1929
Below: South side view of Bagthorpe Military Hospital taken from where Valley Road is now

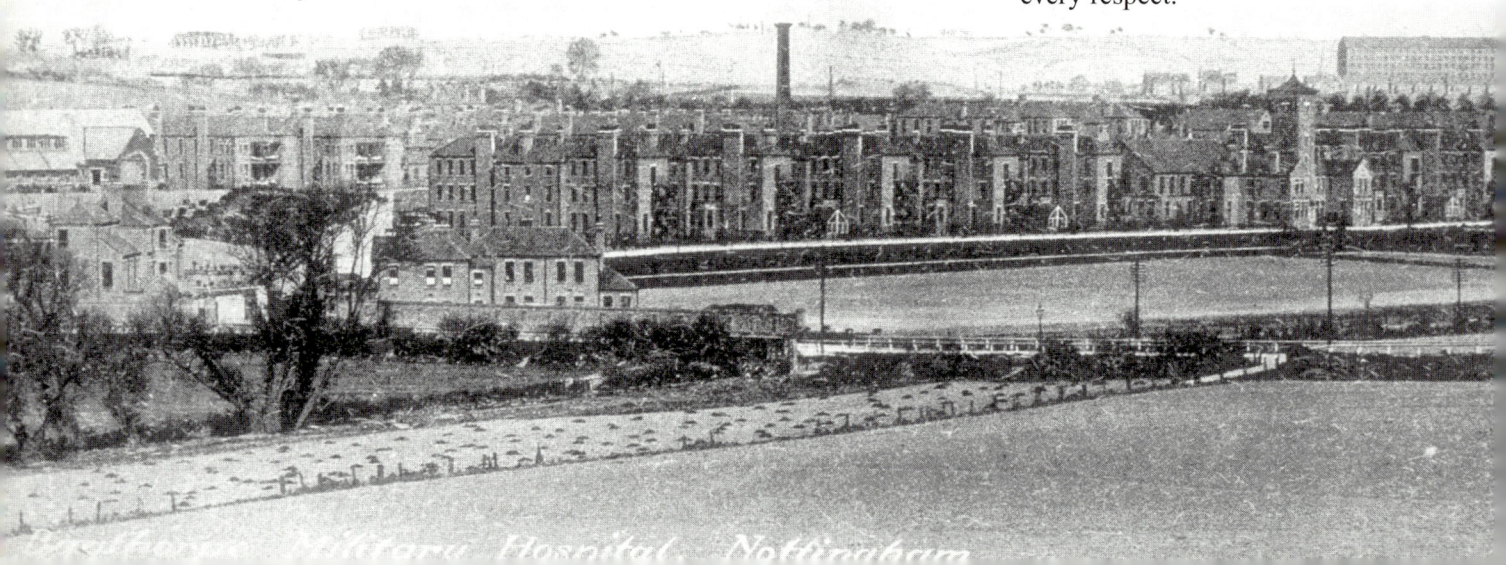

The People's Hospital

"At first the Guardians handed over 500 beds, and subsequently more and more accommodation was given until not only the 750 beds were all handed over but one detached block of the workhouse was also offered and made use of during the emergency of March 1918."

Two significant events happened in 1929. Alderman W Green laid the foundation stone to the hospital's first purpose-built children's wards and in the same year boards of guardians throughout the UK were abolished. Under new legislation introduced in 1930, administrative responsibility for the workhouse passed to the Public Assistance Committee and the infirmary came under the control of the Public Health Committee. It was the end of nearly a century of work by the Board of Guardians in providing food, shelter and relief for the destitute in the Nottingham parish. On average 1,615 patients a day were being maintained at the Bagthorpe Institute and Infirmary and infirmary staff had more than doubled during the previous 20 years from 68 to 148.

The construction of the children's wards, opened in 1930 at a cost of £49,000, was a legacy to the work of Dr Herbert George Ashwell, the 'father' of the City Hospital who retired after 42 years' service as Medical Superintendent. All the wards were south-facing and designed for open-air use with glazed screens opening onto verandas. Two isolation wards had glazed screens to allow observation from the adjoining wards. The two-storey block known as A and B, comprised an entrance hall, rooms for the medical staff, an operating theatre, which in 1931 recorded 592 operations, and separate provision for massage and ultra-violet ray treatment. The site was now like a small town with 785 beds in the infirmary, children's wards (160), mental wards (247), Bagthorpe Institute (639) and casual wards (73).

By 1930 the infirmary's five medical staff, plus four visiting doctors, were treating more than 4,000 patients a year. Now known as the City Infirmary, it desperately needed more space.

Today all that remains of the old children's wards is the block which houses James Ward, named after Dr Sam James, the City Hospital's first Consultant Rheumatologist from 1964 to 1980. On the second floor is the Charnley Suite, named after the famous Orthopaedic Surgeon Sir John Charnley, inventor of the artificial hip joint.

Mrs Marie Quinney, who moved to New Zealand in 2002 from Collingham, near Newark, has vivid memories of her six weeks in the isolation hospital as a four-year-old child in the 1930s. Suffering from diphtheria and scarlet fever, she was treated on an adult ward.

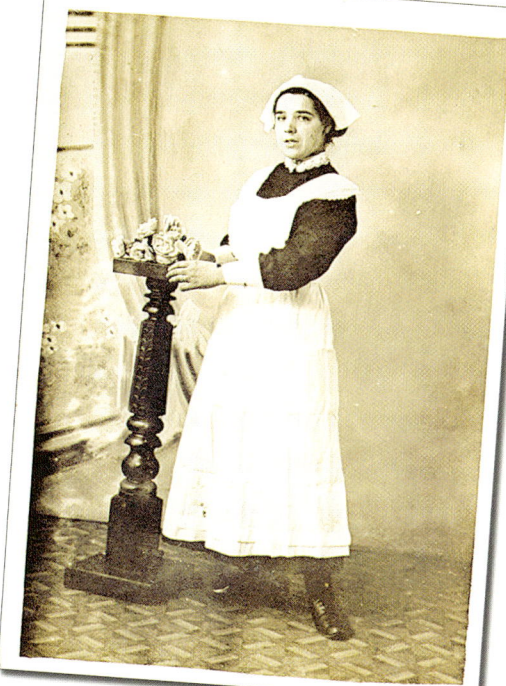

"The other girls seemed quite old," she recalled. "But with hindsight they must have been only 17 or 18. Most of them worked in the Player's factories - tobacco workers who became known as 'Player's Angels.' They befriended me and gave me presents. No visits were allowed. When your family came to see you they had to wave through the window. Lists of patients' conditions were placed daily in the newspaper columns. Those described as dangerously ill could have visits from friends and family.

"Eventually I produced three clear swabs and was well enough to go home. I remember the porter carrying me on his shoulder to the gatehouse, where my parents were waiting to collect me."

Diphtheria and scarlet fever would remain serious diseases. For example the City Isolation Hospital (Heathfield) admitted 22 cases of diphtheria and 82 cases of scarlet fever in 1938. Economically, of course, the whole of the 1930s were harsh times with millions out of work.

Continued on page 11

Above: *A nurse in the mid-1920s wears her uniform with pride*
Left: *Children with tuberculosis being nursed on veranda-style wards around 1950*

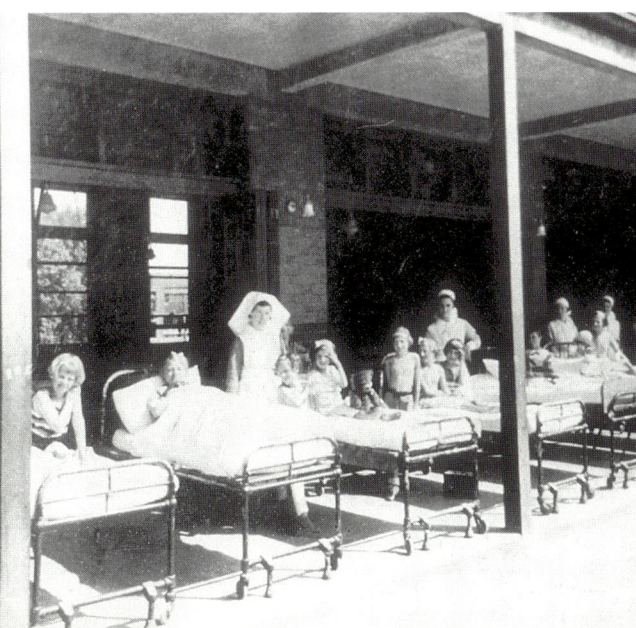

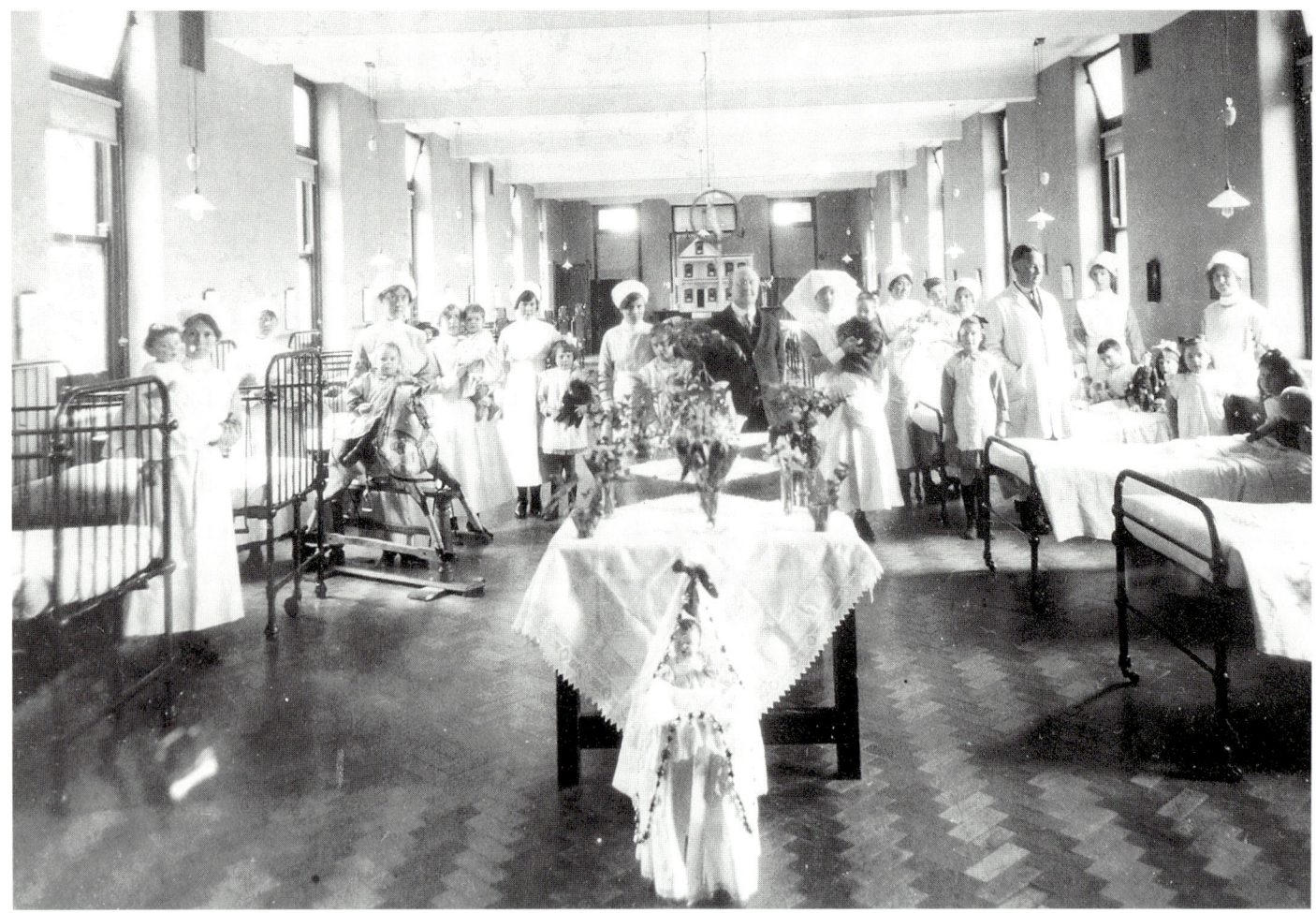

MRS FREDA WALMSLEY recalls:

I LIVED on Park Lane, which runs parallel with Arnold Road, not far from the hospital. In those days there were no council houses around, just fields and allotments.

There were actually three hospitals. The top one was the Isolation Hospital for consumption and scarlet fever patients. The next gate was the City Hospital. From the entrance there was a very long corridor with large wards both sides with upstairs the same. Then the third gate, Bagthorpe, the dreaded 'Baggy', the workhouse.

I remember the days when any brain disorder, epilepsy and palsy were all classed the same. You would see the inmates going for walks two by two, looking so drab in their horrible uniforms, with the same sad look.

Then there were the old folks. In those days the eldest son was responsible for their parents. My husband's father was the eldest in their family and the day came when he had to take his mother. It was not long before there was trouble and she was a nuisance. Then like many more she was shipped off to 'Baggy' to be forgotten. I never met the lady but she existed until the age of 93.

The 'whinging whimsies' of today have no idea how lucky everyone is. I remember before 1948 there was no NHS, no social services, no income support, no child allowance, absolutely nothing, even 'dole' was subject to 'means test'.

Where I came from, if anyone died before the aged of 70, it was case of 'ee didn't they die young?' My grandparents died when they were in their 80s and so did thousands of others. I have an 88-year-old friend; her sister died at 90, her brother has just celebrated his 93rd birthday and the other siblings are in their 70s and 80s.

Their mother died at 96, her husband was a casualty of a mining accident at 50, leaving her with nine children. No handouts or help. She would clean someone's house to get money for a dinner. In fact, she would clean anything to get a little cash.

Mind you, we had no junk food, a penneth of bones from the butcher, boiled and root vegetables added to the stock. A ham hock for 3d boiled and soaked, dried peas added, thickened with flour, pea soup, tripe and onions, cow heel.

I could go on and on . . .

The People's Hospital

Left: A children's ward in 1925

Right: This picture shows the City Hospital's entire medical team in 1939. There were just 10 staff, plus pharmacist Mr Cox, to look after nearly 1,000 patients.

The man seated in the front row (second right) is John Cochrane, destined to become one of Nottingham's best known consultants.

After graduating in medicine from Edinburgh University in 1936, he was appointed house surgeon at the City Hospital in 1937 and the following year became the hospital's first full-time obstetrician and gynaecologist

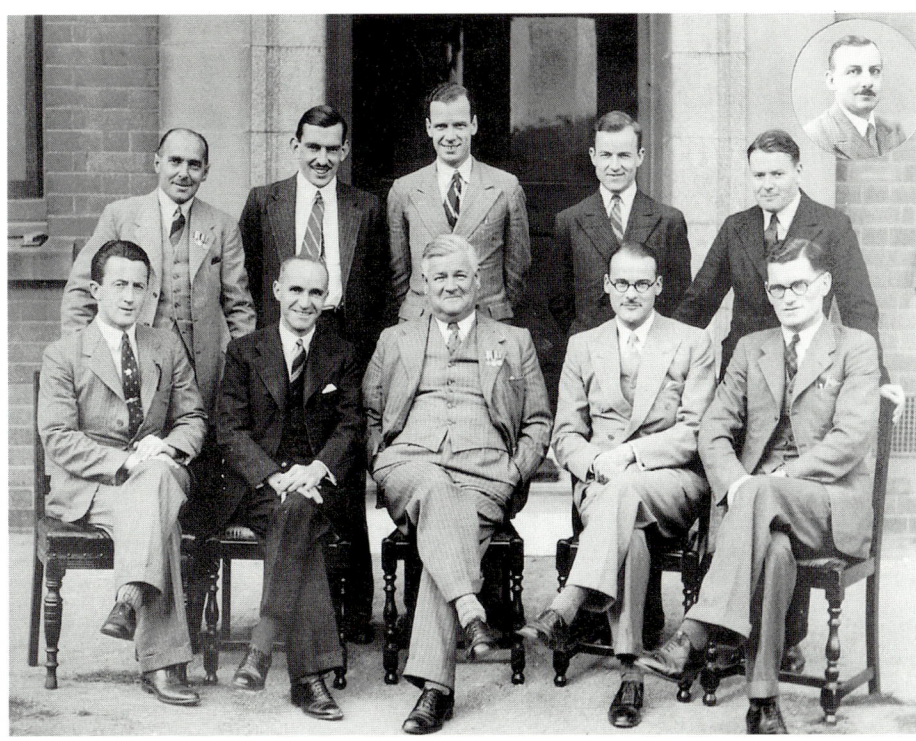

Continued from page 9

An unemployed man with a wife and three children had to survive on 29s 3d a week in 1931. In the same year the universally hated means test was introduced to cut the soaring benefit bill still further. Of course the pound was then worth many times its present value and things were cheap beyond belief. Dressed in his 35-bob 'Weaver-to-Wearer' suit a chap could feel a man about town watching George Robey or Gracie Fields from his 4d seat in the 'gods' at the Empire while smoking Will's 'Wild' Woodbines at five for 2d. On Monday morning the suit probably went back to the pawnbroker.

Domestic staff in the isolation hospital earned £30 a year in 1937, rising by 50s increments to £40, while maids in the main hospital started on £25 a year, rising by 50s increments to £40. A visiting health committee reported: "Since we often take girls of 16 or even under to train as maids, I am of the opinion that the minimum figure is best left as it is, provided we are free to start older and more experienced girls at some point within the scale above this figure."

When she was 16 Marie Quinney was on duty at the hospital as a volunteer, assisting nurses in bathing vagrants when they arrived at the workhouse. As a result of the 1934 Public Health Act, the former workhouse came under the control of the Local Assistance Committee and the Local Health Committee was responsible for the infirmary. In the same year the City Infirmary became a municipal general hospital and was re-named 'The City Hospital'. The institute, or old workhouse, was known as Valebrook Lodge - a title that was to remain up to the inception of the NHS in 1948. Visiting day was altered from Saturday to Sunday in 1938 but the new arrangement could not come into operation until the erection of the new hospital gates. In keeping with a more liberal approach towards patient care, Charity ward was re-named Winifred ward.

These name changes brought wage rises for some staff: a hospital cook's pay increased from £55 to £65 a year and a ward sister's salary went up from £80 a year to £85. A visiting health committee for 1937 makes the first reference to ambulance and receiving room staff. "The numbers of cases, which have had to be fetched by ambulance and dealt with in the receiving room, became so unmanageable during this period that we were obliged to call in extra help if delay was to be avoided. Mrs Mabel Everard - who undertook this work before in an emergency for us - was engaged temporarily at £2 weekly. Her services will be dispensed with as soon as it is consistent with efficiency in this department with the existing staff."

In terms of medical staffing the hospital was still largely dependent for specialist medical and surgical advice on doctors visiting from elsewhere - mostly the Nottingham General Hospital. A visiting committee for 1938 was asked to authorise payments of two guineas each to two consultants who were called in. It was also resolved to put all visiting surgeons on equal salaries of £250 a year.

The city and county local authorities saw the increasing need for skilled surgery in cases of pulmonary tuberculosis and other chest disorders. So in 1936 they appointed the Harley Street consultant Mr Lawrence O' Shaughnessy to conduct a thoracic surgical operating session one long weekend a month, thus establishing the Thoracic department at the City Hospital.

Over the years the number of babies born at the hospital had been

The People's Hospital

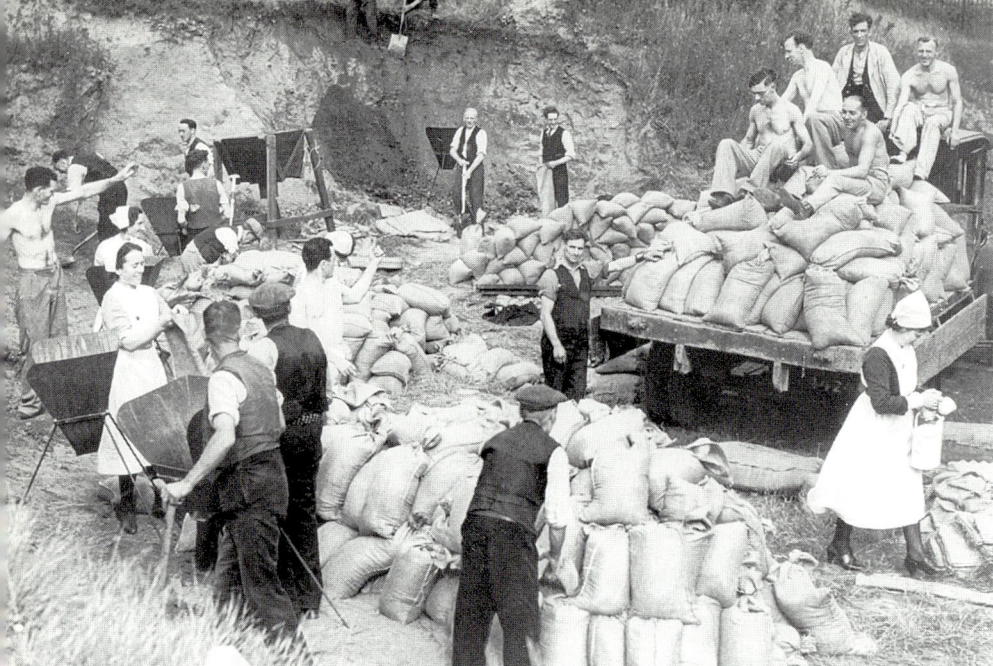

steadily rising and all the medical officers took a share of this delivery work. But in 1938 Dr John Barr Cochrane was appointed as the first full-time resident Obstetrician and Gynaecological Officer. It had been custom for medical officers to carry out the simpler laboratory tests on their own wards until Dr A H Johns opened a clinical pathology laboratory in 1938 with one technician to help him. The scope and efficiency of the tests improved greatly although some specimens were still sent to the General Hospital laboratory.

Recruitment of nurses steadily improved and a new nurses' home was opened in 1938 to accommodate 100 nurses and 20 domestic staff. At that time all nursing staff lived in, including sisters and the Matron Alice Rose. The accommodation also incorporated a training school for 270 nurses. The buildings were repaired to house additional nurses, remedying to some extent the understaffing which had caused critical comment from the Ministry of Health. In a report the health committee warned: "The position has been so acute that accommodation for patients had to be provided by extensions, structural alterations and the erection of wards of a semi-permanent nature for an additional 100 beds.

"In our opinion at least 400 additional beds will be required during the next five years and we have been advised that an additional third storey should be added to the new home to accommodate a further 44 nurses. . ."

But the dark clouds of war were once more gathering and further expansion would have to wait until the inception of the National Health Service in 1948. During the Second World War, military patients as well as some German prisoners-of-war

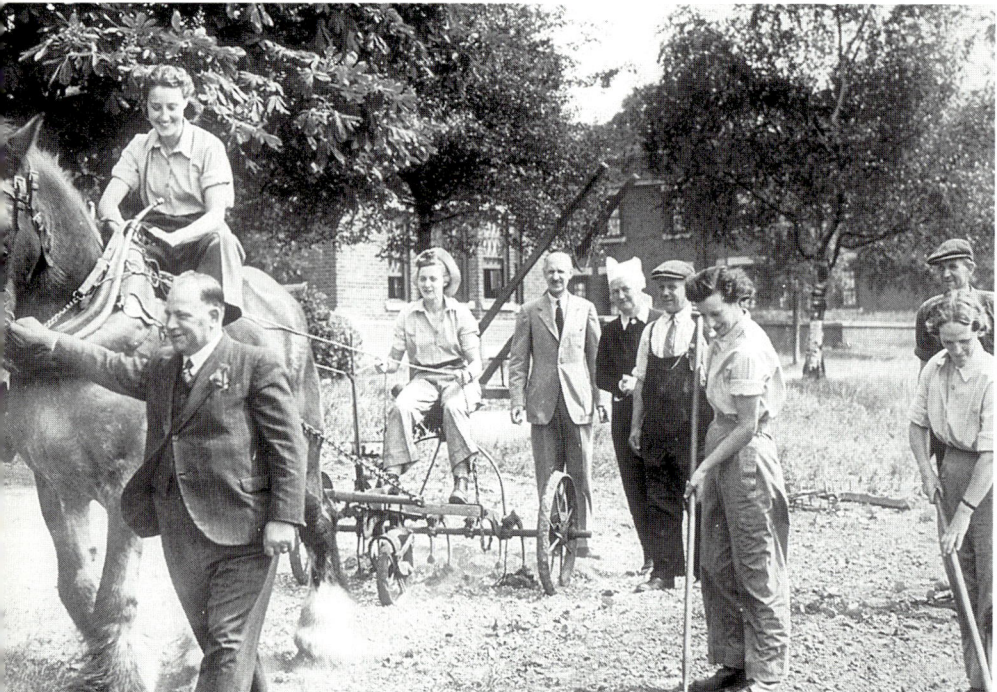

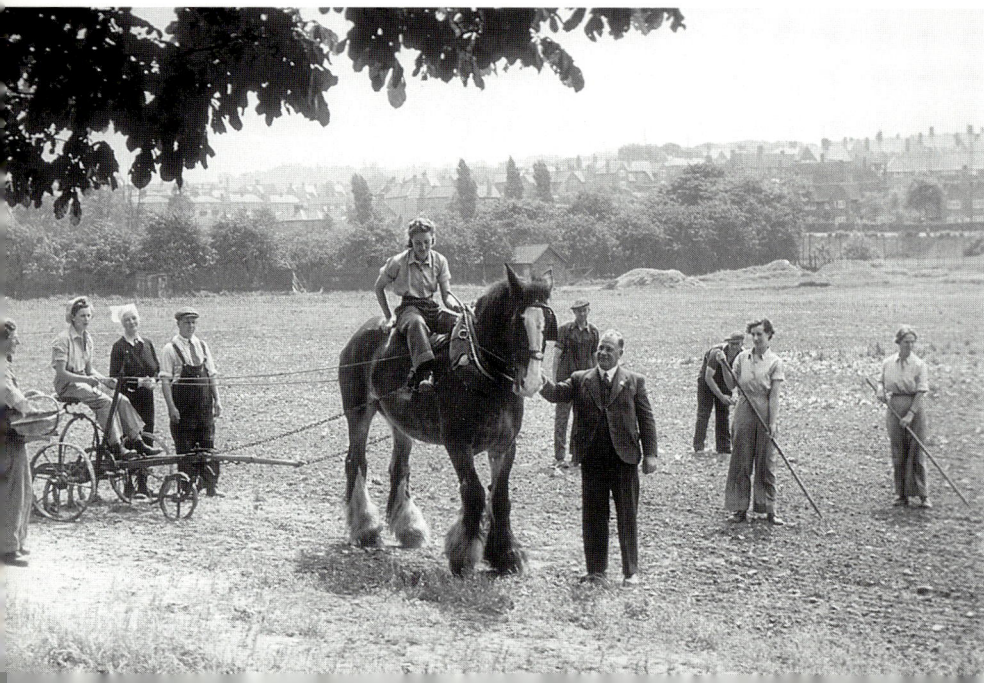

Top: Building air raid shelters on the south side of the campus in 1939

Centre and left: Wartime pictures of Women's Land Army girls 'digging for victory' on City Hospital fields (now the Yellow car park)

The People's Hospital

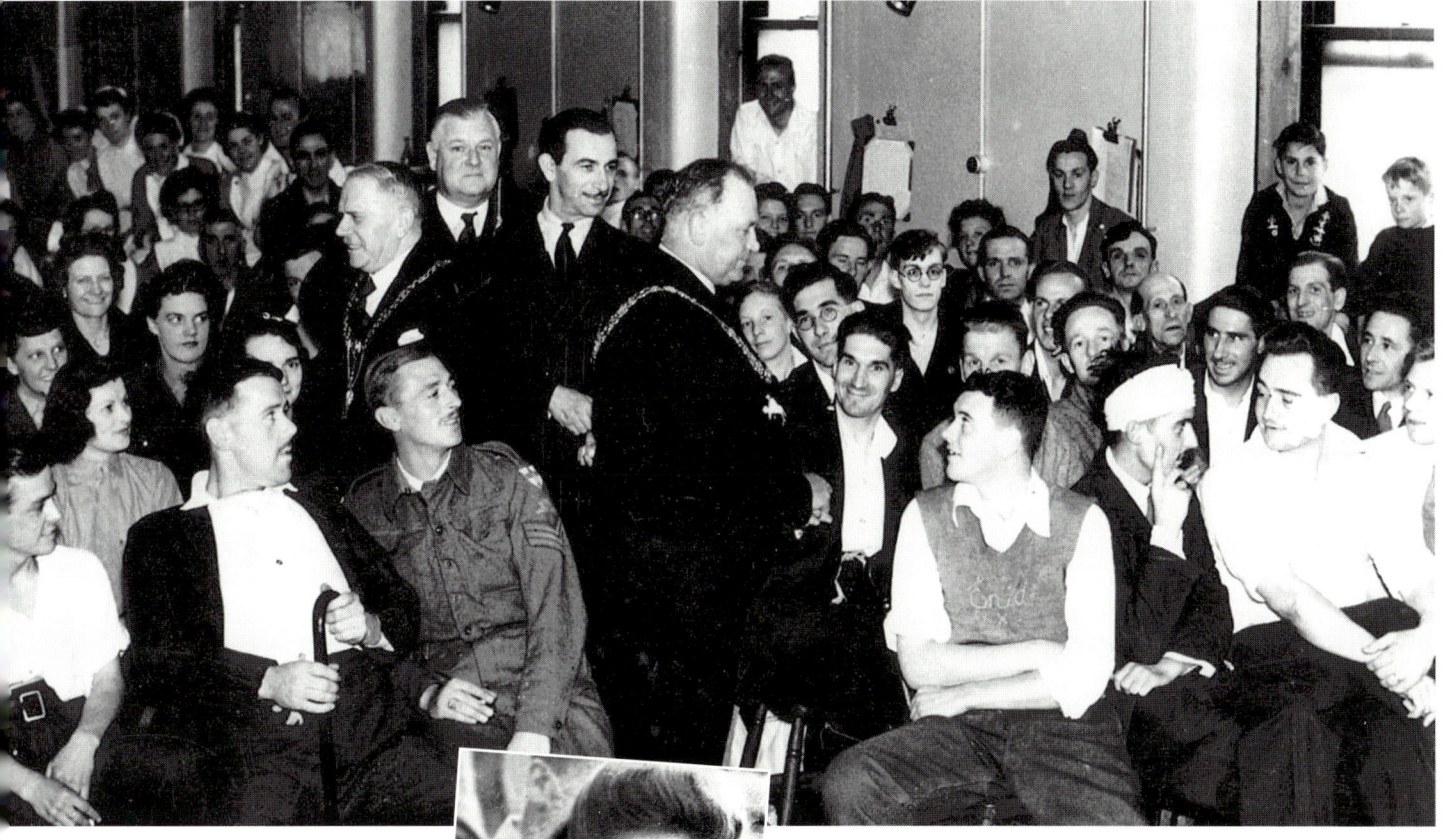

were treated at the City Hospital. It was a time of austerity. For example in 1942 the matron of the neighbouring isolation hospital reported great difficulty in obtaining clothing coupons for nurses' uniforms, and in the same year she also sought permission to purchase a dozen steel helmets for nurses to use during air raids.

One of the wartime highlights for staff and patients was the visit by Vera Lynn, the 'Forces Sweetheart', on July 9, 1943 for an impromptu concert on Lister Two ward. A report in the *Nottingham Evening News* said she had "seldom had a more appreciative audience" in singing her songs to men wounded in the Tunisian campaign.

Following the untimely death in 1946 of Dr Crawford Crowe, a much respected if authoritarian Medical Superintendent, Dr William Morton was appointed as resident Medical Officer. He later developed geriatric medicine at the City Hospital into what is now known as health care of the elderly. He also established the occupational therapy department with a staff of just two.

In his excellent booklet *Bagthorpe to the City: A Story of a Nottingham Hospital*, Dr James Macfie notes that around this time a more democratic atmosphere developed and the Medical Staff Committee, comprising all consultants, came into being.

The City Hospital was preparing for the dawn of a new age... the birth of the National Health Service on July 5, 1948.

Top: Staff and patients await the arrival of the 'Forces Sweetheart' Vera Lynn to sing at the City Hospital's Lister Two ward in 1943
Above: An early picture of Vera Lynn
Right: How the Nottingham Evening News covered the story of her visit

Vera Lynn Entertains Wounded In Nottingham

VERA LYNN, the "Forces sweetheart," has seldom had a more appreciative audience than she did to-day, when she gave her songs in a Nottingham hospital ward in which were men wounded in the Tunisian campaign.

Miss Lynn headed a company drawn from artistes appearing at the Nottingham Empire this week, who, by courtesy of Mr. George Black and the management of the Nottingham Theatre Royal and Empire, devoted their afternoon to giving a variety show to men unable to leave hospital to attend a place of amusement.

Many of those who enjoyed the show cannot yet be moved from their beds.

Other soldiers wounded less seriously, were brought in from other centres, where they are being treated, to the hospital in which the entertainment was staged.

In addition to Miss Lynn and her accompanist, Len Edwards, the artistes who entertained the wounded soldiers were Stainless Stephen, the Sheffield comedian, Murray, the Australian "escapologist," Peter Fannon, and Phil Darbin and Wendy.

The arrangements for the visit had been made by E.N.S.A. acting through Mr. H. Elton, Nottingham representative on the Northern Regional Committee.

Civic recognition was given to the occasion by the presence of the Lord Mayor and Lady Mayoress of Nottingham, Ald. and Mrs. E. A. Braddock, and the Sheriff of Nottingham, Coun. J. E. Mitchell and Mrs. Mitchell, together with Capt. Mills, the area entertainments offic

The People's Hospital

What's in a name?

Great figures behind the ward names

MANY influential figures have shaped the life and times of Nottingham City Hospital during the past century.

The founding fathers, who turned a workhouse and infirmary into a municipal hospital, were followed by distinguished physicians and surgeons, able administrators, notable nurses and generations of staff who contributed enormously to patient care.

Throughout a century of dedicated service, men and women of international standing have been associated with the hospital - and this is reflected in the impressive list of ward names, which read like a medical Who's Who.

This section summarises how those names came to be chosen.

Alexandra ward: (The David Evans Research Centre). At one time this was a locked ward or isolation ward. It took its name from Hattie Elizabeth Alexandra (1901-1968), whose collaboration with immunologist Michael Heidelberger led to the discovery of a cure for meningitis. The Medical Research Centre was renamed the David Evans Research Centre in honour of the man who worked hard to make it a reality. David Evans, *below left*, a former banker and Chairman of the Nottinghamshire Area Health Authority, chaired the £1m appeal to build the centre. The target was achieved in just four years and the building was opened by the Duchess of Gloucester in 1986. Mr Evans

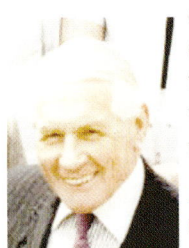

died in November 1996 and the trustees decided it would be appropriate to re-name the building in his honour. A ceremony was held in July 1997 with his son Brian unveiling a commemorative plaque.

Ashwell ward: Named after Dr Herbert George Ashwell, Medical Superintendent of the original Union Workhouse in York Street, Nottingham and later the Bagthorpe Workhouse and Infirmary (City Hospital) from 1888 to 1930. He became known as the 'father' of the hospital, organising the care for wounded soldiers in the First World War and the children's wards were a legacy to his work.

Barclay Thoracic Unit: Named after Mr Robert Christopher Barclay, Consultant Thoracic Surgeon from 1952 to 1981.

Beeston ward: Beeston, near Nottingham was where Jesse Boot (later Lord Trent) made his home after establishing the Boots empire.

Birkett ward: Named after Mr Noel Birkett, Consultant Orthopaedic Surgeon at the City and Nottingham General Hospital from 1947 to 1970.

Bramley ward: Takes its name from the Bramley Apple first grown in an orchard at Southwell, Nottinghamshire.

Bonington ward: This ward takes its name from Richard Parks Bonington, the 19th century romantic artist from Arnold, near Nottingham, who was renowned for his landscapes and historical scenes.

Carrel ward: Named after American surgeon Alexis Carrel (1873-1944), who won the Nobel Prize for his work on transplantation and suturing blood vessels in transplantation.

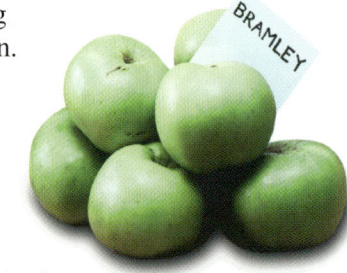

Cavell ward: Takes its name from Edith Louisa Cavell, *above*, (1873-1915), the brave English nurse who cared for friend and foe in Brussels in 1914-15. She was executed by the Germans for helping Allied prisoners-of-war.

Charnley Suite: This department is named after Orthopaedic Surgeon John Charnley (1911-1982), who invented the artificial hip joint, bringing relief to thousands of arthritis sufferers throughout the world.

Edward One and Two wards: These two wards take their name from King Edward VII (1841-1910), who married Princess Alexandra of Denmark in 1863. He succeeded his mother, Queen Victoria, to the throne in 1901.

Fleming ward: Named after the eminent Scottish bacteriologist Sir Alexander Fleming (1881-1955), who discovered the antibacterial enzyme lysozyme in 1922 and pencillin in 1928. Fleming was knighted in 1944. In 1945 he shared the Nobel Prize with Australian scientist Howard Walter Florey and German-British pathologist Ernst Boris Chain for their contributions to the development of penicillin.

Fletcher ward: Named after Professor John Fletcher, who treated thousands of leukaemia patients during 27 years at Nottingham City Hospital from 1971 to 1998. Sylvia Bishton, of the Nottingham Leukaemia Appeal said: "He is a very dedicated man - not just in the hospital but behind the scenes - to make sure that the treatment of leukaemia patients in Nottingham is the among the best in the country."

Fraser ward: Named after Nottingham's first Consultant Radiologist Dr William Fraser from 1955-1981.

The People's Hospital

Gedling ward: Takes its name from the district on the outskirts of Nottingham.

Gervis Pearson ward: Named after Lt Col Noel Gervis Pearson (1884-1958), a distinguished soldier and Chairman of the Nottingham General Hospital's Monthly Board when the hospital became part of the NHS in 1948.

Gillies ward: Takes it name from Sir Harold Delf Gillies (1882-1960), a pioneer in the development of plastic and reconstructive surgery.

Harvey One and Two wards: Named after the distinguished physician Sir William Harvey (1578-1657), who discovered the circulation of the blood.

Hogarth ward: Takes its name from Robert George Hogarth, Honorary Consultant and founder of the radiotherapy department at Nottingham General Hospital, long before it transferred to the City Hospital in 1993.

James ward: Named after the City Hospital's first Consultant Rheumatologist Dr Sam James.

Jenner ward: Named after the pioneering physician Edward Jenner (1749-1823), whose discovery of vaccination against smallpox in 1798 helped lay the foundations of modern immunology.

Lambley ward: Named after the village of Lambley, near Nottingham.

Lawrence ward: Named after the famous English writer D H Lawrence, (1885-1930), who was born at Eastwood, Nottinghamshire.

Linby ward: Named after the Nottinghamshire village.

Loxley ward: Named after Nottingham's folklore hero Robin Hood of Loxley.

Lister One and Two wards: Named after Joseph Lister (1827-1912), founder of antiseptic surgery in 1865 which greatly reduced the mortality rate in hospitals.

Millard ward: Named after American professor David Ralph Millard, the world's leading specialist in cleft palate and harelip surgery.

Morton ward: Named after Dr William Morton, who was appointed Physician Superintendent of the City Hospital in 1946. He established psycho-geriatric nursing at the St Francis Unit and was also responsible for the creation of the City Hospital's occupational therapy department.

Nightingale ward: Named after the famous nurse and hospital reformer Florence Nightingale, *above*, (1820-1910). During the Crimean War she encountered considerable official opposition towards organising a nursing service for British soldiers, who called her "the lady of the lamp."

Oxton ward: Named after the Nottinghamshire village.

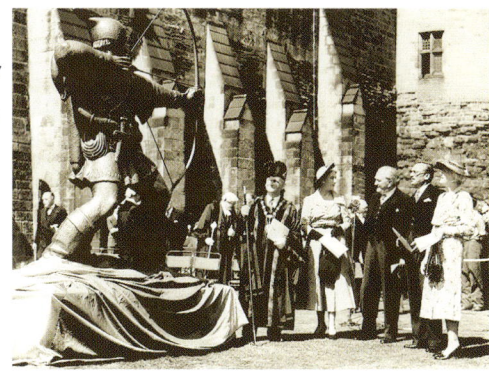

Right: Studying the Robin Hood statue immediately after its unveiling, are the Duchess of Portland with the sculptor and city dignitaries. Loxley and Winifred wards owe their names to Robin Hood and the Duchess of Portland

Papplewick ward: Takes its name from the Nottinghamshire village where England's first steam powered mill was built in 1785.

Patience One and Two wards: Named after Sister Patience, a ward sister during the early days of the Bagthorpe Workhouse and Infirmary.

Robert Jones ward: Named after the famous Welsh Orthopaedic Surgeon Robert Jones, He was responsible for the health of the 30,000 navvies who built the Manchester Ship Canal.

Simpson One and Two wards: Named after the Scottish Obstetrician James Young Simpson (1811-1870), who initiated the use of chloroform in childbirth.

Southwell ward: Named after the Nottinghamshire minster town where Charles 1 spent his last night of freedom before being captured by Roundheads near Newark.

Toghill ward: Named after Dr Peter Toghill, one of Nottingham's most influential physicians. He worked at the City Hospital from 1968 to the early 1970s and was a popular clinical sub dean for three years. Based at University Hospital, he has special interest in lymphoma and liver disease. When he 'retired', he founded and ran the continuing medical education department at the Royal College of Physicians in London. President of the Nottingham Hospitals' Choir, past president of the Nottingham Medico-Chirurgical Society and the Nottinghamshire Medico-Legal Society. Author of many academic papers, three popular textbooks and articles on W G Grace and C B Fry.

Victoria One and Two wards: These wards, housing the assessment unit, cardiac intensive care unit and the adult intensive care unit, were named after Queen Victoria.

Warren ward: Named after the American surgeon John Collins Warren (1778-1856), who took part with dentist William Morton in the first public demonstration of ether as a surgical anaesthetic in 1846.

Winifred One and Two wards: Named after Winifred the Duchess of Portland, founder member of the City Hospital League of Friends in the early 1950s.

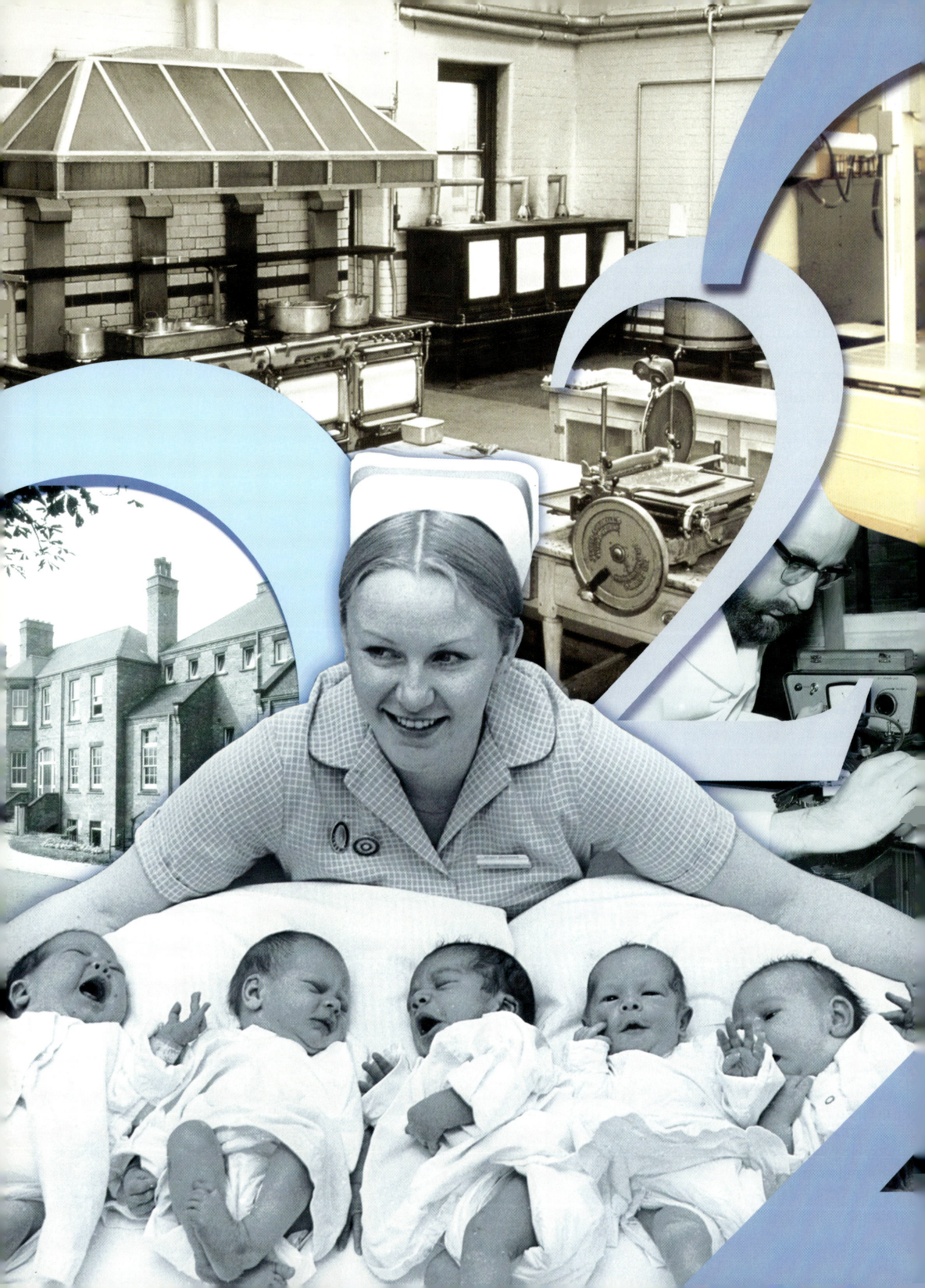

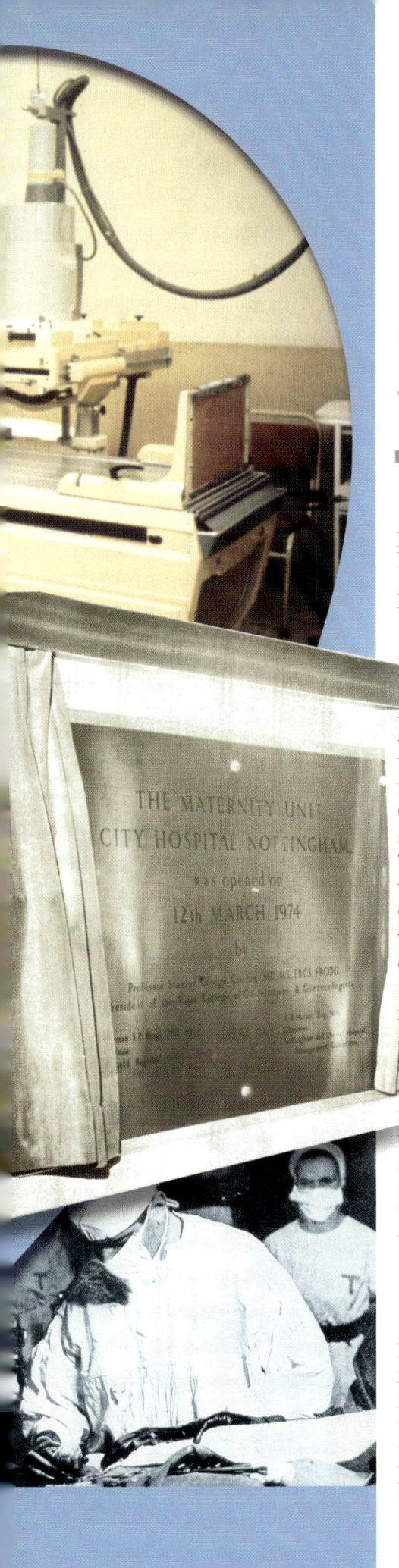

Exciting times — and real progress

The growth years (1948-1982)

THE next stage of our journey takes readers through the growth years - a remarkable period of progress that transformed Nottingham City Hospital from a general infirmary into a leading teaching hospital.

This transition was boosted by the inception of the National Health Service on July 5, 1948. Generally the new state-funded system was eagerly awaited but many senior consultants viewed it with trepidation. They feared Government interference and GPs were worried it would lead to state access of their patients' records. Transferring day-to-day running of the hospital from the Local Health Committee to the NHS brought teething problems and delayed development plans.

Extra facilities were urgently needed to meet rising demands on services; in less than two decades the number of patients had more than doubled, from 4,189 in 1930 to 9,100 in 1947. Operations performed during this period rose nearly six-fold from 592 to 3,098; X-ray examinations increased dramatically from 498 to 7,724 and the maternity department was working at full stretch, delivering 1,644 babies in 1947 compared with 159 in 1930.

The birth of the NHS also brought a change in administration. The City Hospital came under the direction of Nottingham No 2 Hospital Management Committee, chaired by Alderman Robert Shaw. Overall control passed to the regional hospital board based in Sheffield.

The hospital made a real effort to sweep away the gloom of the war years. Drab brown and olive green walls were replaced with creams and ochres and the black iron bed frames were painted in pastel hues.

Mary Beers, former Secretary to the Medical Committee, recalls:

"My first memory of the Nottingham City Hospital was as a patient in August 1945. My 31-year-old mother had been admitted with diphtheria, followed a few days later by me. I was a carrier and had apparently given the disease to her. I was not ill and was discharged after two weeks following three negative swabs. However my mother, who had not been immunised, was very unwell and hospitalised for eight weeks. During her incarceration six children with diphtheria died on the ward she was on. I guess it must have been a Heathfield ward, a dreadful place with even more dire senior staff."

It should be noted that at the inception of the NHS in 1948, the Heathfield Wards (the City Isolation Hospital) came under the Nottingham No 1 Hospital Management Committee and were controlled from the General Hospital. The wards didn't become part of the City Hospital until 1968. Later re-designated as convalescence wards, they remained in use until the early 1990s when they were closed to make way for the building of a new maternity unit.

Recalling girlhood memories in 1945, Mary reflects:

"Some of the nurses were lovely but lacking in enough seniority to alter

Continued on page 19

The People's Hospital

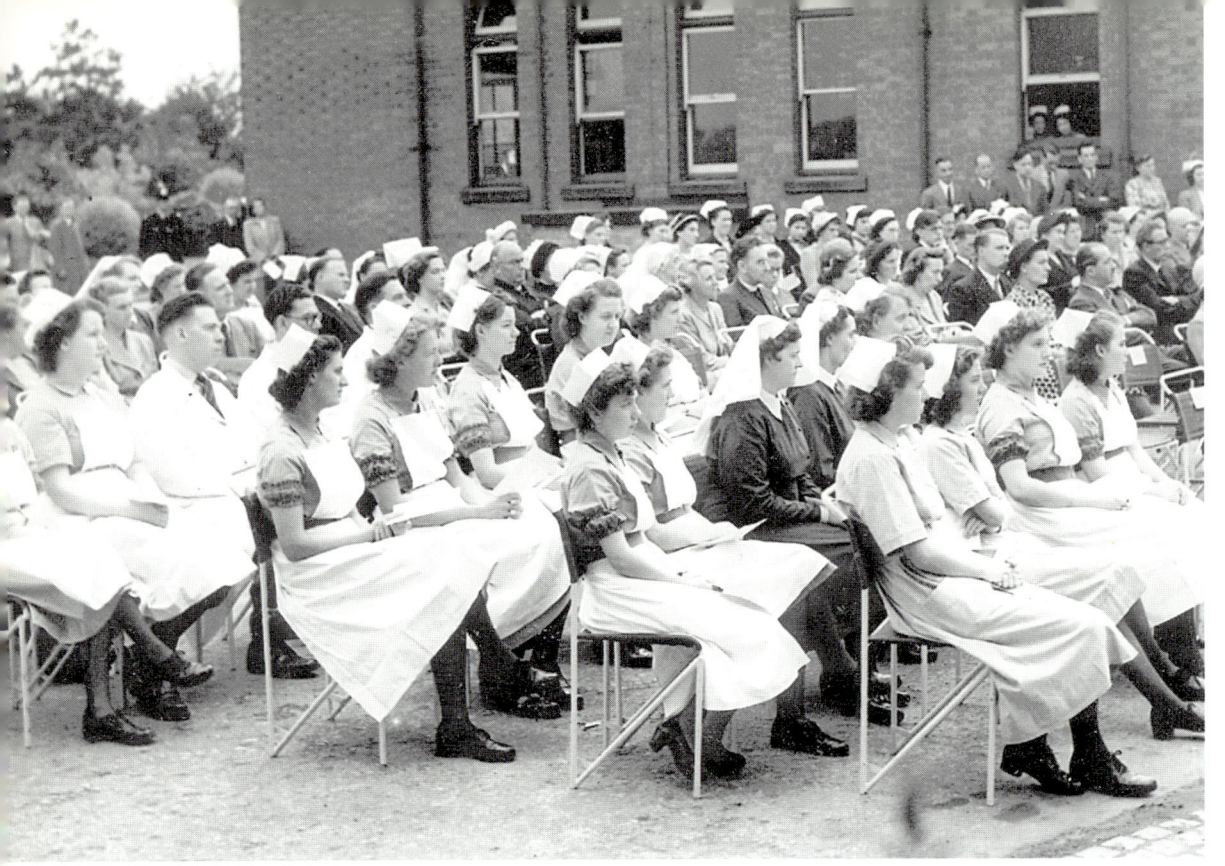

Left: *Nurses and other staff attending the foundation stone laying ceremony for new twin theatres at the City Hospital on July 28, 1951*

THE VERANDA BELLES

MRS JOAN TOMLINSON (nee Lowe), of Old Basford, has vivid memories of the two years she spent at Nottingham City Hospital as a TB spinal patient in 1951/52. She was 19 at the time and nurses and patients soon nicknamed her one of the 'Veranda Belles' on Victoria Two orthopaedic ward, where all the beds were sited under outdoor verandas.

Joan went into the hospital just after being chosen as the Bestwood Estate May Queen. So as a consolation for missing out on the honour, the matron arranged for Joan to receive a visit from the newly-elected May Queen and her retinue, who presented a bunch of flowers and a basket of fruit to every patient on the ward.

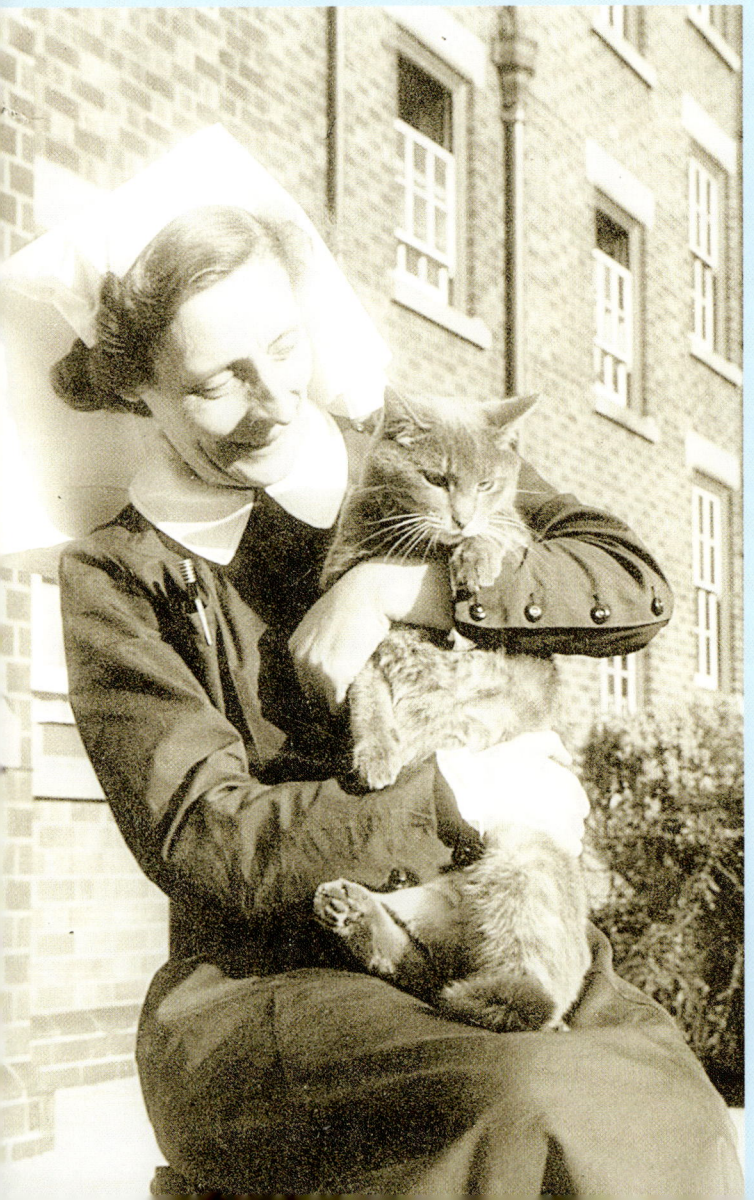

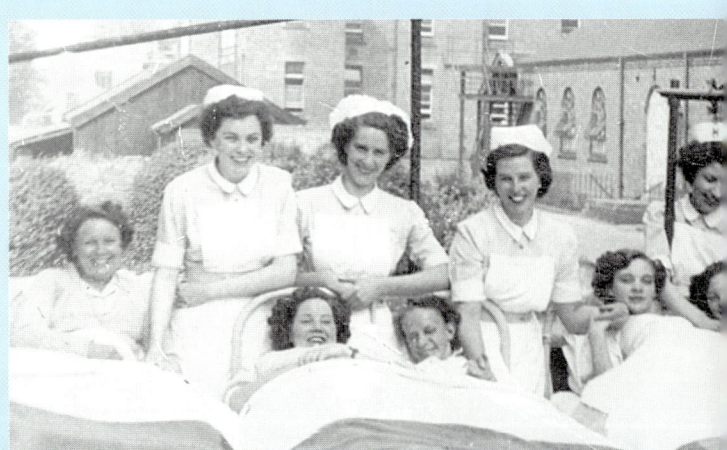

Above: *Nurses and patients - nicknamed the Veranda Belles - on Victoria Two ward in 1952*
Left: *Sister Jew, who had hundreds of student nurses in her care, is seen sitting outside the nurses' home in the 1950s with her pet cat*

The People's Hospital

Continued from page 17

the regime. Visiting was not allowed for one's first three weeks inside, and when visitors came they were forced to stay outside and talk to us through the windows. In that case why the three-week rule? On a lighter note, Britain celebrated VJ Day during our stay and we watched the celebrations and fireworks as patients from other wards had a whale of a time outside."

In 1937 the hospital had approved plans to add verandas to certain wards. Now this scheme was extended to add sun lounges and single room cubicles to more wards. Outdoor surroundings were brightened too by laying lawns, planting trees and creating colourful flowerbeds. A former nurse, recalling that time, said:

"It was like living and working in a lovely park."

Like the NHS itself, many hospital departments were still evolving. For example the hospital's two physiotherapists worked in 1949 in a converted sewing room fitted with wall bars and walking aids. The first attempts were made in 1950 to establish a dietetic service and the Medical Superintendent Dr William Morton instigated an occupational therapy service in the same year. The first qualified OT worked part-time and her base was the bathroom of a disused ward. When a full-time therapist was appointed in 1951, the department had acquired its own hut to which a kitchen unit was added in 1957. An OT department was opened in Sherwood Hospital in 1959 and occupational therapists gratefully accepted a gift from Barton Transport — turning the back end of a bus into a training unit, where disabled people could practice getting up and down steps. The converted bus saw sterling service for many years until the department transferred to modern premises in the late 1980s.

The first major advance following the creation of the NHS was the opening of the new twin operating theatre suite by the Duchess of Gloucester in 1954. The hospital had been waiting for these facilities since 1937 and once the new building was ready it was brought into use at once. By the time the Duchess carried out the official opening, 1,500 operations

Visiting was pretty restrictive in those days, Joan recalls. "It was just one hour from 7pm to 8pm on Monday, Wednesday and Friday nights and two hours on Sunday afternoons from 2pm to 4pm.

Visitors had to show their visiting card at the gate to admit two visitors. Children were excluded as no visitor could be under 12."

But nurses did their best to make Christmas a happy time for patients. Joan recalls the matron and the nurses turning their cloaks to the red side to tour the wards on Christmas Eve, carrying lanterns and singing carols.

"All diets were abolished on Christmas Day and we tucked into an eggs and gammon breakfast. Dr Slack came round to carve the turkey in the middle of the ward and we also had Christmas pudding. Off duty nurses even came in to have a festive drink with us."

Joan looked forward to visits from her boyfriend Colin, later to become her husband. They got engaged on the ward on May 9, 1951 and Colin brought in a gramophone player to keep the patients entertained. Joan recalls: "Colin bought the gramophone for £3 from Sneinton Market. It was the wind-up type and if we wanted a record on we had to wait until a nurse was free. I also remember Rediffusion being installed in all the wards and listening to Valentine Dyall (The Man in Black) on the radio."

During her long stay in hospital, Joan underwent a bone graft operation performed by Consultant Orthopaedic Surgeon Mr Noel Birkett. Recalling the chilly conditions on the ward, she explained: "The verandas were totally open. It was cold because we only had two blankets. I wore a nightdress cut down the back because I was swathed in plaster and lay on top of the bed on a frame."

Joan was eventually discharged in October, 1952. She

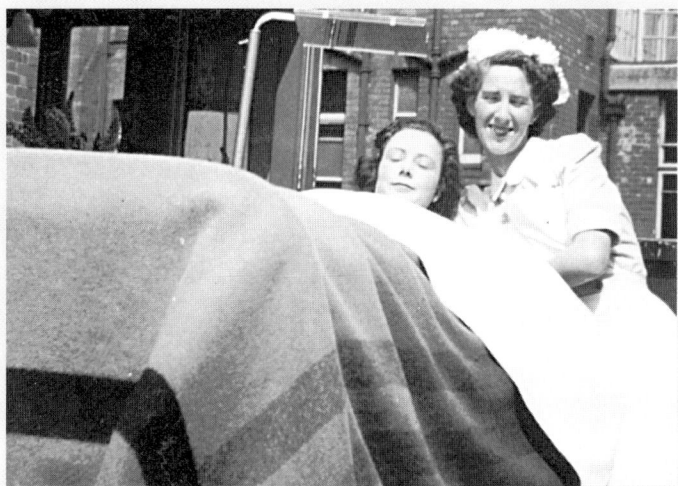

Joan Tomlinson (nee Lowe) with Staff Nurse Mary Parker following her operation in June 1952

married on her 22nd birthday on February 20, 1954 and went on to have two children. She has since returned to Nottingham City Hospital 10 times and is full of praise for the care she has received. As a patient of Consultant Dr Keith Morris, she was referred to St Bart's Hospital, London for an operation in 1986 and had an artificial heart valve fitted at Groby Road Hospital, Leicester in 1993.

■ *The practice of putting beds on chilly verandas to treat TB patients continued well into the 1950s. Colleagues told a retired hospital consultant of the time that snow drifted into one of the open-air wards during the bitterly cold winter of 1947.*

Treatment of many infectious conditions changed once drugs such as streptomycin and penicillin (manufactured on the hospital site) became more widely available.

The People's Hospital

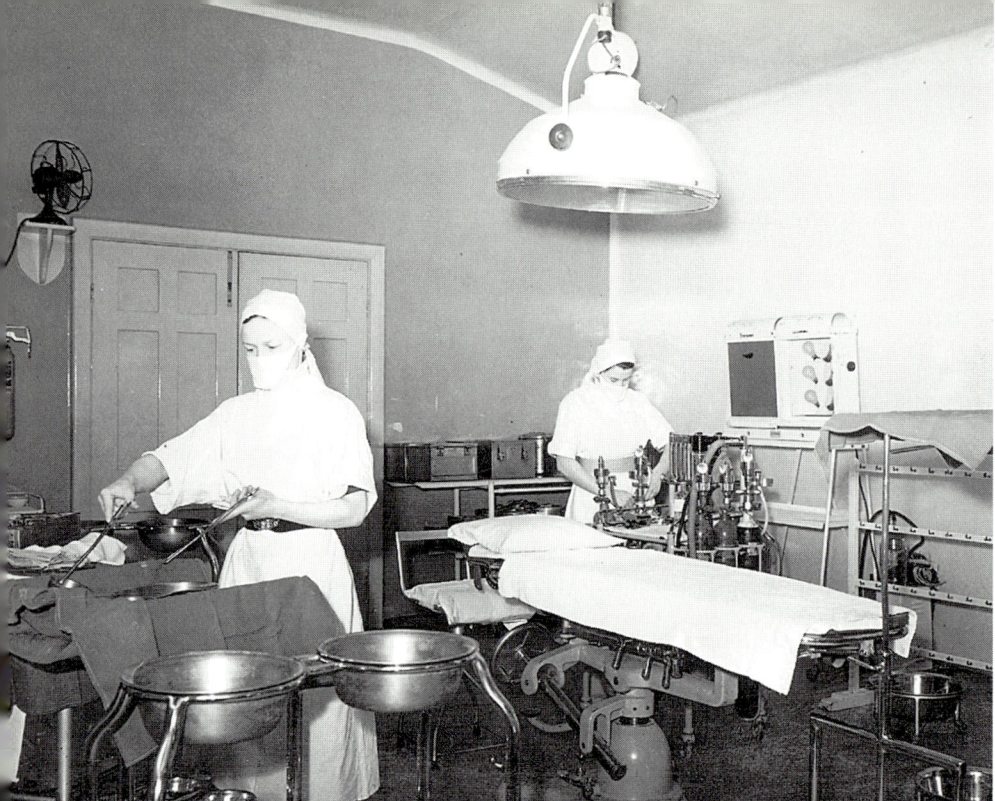

New twin theatres were officially opened in April 1954

THE VERANDA BELLES

MRS Mavis Astill, of Mapperley, was only nine when she became a City Hospital patient in 1946.

She recalled: "I went in for an appendicitis operation. I remember laying on the operating table and looking round the room. On the shelves were jars of pickled parts - appendix I assume!

"There was no injection to put you out. They just came behind you with a cloth of ether."

Mavis has a photograph of her Aunt Betty who spent three years and four months in the hospital from the late 1940s onwards receiving treatment for a TB spine.

"She had to lay on a plaster cast. Her back was bare on the cast and as the photo *(right)* shows, they were out on the veranda for fresh air even in very cold weather.

"As I was under 12 I was not allowed to visit officially. A man sat at the main gate in the office on Hucknall Road checking everybody's

continued from page 19

visiting cards. I was supposed to sit in the waiting room. It was usually Sunday afternoons when my family visited and I used to play on the grass opposite. There was a slight bank down the other side and when the man wasn't looking I would creep down the bank and run along to the veranda to see my aunt. One day I slipped on the bank, badly spraining my ankle, which I suppose was judgement on me!"

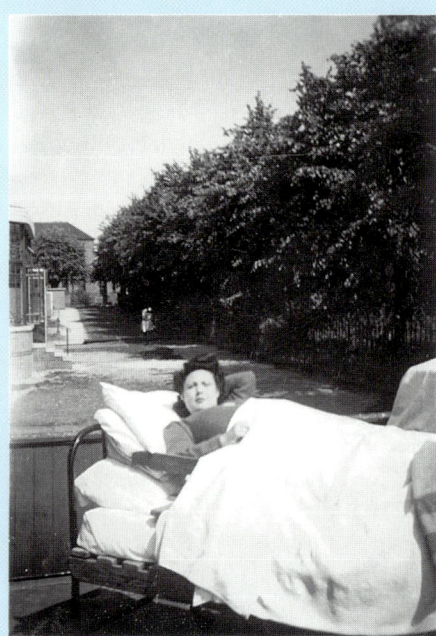

Right: *Aunty Betty pictured outside on the veranda during her very long stay in the City Hospital in the late 1940s receiving treatment for a TB spine*

Continued from page 19

had been performed by a team of 13 surgeons.

A feature article in the *Nottingham Guardian Journal* described the new theatres as the most modern in the Midlands. The windows in the building were never opened. All the air was washed, sterilised and heated before being pumped into the theatres through vents near the ceiling and extracted by fans at floor level.

The writer explained: "The first thing that strikes the visitor in these shining temples of surgery is the air of quiet. Not only is the floor noiseless but the walls are coated with rough faced sound-absorbing plaster.

"The theatres stand on either side of a central sterilising room, which contain three built-in autoclaves. Two of these are used for sterilising instruments and the central one is used to sterilise dressings, gowns, masks and the like.

"All is chrome and white, with the black face of the autoclaves standing out in sharp contrast. As in the two theatres the walls are of a pale blue duck-egg finish to avoid light reflection.

"Above each operating table is suspended the large mushroom head of the scialytic lamps, mirror-lined, so that they cast a shadowless brilliance."

Other refinements included automatic shutters which could be snapped down over eastward facing windows when ophthalmic or ear, nose and throat surgery was being carried out. Each theatre also had illuminated panels for viewing X-ray plates and the unit was equipped with its own dark room so that plates could be exposed, developed and viewed while an operation was in progress. Alongside the theatres were two recovery rooms for patients.

The development brought the number of main operating theatres available to four and by this time the hospital had 804 beds.

But the 16 main wards badly

The People's Hospital

needed updating. They were still 'Nightingale' in style with 14 beds down each side of the open ward with washing and toilet facilities at one end. The ward corridor was of grey stone with white tiled walls; a large linen store, kitchen, clothing store and sister's office led off this corridor. The kitchen was used for heating up patients' food and also contained a large, noisy steriliser which was constantly in use. There was one lift for each pair of four-ward blocks, so patients for two wards had to cross an open bridge without protection from the weather. Work started in 1963 on a major reconstruction scheme to divide the wards into four-bedded bays with three single-bed rooms and a lift to all wards. The steriliser was removed. Washing and toilet facilities were re-sited half way down the length of the ward and there was a day room for patients. Consultant Dr James Macfie described the changes as dramatic. "Unfortunately," he added, "the work was completed on only eight wards from 1965 onwards; the money allocated for the purpose being used to build the H Block. The remaining wards in later years were refurbished and became quite acceptable, if still a little dated."

Another senior consultant commented: "Some years previously a programme of upgrading the main wards had been agreed as being cheaper than knocking blocks down and building modern hospital structures. In retrospect this was the wrong decision. Upgrading was a poor compromise, cost much more than originally identified and became progressively delayed. In fact the programme was never completed."

He added: "Post 1963 it took some time to get attitudes changed. The old voluntary hospital (General Hospital) was the dominant player and had most of the medical representation on regional committees. However, once the regional office had accepted the equal role of the two acute general hospitals (before University Hospital was running) then the whole ethos changed.

"Gone was the 'Poor Law' hangover and money for capital projects and revenue came in increasing amounts to the City Hospital for desperately needed advancement.

"The commitment of the City Hospital consultants to fight for their share of resources was almost universal among the increasing numbers of consultant staff. Furthermore, relationships with administration were good and the very friendly atmosphere in the hospital (which I had immediately noticed on arrival) was preserved. It was a very happy place in which to work and teamwork was excellent. There was a very loyal and enthusiastic staff at all grades. Considering the less than good workplace facilities which persisted for many for a very long time, the fact that things were progressively improving was very important for morale."

Meanwhile the development of more powerful drugs made biochemistry a vital discipline in the treatment of diseases. This was recognised in 1952 by the opening of three new biochemical laboratories to analyse 10,000 specimens a year. During an open day, invited guests

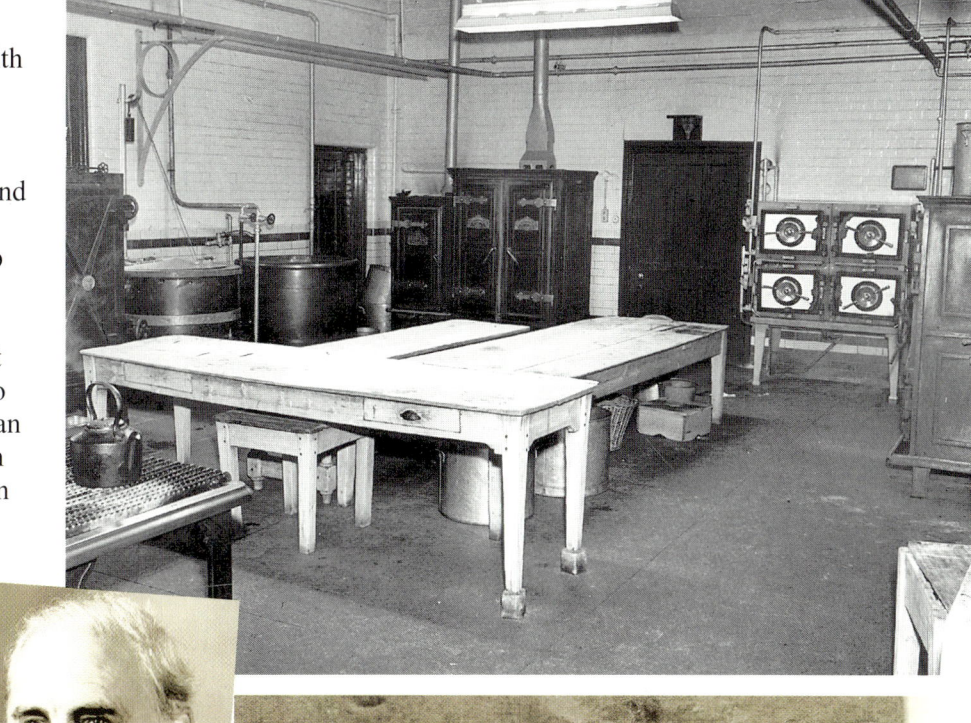

Top: Sherwood Hospital kitchen in 1954
Above: Consultant Dr James Macfie

The Daykin triplets - born January 23, 1954. The first full set of triplets to survive at the City Hospital were shown round the new laboratories by Dr A H Johns, Director of the pathology department and Dr J B Foote, Director of the biochemical section.

The role of volunteers in hospitals was beginning to be recognised and the City Hospital League of Friends was formed in 1954 with the Duchess of Portland becoming the first President.

A year later the plastics and reconstructive unit was established, following the appointment of Mr David Wynn-Williams as the hospital's first plastic surgeon. The late 1950s saw two major improvements - the opening of a large purpose-built outpatients department in 1958 and about 18 months later a new X-ray department came into use.

The £50,000 X-ray unit, containing the latest diagnostic equipment to give clearer, faster films, was opened by Mr A V Martin, Chairman of the Sheffield Regional Board. In charge of the department was Consultant Radiologist Dr C H Wood and Superintendent Radiographer Leslie Hall. The 14 staff wore heavy gloves and large protective rubber and lead aprons, weighing about 25 lb.

The new £100,000 outpatient department was described as one of the most modern in the country. When the outpatient service started on Jenner Ward in 1947 it was possible to run only one clinic. By 1957 attendances topped 30,000 and bigger, better facilities were desperately needed. Twenty four outpatient sessions a week were going ahead in the new department and each of the three clinical suites had rooms for consultation, examination, minor surgical procedures and special investigations. Accommodation was also provided for almoners (social workers), chiropodists, speech therapists, an area for pathology investigation and an outpatient pharmacy. There was a waiting room with canteen, a small lecture room, a plaster theatre, a dental clinic room with a theatre, plus adequate office and patient appointment space. Sister in charge of the new department was Sister J Thompson.

A children's playroom and area for storing teaching equipment at the City Hospital School was officially opened by the Lord Mayor Alderman John Llewellyn Davies in 1961. Cost of the £5,000 pre-fabricated building was shared by Nottingham Education Committee and the City Hospital League of Friends. An Evening Post report said the project was a reminder that a youngster's education does not stop when they are admitted to hospital.

"Classes were held in the wards and

Below: Opening of the X-ray department at the City Hospital in 1959

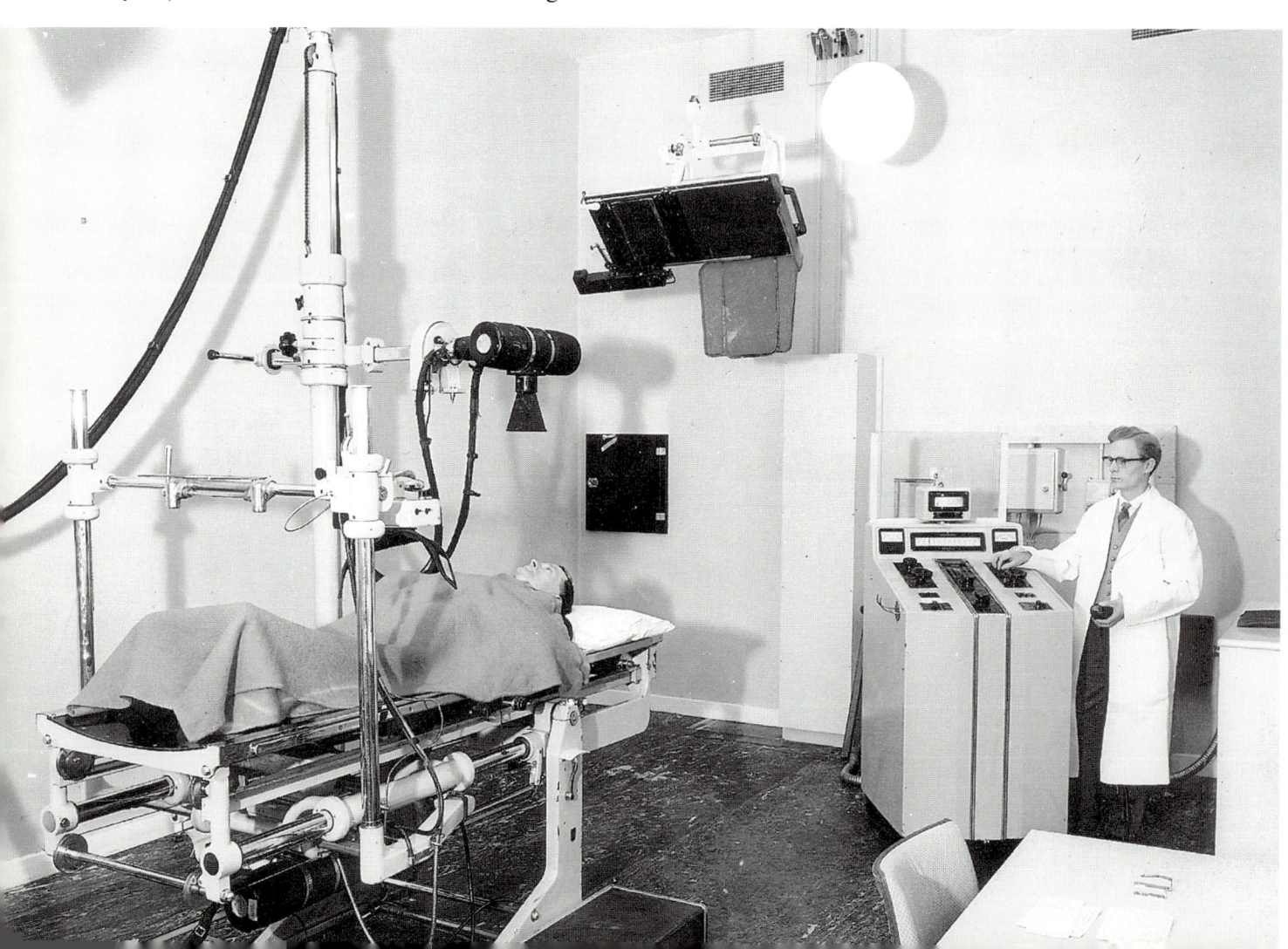

The People's Hospital

the 'school' had full time teaching staff supervised by head teacher Miss A V Williams. Children confined to beds use portable desks. The school roll is never less than 50 and each child gets individual attention. There are several cases of children compelled to do all their 11-plus preparations while in hospital and getting through to grammar school. Some have even passed their GCE examinations while still in hospital."

A children's nursery opened in December 1963 to help former City Hospital nurses with young children who wanted to return to their careers. It was hoped the 'nursery for nurses' scheme, housed in the John Robb Playroom, would go a long way to solving the shortage of trained staff, especially among midwives.

The *Guardian Journal* featured the project and published a photograph of Matron Miss G Hayre talking to children and staff in the playroom.

After Dr Johns retired in 1963, the pathology department was reorganised. A specialist histopathologist was appointed and one of the responsibilities of Dr (later Professor) Roger Cotton was to start a diagnostic cytology service. The microbiology service was taken over by Dr E R Mitchell, Director of the Public Health Laboratory Service.

The hospital's quarter mile long main corridor was spruced up around 1965. Its shape and length could not be altered; but laying sound-deadening flooring to replace the white and brown marble effect tiles, plus the addition of a false ceiling, cheerful decoration and better lighting altered the whole atmosphere.

In the same year Group Captain Douglas Bader came to the City Hospital site to open the Nottingham School of Physiotherapy in a building that had previously been used as admission dormitories for the former workhouse.

Another significant development destined to have a major impact on the future shape and scope of the City Hospital was the decision to create a

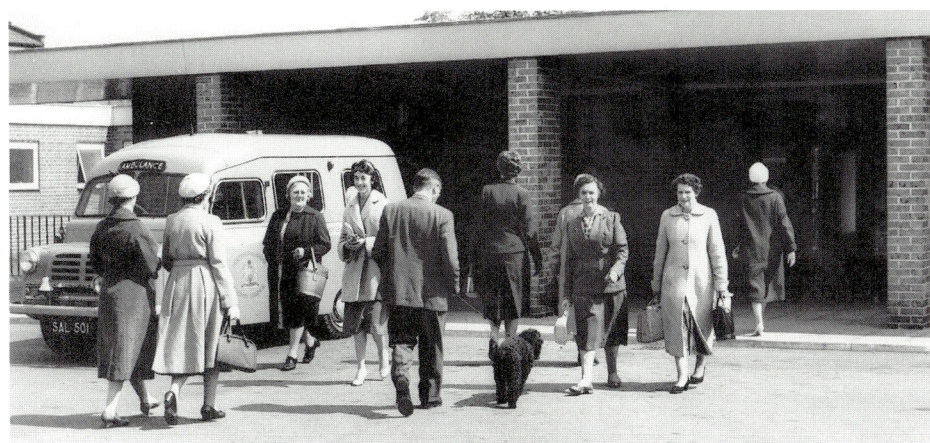

Above: A view of the entrance to the new Outpatients department at the City Hospital which was opened in 1959

Right: Patients waiting to be treated at the new Outpatients department

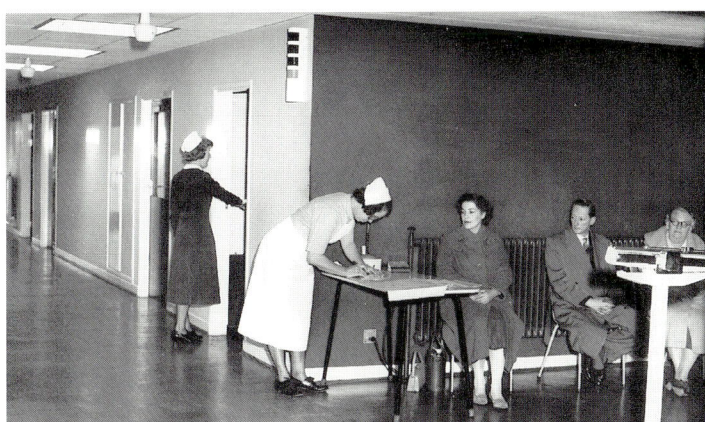

new integrated teaching hospital for Nottingham. The project came to fruition in 1977 when the Queen visited Nottingham as part of her Silver Jubilee celebrations and performed the opening ceremony of the new University Hospital and Medical School, naming the whole complex the Queen's Medical Centre. Built at a cost of about £70m - equivalent to two Concordes - it was described in 1979 as the largest group of hospital buildings in the world.

Professor David Greenfield, Foundation Dean of Medicine from 1966 to 1981, describes the development of relations between the Medical School of the University of Nottingham and the Nottingham City Hospital.

He writes: "On 27 July, 1964 the Minister of Health informed Parliament that a new medical school was to be established in Nottingham with an intake of 100 students a year, in conjunction with a new hospital of 1,200 beds. On the advice of Sir Robert Aitken, Vice Chancellor of the University of Birmingham, the University of Nottingham set up a Medical School Advisory Committee under the Chairmanship of Sir George Pickering. This reported to the university in April 1965; the report was published in June 1965. It recommended that undergraduate teaching should largely be concentrated in the new Medical Centre, but that the City Hospital and the General Hospital would be indispensable for the provision of house appointments in the pre-registration year, and that they would need suitable facilities for graduate education.

"In 1966 the university planned to admit medical students in 1970, using the Medical School part of the new Medical Centre to accommodate them, and it expected them to proceed to clinical work in the new hospital part of the Medical Centre.

"However, the site for the Medical Centre had not been purchased by the

Continued on page 25

MEMORIES OF JOHN COCHRANE

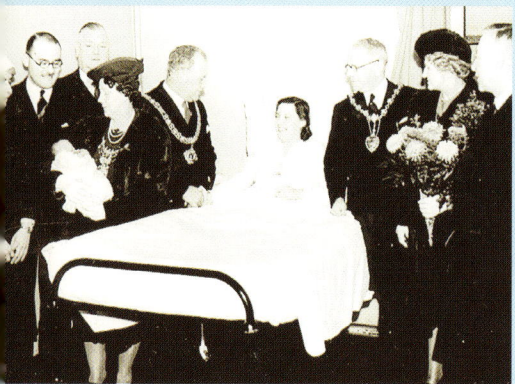

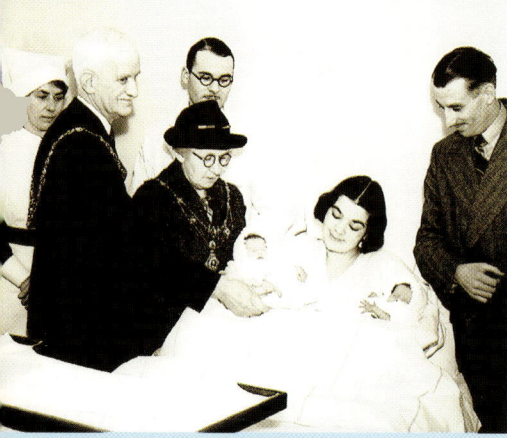

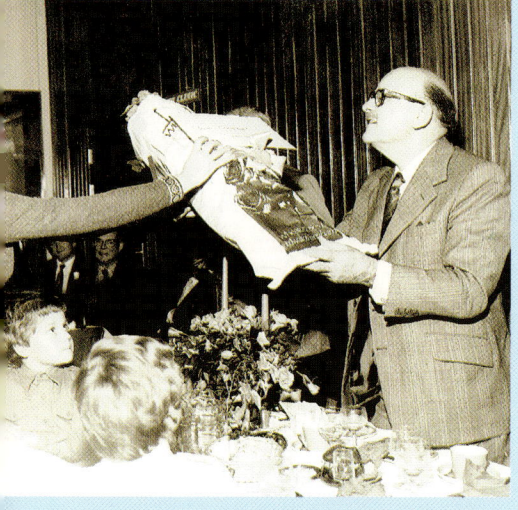

Top: Mrs White is congratulated on the birth of her son Peter (held by the Lady Mayoress) at the Firs Maternity Hospital on Christmas Day, 1943. Also pictured are the Matron Miss M Hooley, Dr John Cochrane (Obstetric Officer) and Dr Crawford Crowe (Medical Superintendent)

Centre: Consultant Harold Malkin, Sister M Hooley and Dr John Cochrane pictured in the late 1930s with civic heads after the birth of twins at the City Hospital.

Above: Sister Audrey Wade presents a bouquet of roses to Consultant Obstetrician Mr John Cochrane when he retired in 1976

WHILE compiling this book joint authors Paul Swift and David Lowe appealed through the local media for City Hospital memorabilia from the war years to the 1970s. They received a very enthusiastic response from people wanting to tell their City Hospital stories, especially their experiences of Mr John Barr Cochrane *(pictured)*.

'JB', as he was later known, was appointed House Surgeon at the City Hospital in 1937 and the following year became the hospital's first full-time Obstetrician and Gynaecologist.

He spent the rest of his professional life at the City Hospital being made Consultant at the inception of the National Health Service in 1948.

A man of immense energy with a prodigious workload, he set high standards in the personal care of his patients and the administration of his department.

Until he was appointed, maternity patients were looked after by a sister and whichever of the medical officers had particular experience of, or interest in, obstetrics. There was no blood transfusion service and no antibiotics.

Mr Cochrane and his colleague Mr H J Malkin helped spearhead improvements. Antenatal clinics and a blood transfusion service were soon set up and a 'flying squad' was established to go out from the hospital to deal with major problems that arose in home confinements.

Mr Cochrane's heart and soul was dedicated to the City Hospital and he took a major role in its development from a local authority hospital with just a handful of house staff into a leading teaching hospital with more than 100 medical staff.

A former trustee of the Nottingham Medico-Chirurgical Society, he worked tirelessly on behalf of Cancer Research and the Convent Hospital.

In his younger days he was a very competent jazz drummer and a keen cricketer, leading the City Hospital's team for many years. In 1985 he became President of the Nottinghamshire County Cricket Club and Nottinghamshire Cricket Association.

One of Paul Swift's favourite photographs *(top left)* shows a civic party grouped around the bedside at the Firs Maternity Hospital in Mansfield Road. They were congratulating Nottingham mother Mrs White on giving birth to a son, Peter Noel White, on Christmas Day 1943. Among those pictured are Mr Cochrane, Medical Superintendent Dr C L Crawford-Crowe and the Matron Miss M Hooley.

Margaret Lander (nee Halls), of Beeston, was among those who responded to an Evening Post article about the City Hospital's centenary. She trained to become a midwife at the City Hospital in 1953-54 and sent in a photograph showing the training group with Mr Cochrane and their sister tutor.

A Cinderhill mother writes: "In 1954, after suffering four miscarriages, I was put in the care of 'JB' at the Firs. Although some patients found him rather brusque on occasions, most of us thought he was a wonderful gynaecologist. He took me into the Firs Maternity Hospital. I

The People's Hospital

was in a two bed 'amenity ward' and had to stay in bed for three months, being visited every week by Mr Cochrane, who would greet me with the remark: "Well, lassie and how are we today?" until finally my son was born safely, seven weeks prematurely. He is now 48.

"How different hospital procedures were in those days. We were only allowed one visitor - our husband - from 7pm to 8pm each evening. Because my husband was unable to visit on Fridays, as a very special concession my mother was allowed to come then.

"The babies were kept in the nursery and only brought out for feeding, although in my case, my son was tube fed and kept in a constant temperature and so I wasn't allowed to see him until after seven days, since new mums had to stay in bed for that length of time.

"But the care and all aspects of the nursing could not have been better and I shall never cease to be grateful for it."

Keen amateur photographer Mr Kenneth E Adams, of Littleover, Derby, who submitted two splendid prints he took at the City Hospital in 1953, recalled: "Both my children were born at the Firs Maternity Hospital when the obstetrician was Mr Cochrane - my daughter was born on April 21, 1937 and my son John on July 26, 1948 so he was one of the first Health Service babies.

"I worked at the City Hospital from May 1949 until January 1954 firstly as a trainee administrator in the General Office and then as Deputy Medical Records Officer. I studied for four years and having passed the finals of the Institute of Hospital Administrators in June 1953 I moved to Derbyshire where I was a hospital secretary for 21 years before retiring in 1975."

Mr Cochrane helped plan the City Hospital's new maternity unit which opened in 1973. He died in 1985.

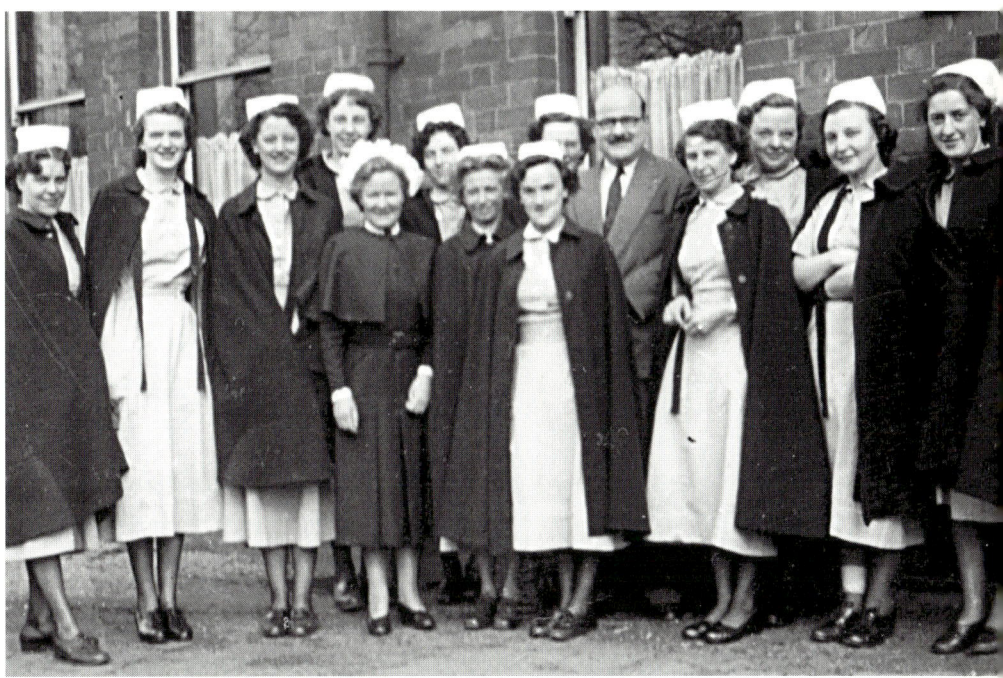

Mr John Cochrane is pictured here with midwifery staff including Margaret Lander (nee Halls). Picture dated 1953/54

Continued from 23

university and the Regional Health Authority and building could not start on it until 1970. The Medical School was unable to use the medical services component until 1974 and the hospital facilities became available in stages from 1971.

"In the face of these difficulties, the first intake of medical students, 48 in number, was admitted on time in 1970. Their clinical courses were inevitably provided by existing hospitals, mainly the City Hospital and the General Hospital, starting in 1973. All consultant staff in Nottingham were appointed as part-time clinical teachers. It was a great help that the City Hospital was willing to accept one half of the clinical students, and that Dr J S P Jones was willing to accept appointment as the Foundation Clinical Sub-Dean.

"Thus the delays in the building of University Hospital led to the teaching of one half of the clinical students very much earlier than was initially expected, and long before the City Hospital had received the great improvements to facilities and the addition of academic accommodation which it now has.

"While I was Dean the relationship between the university and the City Hospital was cordial and I believe it has remained so. The City Hospital staff were enthusiastic collaborators and excellent colleagues."

In his book *Bagthorpe to the City: Story of a Nottingham Hospital*, James Macfie explains why Nottingham's new Medical School was a great spur to the development of the City Hospital.

"At last an adequately funded building programme was about to be launched and over the next 10 years the campus was transformed. At the same time, with the active support of the new Dean of the Faculty of Medicine, Professor A D M Greenfield, medical staffing numbers were drastically revised and a large number of appointments of all grades in all disciplines were made."

The presence of the Nottingham School of Physiotherapy on the site from 1965 also gave a welcome boost to staff recruitment and by 1970 a new purpose-built physiotherapy department - one of the largest in the country - was opened at the City Hospital by Lady Hamilton, President of the Disabled Living Foundation. An

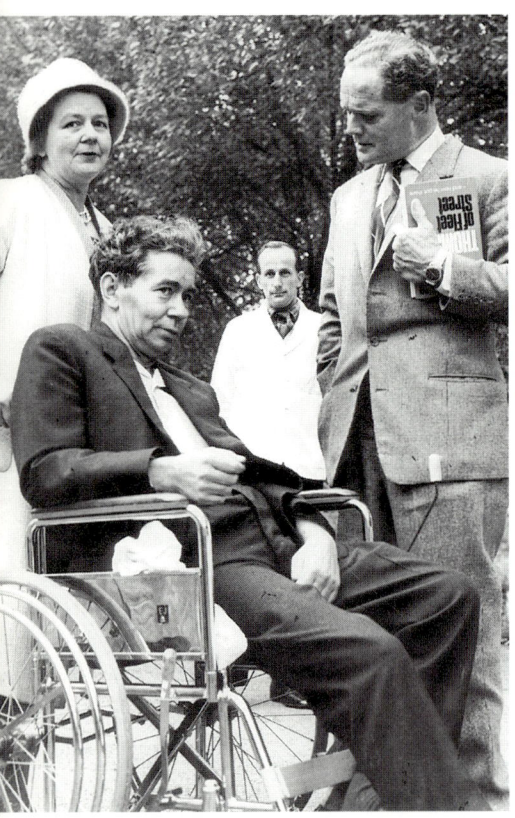

Group Captain Douglas Bader visiting patients during the opening of the physiotherapy department in 1965

eye-catching feature of the design was a pyramid-shaped roof over the waiting area intended to create the impression it was floating on air. The department also housed the outpatient clinics in rheumatology and rehabilitation and provided excellent facilities for treatment and consultation. It had 24 treatment cubicles with an adjoining exercise area, a clinical wing with two consulting and examination rooms, a gymnasium and a hydrotherapy pool.

It was the first of a number of new buildings costing about £5m to establish the City Hospital as a full district general hospital.

Teaching hospital status was awarded in 1970 and the hospital welcomed its first group of 44 clinical students in April 1973. They assembled in the lecture theatre in the Post Graduate Education Centre, opened a year earlier by Professor John Butterfield (later Lord Butterfield), Vice Chancellor of the University of Nottingham.

The Post Graduate Education Centre has always been a model of its kind. It was purpose-built in 1972 by Trent Regional Health Authority to be a Nottingham district-wide facility for the teaching of dental and medical staff, including general practitioners and hospital doctors. It later came under the direct supervision of the City Hospital.

As part of the original plans, accommodation was incorporated for the headquarters of the Nottingham Medico-Chirurgical Society, founded in 1828. One of the oldest medical societies in the country, it moved to the City Hospital from its building in St James' Street. Current membership is around 780, about half of whom are GPs and half are hospital consultants.

Input also came from the University of Nottingham to provide for the teaching of medical students (a research room, teaching room, student common room and contributions to the medical library). The daily running of the centre was for 14 years undertaken by an administrator (Mrs Cayley) together with a part-time assistant. The centre was overseen by a council comprising representatives of all the user groups, chaired by Dr David Banks.

The tiered lecture theatre, seating 152 and equipped with excellent, state-of-the-art projection equipment, was a much sought-after resource, not only for the medical staff and students but for paramedical groups, for charities and self-help groups, coming from all over the Trent region. In addition there were lecture and seminar rooms, and a lounge which was used for refreshments and medical exhibitions.

Mr (later Professor) Roger Blamey arrived in 1973 to open the City Hospital section of the university department of surgery. He established a breast cancer unit, which would later become internationally known.

Around this time six new operating theatres were opened. Included in the capital developments, and built alongside the operating theatres, was the central sterile supplies department (CSSD), providing a vital service for the City Hospital and other hospitals in the Nottingham area. Both departments were officially opened by leading heart surgeon Sir Thomas Holmes-Sellors in 1973.

Another major project was the construction of a new 168-bed maternity unit, described as one of the best in Britain. It was officially opened in 1974 by Professor Stanley Clayton, President of the Royal College of Obstetrics and Gynaecologists, who congratulated the hospital on completing the building before a predicted financial 'ice age' for the NHS arrived. The four storey unit housed wards, reception area, ante-natal clinic, admission, labour and operating theatre suites, a 46-bed special care baby unit and professorial accommodation for the department of obstetrics and gynaecology. A bridge corridor at first floor level linked the teaching unit with laboratory and lecture facilities for University of

The People's Hospital

Nottingham medical students.

It was a far cry from the old maternity unit's 'lying in wards', originally housed where Oxton and Gedling wards are now located. The City Hospital, in common with others, developed through a process of adapting or demolishing old buildings and redeveloping new ones. For example the former maternity 'labour suite' would later become the coronary care unit. Until purpose-built facilities were created, the special care baby unit was sited in what would later become the renal unit - opened in 1975 after a successful public fundraising campaign launched in 1966.

Even before the new maternity unit opened its doors, hospital authorities were clamping down on gift packs to mothers about to be discharged with their newly born babies.

The gifts were designed to advertise various proprietary products. But the practice was curbed after samples of soap flakes, baby cream, infant medicines and even beer were found in mums' lockers.

Meanwhile the hospital was making positive headlines too by winning the National Hospital Service Reserve Forward Medical Aid Unit competition at Grantham. Watched by more than 300 spectators, the City Hospital team, led by Dr J V Jeffier and Sister A Wesson, treated 30 casualties for injuries ranging from a broken leg to minor cuts and bruises.

In 1964 Victoria Two and Winifred Two became the first wards to benefit from an £800,000 upgrading scheme. The improvements would mean space, additional bathrooms, a new nurses' station, sister's office, better kitchen facilities and better sluicing facilities.

But around this time, warnings were being sounded of a hospital staffing crisis in Nottingham. As well as shortages of nursing and medical staff, hospitals were struggling to recruit sufficient porters, ward staff, cleaners, gardeners, kitchen staff and cooks. Unions said poor wages lay at the heart of the problem.

In 1967 the first 'artificial kidney' dialysis machine was presented to the hospital and was housed in a former operating theatre off the main corridor. The Lord Mayor set up a fund to provide further equipment and by the time Dr Martin Knapp was appointed the first Nephrologist, the renal unit had several machines housed in the old maternity block. The first kidney transplant operation was performed at the City Hospital by Mr Blamey early in 1974.

By then work had started on a new ward block, incorporating paediatric facilities and a 10 bed unit specialising in the treatment of chronic kidney disease. Burns and plastic surgery facilities were also to be improved with more beds and better equipment. In the same year the urology department was established following the appointment of two consultants Mr William Matthew Grey and Mr Patrick Bates.

The 1970s saw greater changes than in any other decade since 1903. A temporary coronary care unit opened in Winifred ward and four new 30-bed wards were built and opened in Sherwood Hospital. A block of six new operating theatres opened in 1973 and the old twin theatres were converted into a genito-urinary unit with operating, X-ray, outpatient and day case facilities.

In 1974 the staff Leisure Centre opened its doors and a large car park was completed nearby. An appeal was launched by the Lord Mayor Alderman Eric Foster and the City Hospital League of Friends played an important part in fundraising. Built at a cost of £100,000, it was welcomed as a place where hospital staff could relax and socialise. There was a licensed lounge bar and facilities for squash, badminton, archery, snooker, indoor bowls and dancing.

Meanwhile the demand for outpatient services was spiralling. So a large extension, virtually doubling the facilities created 15 years earlier, was opened in 1973. Three more clinics were created, an outpatient

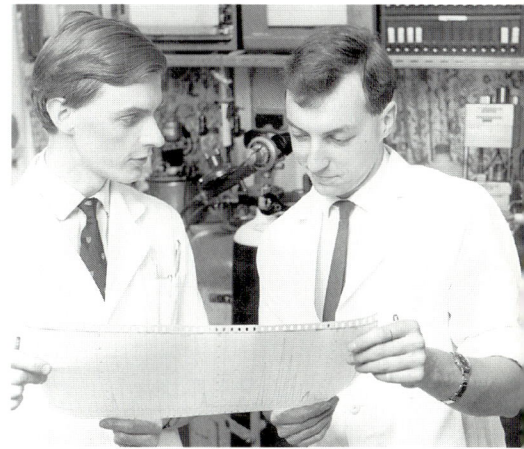

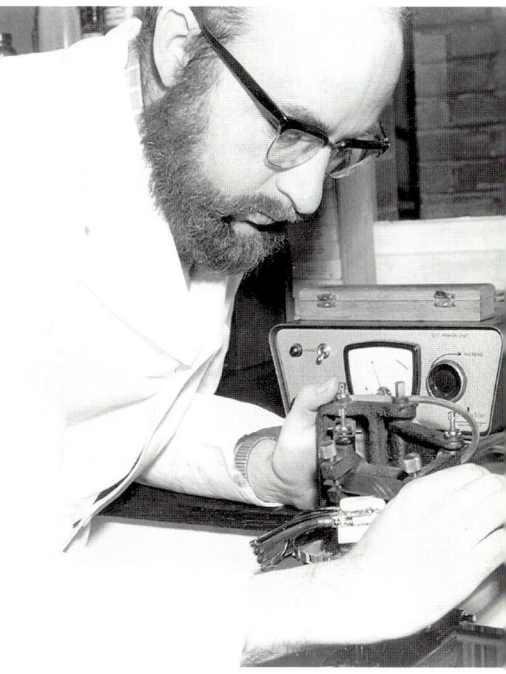

Top: Mr Colin Selby (left) and Mr Gordon Masson discussing a graph of results taken from an auto-analyser (in the back ground), which analyses chemical constituents in blood

Above: Mr K Gordon, in the histopathology section, cutting a frozen section of tissue to obtain or confirm rapid diagnosis. Both pictures were taken in 1967

pharmacy was added and the laboratory was enlarged. Nottingham's chest clinics had now closed and all their services were provided from the outpatient department. In 1958 there were 10,831 new attendances and 24,270 follow-up visits. By 1982 these corresponding figures would soar to nearly 28,000 new attendances and more than 111,000 follow-up visits. A £300,000 scheme was also approved for four additional X-ray

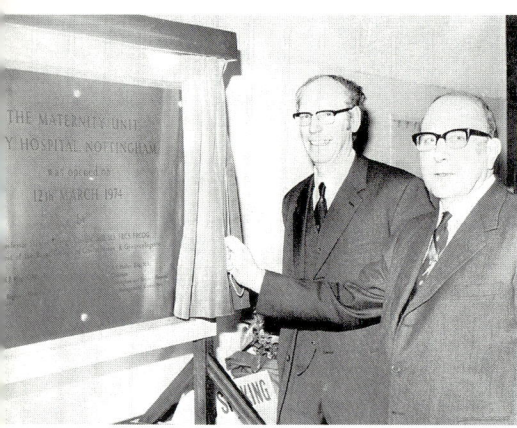
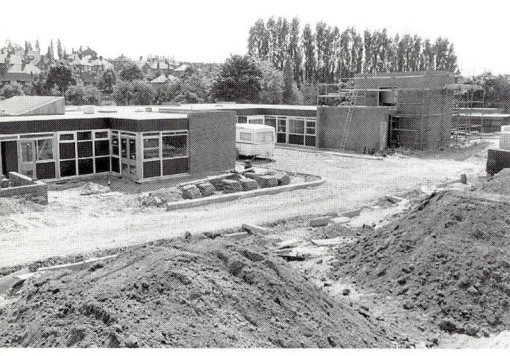

Top: Prof Stanley G Clayton (right) unveils a plaque at the opening of the maternity unit on March 12, 1974. Looking on is Mr Hurley

Above: Work in progress on Nottingham City Hospital's Hayward House in May 1978

rooms, together with ancillary and teaching accommodation.

With all the building work going on it was felt the City Hospital campus should be renamed. Two titles were suggested - The Royal Nottingham Hospital and the City of Nottingham Hospital. But at this time the City Hospital couldn't produce proof of Royal patronage and the renaming idea was dropped.

However by 1972, there were four hospitals on the same site - Sherwood Hospital, St Francis (a unit for the elderly mentally ill under the direction of Mapperley Hospital), Heathfield Hospital (the former isolation hospital) and Nottingham City Hospital. It was time for rationalisation and the Hospital Management Committee voted in favour of dropping the name Sherwood from the City Hospital title. It ended once and for all the old workhouse stigmas and fears of admission. For a short time the name Bagthorpe was revived - it was the name chosen by a group of doctors for a newly formed wine society in 1979. Alas, this was short-lived, the Bagthorpe Wine Society folded when the drink-driving laws were introduced. But at least one member continued with his wine tasting. Ian Ellis went on to achieve honours in the Sunday Times Wine Taster of the Year competition and he often gives talks on the subject to various groups of colleagues.

The university department of microbiology was established in the basement of what had been the vagrants' block near the entrance to Sherwood Hospital. In 1975 the kidney unit was established in reasonable premises in the old maternity department and it offered facilities for long term dialysis. There were extensions to the X-ray department and an adequately equipped coronary care unit was created in the old labour ward. A new haematology laboratory was opened and heating was installed in the corridors leading from the main building. Part of the long-delayed H Block was opened in 1980 for renal dialysis, soon followed by the department of clinical genetics and by the burns unit. Hayward House, a specialist palliative care unit, also opened in 1980.

The younger chronic sick had never had any suitable hospital accommodation: most 'chronic wards' were occupied by the elderly and beds for younger patients were normally needed for treatment of acute illness. In 1981 Linden Lodge was opened on the site of two former maternity wards, providing excellent facilities for nursing 26 younger chronic patients.

Rodney Cove-Smith, a former junior doctor who went on to become a Consultant, remembers the 70s as a 'golden era' for the City Hospital.

"It was changing from being a district general hospital into a major teaching centre. It was a time of great expansion in buildings and staff. The new maternity unit, designed by Mr Cochrane some 25 years earlier, was finally completed, just in time for him to retire! In 1971, when I arrived in Nottingham as a Medical Registrar, a typical medical 'firm' had 54 beds manned by one pre-registration house officer, one senior house officer, one registrar and two consultants. By the time I left in 1978, with no change in bed numbers, there were two pre-registration house officers, three senior house officers, a registrar, a research fellow, a senior registrar and three consultants.

"In the early 1970s the workload for junior doctors was very heavy but there was a fantastic team spirit and a very lively doctors' mess. Also, and unusually for that time in the NHS, the relationship between the doctors and the hospital administrators was excellent. In 1971 junior doctors mostly lived in the hospital grounds and spent several nights a week on-call, so it was felt important to have good facilities. The then Mess President and Secretary, David Parr and Ian McLachlan (the latter a GP in

The People's Hospital

Nottingham) suggested that the hospital build two squash courts in the hospital grounds, for the use of the doctors. They persuaded all the junior doctors and many of the consultant staff to contribute money to a fund to raise £10,000. Expecting a cool response when they approached the Hospital Administrator Roy Batterbury, they were surprised to find him very enthusiastic. In fact he decided to improve the facilities for all the staff and build a leisure centre. Architects were appointed and with the help of the Boots Company, the leisure centre was built, comprising lounge bar, snooker/table tennis room, a large hall for dances and badminton, changing rooms and two squash courts. It was a huge success and certainly contributed to staff morale. The opening night saw a splendid party with Leslie Crowther performing the opening ceremony.

"In those days doctors needed somewhere in the hospital to relax at the end of the day and to meet and socialise. The doctors' dining room had been closed (too exclusive). We eventually had a system whereby the young doctors would meet their senior colleagues there in the evening for informal teaching sessions.

"The early 1970s were also a great time for mess dinners and parties. Again the hospital staff entered into the spirit. The catering staff decided to help plan 'dinners with a theme', perhaps the most memorable being a medieval dinner, with barrels of real ale provided by Shipstones and a top table where all those 'below the salt' had to come and beg for it! There was music, singing and dancing and a pillory! And the first person in the pillory to have rotten eggs and tomatoes hurled at him was the Catering Manager Lee Soden. In those days there was a strong Australian contingent, mainly obstetricians coming to gain experience in the UK, who were lively members of any party where alcohol was consumed, and laid on wonderful barbeques in the summer. After one particularly lively mess party I was summoned to see Roy Batterbury because there had been a complaint about the noise keeping the patients awake. I had to apologise on behalf of my colleagues, and was told there were to be no similar parties 'at least until next year!' Because of the extensive grounds at the City Hospital we were able to enjoy a variety of sporting events. As well as squash, badminton and tennis, there was an active cricket team featuring several doctors, which played in the Nottingham Sunday and evening leagues. There were football, cricket and hockey matches against the General Hospital, often followed by a party in the evening; and there were several very successful summer balls.

"In the winter, the junior doctors mounted a series of memorable Christmas shows, following the usual tradition of mocking their colleagues and mimicking their seniors. Great fun for the participants if not always the audience! All the doctors who worked at Nottingham at that time look back on it as a golden era. We worked hard, we played hard and we learned an enormous amount in a very friendly environment.

"The enthusiasm for teaching and learning was immense. As a 'young' medical school, Nottingham attracted consultants keen to teach, who encouraged and befriended the junior

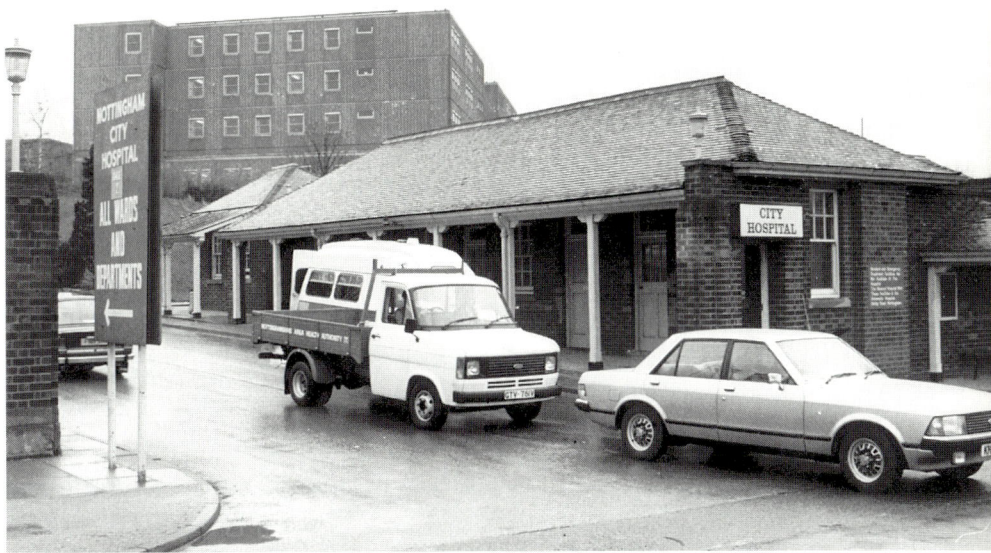

One of the main entrances to Nottingham City Hospital taken in March 1980

doctors, making an excellent learning environment. A new education centre was built at the City Hospital, where regular lunchtime teaching sessions were established - and with free food for the impoverished doctors, attendance was always excellent.

"The first medical students arrived in 1973 and in their very first week came to the hospital, all wide-eyed and enthusiastic. Five years later, the same individuals, now qualified, had adopted the rather callous, cynical and world-weary affect of the junior doctor, and it was our job to re-instil in them the enthusiasm for medicine, for treating patients, for learning their craft. The Nottingham Medical School in the early days was an exciting place, and attracted some very bright individuals to the City Hospital. Many of the young doctors who worked there in the 1970s are now eminent in their field; eight or nine professors, many well known consultants and excellent GPs, working all over the world and sometimes meeting at national or international meetings, where inevitably talk turns to Nottingham, the fun and camaraderie, but also the high standard of teaching and learning which it inspired. It really was a golden era."

The People's Hospital

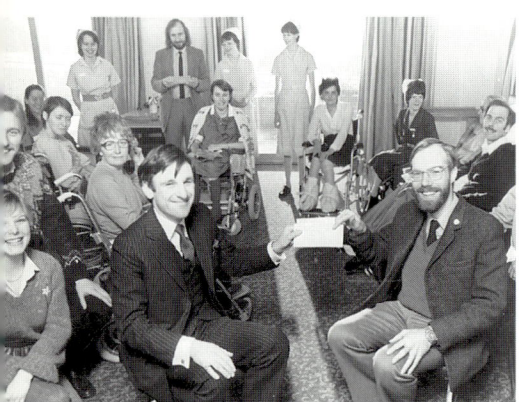

Dr Alan Whitely (centre left), Consultant Neurologist at the City Hospital's Linden Lodge unit, receives cheques for £618 from Dr John Cooper, Secretary of the Boots Table Tennis Club who raised the cash in a sponsored tournament. Picture taken January 23, 1982

Professor John Fletcher, who started work at Nottingham City Hospital in 1971, recalled: "I was the first Consultant Physician appointed in Nottingham as part of the expansion required by the establishment of the new medical school. In other words I did not replace a retirement or death.

"Martin Knapp had been appointed a few months earlier with the remit of developing a renal service. I worked with James Macfie on Patience wards. Martin was teamed with Alfred Thomas on Fleming wards, which later became the department of therapeutics, then respiratory medicine and now offices. The other medical firm, on Winifred wards, was Robert Duff with the medical unit which meant that Tony Mitchell, Michael Langman and John Hampton took consultant responsibility in turns, I think two months at a time. There were also three medical firms at the General Hospital so that each firm was 'on take' one in six and each consultant one in 12.

"Tony Mitchell was responsible for the thinking behind these arrangements. The Pickering Report, the blueprint for the new medical school, envisaged a teaching hospital on or near the university campus which was to be an academic centre of excellence for teaching and research but unfortunately, Pickering completely ignored the City Hospital and with it, both the needs of the people of Nottingham and the likely future need to increase the number of medical students.

"Tony saw that services at the City Hospital had to be built up so that it could become an equal partner with the University Hospital, when built, for clinical care and teaching if not for research. A two-tier hospital service would have been a distaster, hence the involvement of the medical unit and the appointments of Martin and I at the City.

"The early 1970s were very exciting. Everything was new and up for grabs. The physicians, led by Tony, discussed and laid down the principles of how we would teach the medical students who first arrived on the wards in September, 1971. There was to be core knowledge of common medical conditions, for example, heart attack, stroke and pneumonia, to be taught on the wards while in the outpatient department we would concentrate on how patients actually present. There was no shortage of material as we were all incredibly busy dealing with the floods of patients coming through the doors on take, usually more than 40 in 24 hours, as well as very busy outpatients.

"We were all general physicians, nowadays a dying breed, dealing with every sort of medical condition but each having a special interest. There were no other specialist units. Sam James practised 'physical medicine' but there was no specialist rheumatologist, no chest physicians. Dr Don ran the infectious disease unit on the Heathfield site but was mainly concerned with childhood diarrhoea. Neurosurgical cases had to be referred to Derby and cardiac surgery to Leicester.

"There was a small neurology department at the General Hospital but we looked after both long term and emergency neurology cases. To help us, James and I originally had a registrar, who was the only one in the hospital with the MRCP (Member of the Royal College of Physicians), a senior house officer and a houseman. "However the number and competence of the junior staff changed quickly as the reputation of Nottingham spread and very soon we were attracting the very best young doctors, particularly from London.

"Some of the wards on the main corridor had been upgraded and extended while others were still the old Nightingale wards. James and I were lucky as we had upgraded wards with 54 beds, six four-bedded bays and three side wards on each side. A big difference between then and now was the medical team as nobody

The People's Hospital

worked shifts. The junior staff worked with and were responsible to a single consultant whose ways of working they understood, while the consultant knew his juniors and took responsibility for their clinical work, teaching and the development of careers. This may still be the situation on specialist units but not in general medicine. Each consultant was autonomous. For example, if James Macfie wished for my opinion about a patient then he wrote in the patient's notes and I replied in the same way.

"At the same time communications between different consultants and the hospital secretary were easy as we all met over lunch in the doctors' dining room and were able to discuss problems privately among ourselves and particularly with our surgical colleagues. This continued after the new dining room opened as we then used the waitress service area but it did not last.

"Another very important feature of the City Hospital was its almost unique management structure. This had been set up before I arrived by Roger Cotton. It revolved around a medical executive and the medical staff meeting. The executive consisted of five or six consultants representing different specialties together with Roy Batterbury (the hospital Secretary), Tony Needs (the Treasurer), the chief nurse and a representative of the junior doctors. The executive met every two weeks and then reported once a month to a well attended staff meeting.

"The chairman of the medical staff was elected by his peers which gave him real authority. Through this structure medical staff were involved in all important decisions. For example, soon after I arrived we had to decide whether the remaining wards on the main City Hospital corridor should be extended and upgraded or wait for a new building. We decided on the upgrade, which in hindsight was probably correct as the older parts of the hospital have not yet been replaced.

"In 1976 the new maternity unit was opened by the Duchess of Gloucester. During its construction Stephen Jones had carefully documented the use of asbestos lagging around pipes. As the building became older the lagging started to wear out and leak dangerous asbestos fibres. The building was then condemned and had to be demolished. What a waste of money.

"In 1978 the City Hospital was visited by the Minister of Health. We showed him the appalling facilities used by the plastic surgery and burns unit including the kitchen sink into which wounds of burns patients were debreeded. He was obviously impressed as funding became available for the new H Block in which plastic surgery and the burns unit are now housed.

"Looking back, many of my generation think of the 1970s at the City Hospital with great affection. It was an exciting time. Every year there was progress although its pace varied.

"We knew we were involved in the important project of developing Nottingham as a whole and the City Hospital in particular as a major teaching and research centre, a centre of excellence. We are grateful to have been consultants at that time."

So as readers have seen, the post-war years to the early 1980s were a remarkably dynamic period in the development of the City Hospital - and nowhere was the progress more marked than in health care of the elderly.

Much of the credit for this was due to two pioneering physicians. In 1948 Dr William Morton established one of the earliest geriatric units in two acute admission and assessment wards in the City Hospital, supported by long stay wards in Sherwood Hospital. This became an accepted pattern of service but at the time it was visionary. For until the mid-1940s the care of the elderly in Bagthorpe, as elsewhere, was largely custodial. There was then a slow but steady swing towards the application of the principles of general medicine.

Dr William Morton published two key papers, one on the use of wards in a general hospital for assessing elderly ill people and the other on the provision of respite care accommodation for the chronically ill so that relatives could have a break.

After his untimely death in 1960, the service stagnated until Dr Eric Morton was appointed full time physician in geriatric medicine in 1964. Sherwood Hospital at this time was a dreary red brick edifice with a long, cold, brick-lined corridor. It was the route to eight, sub-standard three-storey blocks, five of which were occupied by hospital patients and three were used by the local authority for what was known as part-three residential accommodation. A day hospital, which opened in 1969 in a new building on spare land between Sherwood Hospital and Valley Road, meant that inpatients could continue to have supervised treatment after being discharged home.

But it wasn't until 1970, just as the City Hospital was entering a new age of clinical teaching, that the local authority finally relinquished control of the old Sherwood Hospital wards. It brought to an end nearly 70 years of local authority control that began when the hospital opened as a workhouse and infirmary in 1903.

Seven decades on, many of the older local people still thought of it as Bagthorpe Workhouse or 'Baggy' and feared the name. There were 300 people on the waiting list either at home awaiting admission or in other hospitals awaiting transfer. There was no resident medical staff and day-to-day cover was provided by three general practitioner clinical assistants. By the end of 1982 the waiting list was down to under 20, largely because of the more active style of service and because facilities for the elderly had opened elsewhere.

Nottingham City Hospital had finally laid to rest its workhouse origins and was gearing up for even more exciting times ahead . . .

Emergency X-Ray

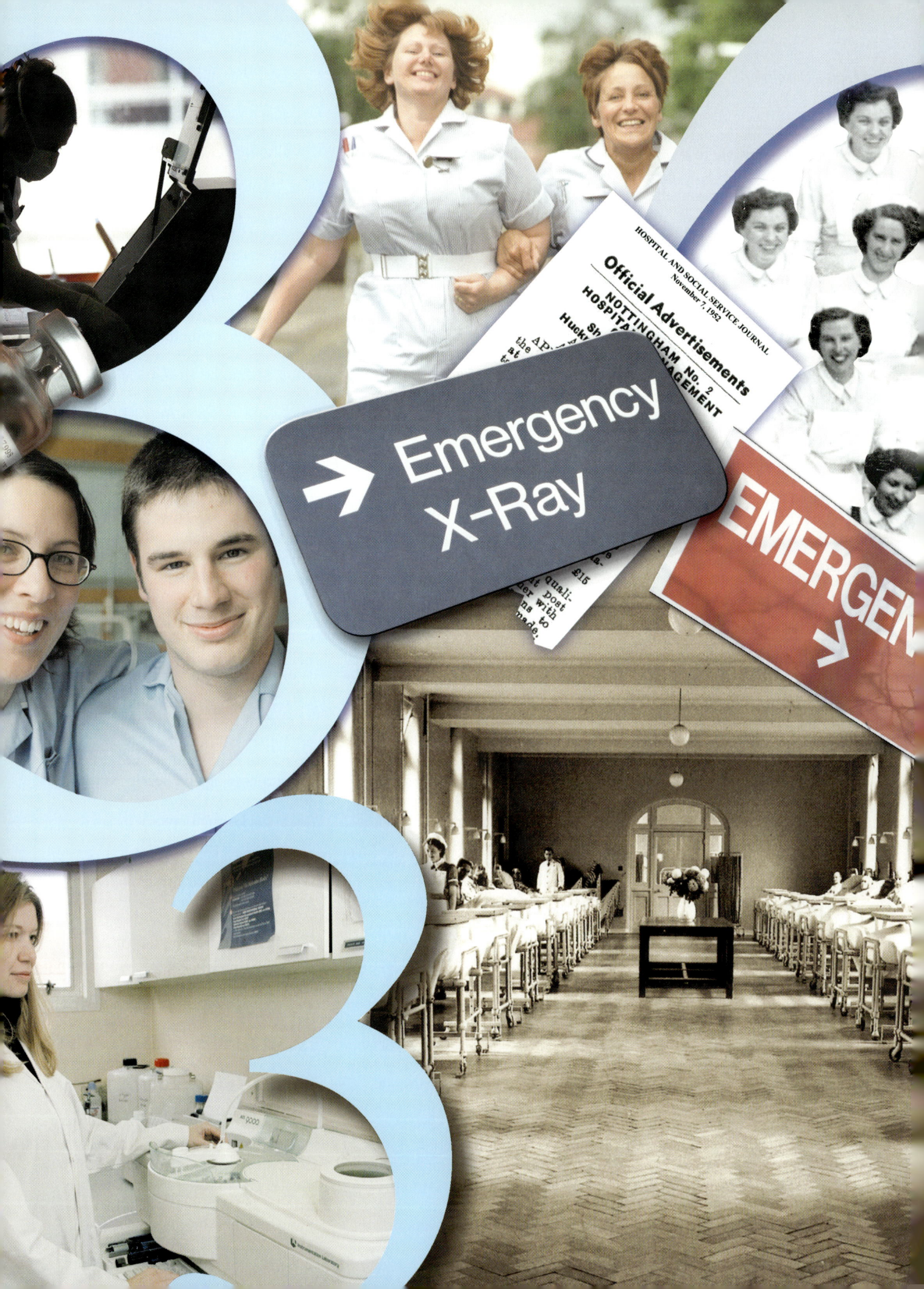

EMERGEN

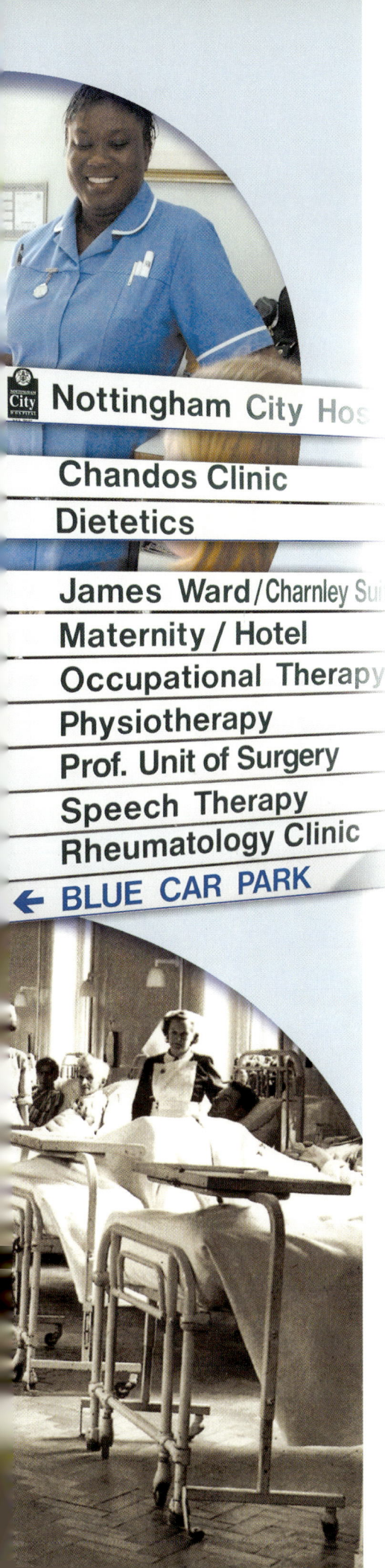

The spirit of nursing

A century of memories from the front line

NURSES, working with a host of support services at the front line of patient care, are close to the heart of a hospital's unique spirit. So it was fitting that the historic announcement to change the name of the Nottingham City Infirmary to 'The City Hospital' in 1935 was made at the nurses' annual distribution of prizes and certificates. Matron, Miss Alice Rose, said she was pleased with the year's examination passes but felt nursing was tending to become a little too academic. At that time each nurse had a 12-week spell in the Preliminary Training School, followed by an eight-week introductory course to give an insight into hospital life.

Ever since the earliest days of the infirmary there has been a strong tradition of nurse training on the campus. Successive generations of nurses who trained firstly at the Bagthorpe Infirmary School of Nursing and later Nottingham City Hospital School of Nursing wore their distinctive badges with pride.

The school opened in 1929 in one large classroom in Nurses' Home One. There were two full-time nurse tutors and matron gave many of the lectures. It was one of the first schools to accept young men for training.

But what was nursing really like in those days? An amusing insight into the profession appears in the novel *A Nurse in Our Time* (Hutchinson) by Evelyn Prentis. She came from her Lincolnshire home to train at Nottingham City Hospital in 1934 when a nurse's salary was £20 to £25 a year.

Working alongside a nurse named Davies from Neath, Evelyn relates her first encounter with bedpans. "As I took the bedpans from her and emptied the contents down the sink there went most of the romantic dreams of cool hands on fevered brows I had imagined nursing was all about. There had been no mention of bedpans in *Peg's Paper*. Only noble sacrifice and burning glances exchanged between doctors and nurses. I had to re-adjust my ideas quite a lot.

"You'd better do that one again," said Davies, throwing a reject back at me. "Matron looks down the handles when she does her round and she'll have you in the office if she finds a dirty one."

Evelyn adds: "The patients we nursed had their own trials and tribulations. They were posseted, plastered, poulticed and purged until they either got better and went home to escape our attentions, or they wilted away in spite of them." She dedicates her book to her grandchildren and the "countless nurses who have worn their feet to the bones since the days of Florence Nightingale."

Before delving into nursing past and present, it's worth recalling that the profession had its roots in the values of the Church, and to lesser extent, the Army. Both traditions strongly influenced the development of nursing long after it became a secular profession. Titles such as 'sister' and 'almoner' stem from the Church whereas terms such as 'duties' and 'orderly' show the military influence.

The People's Hospital

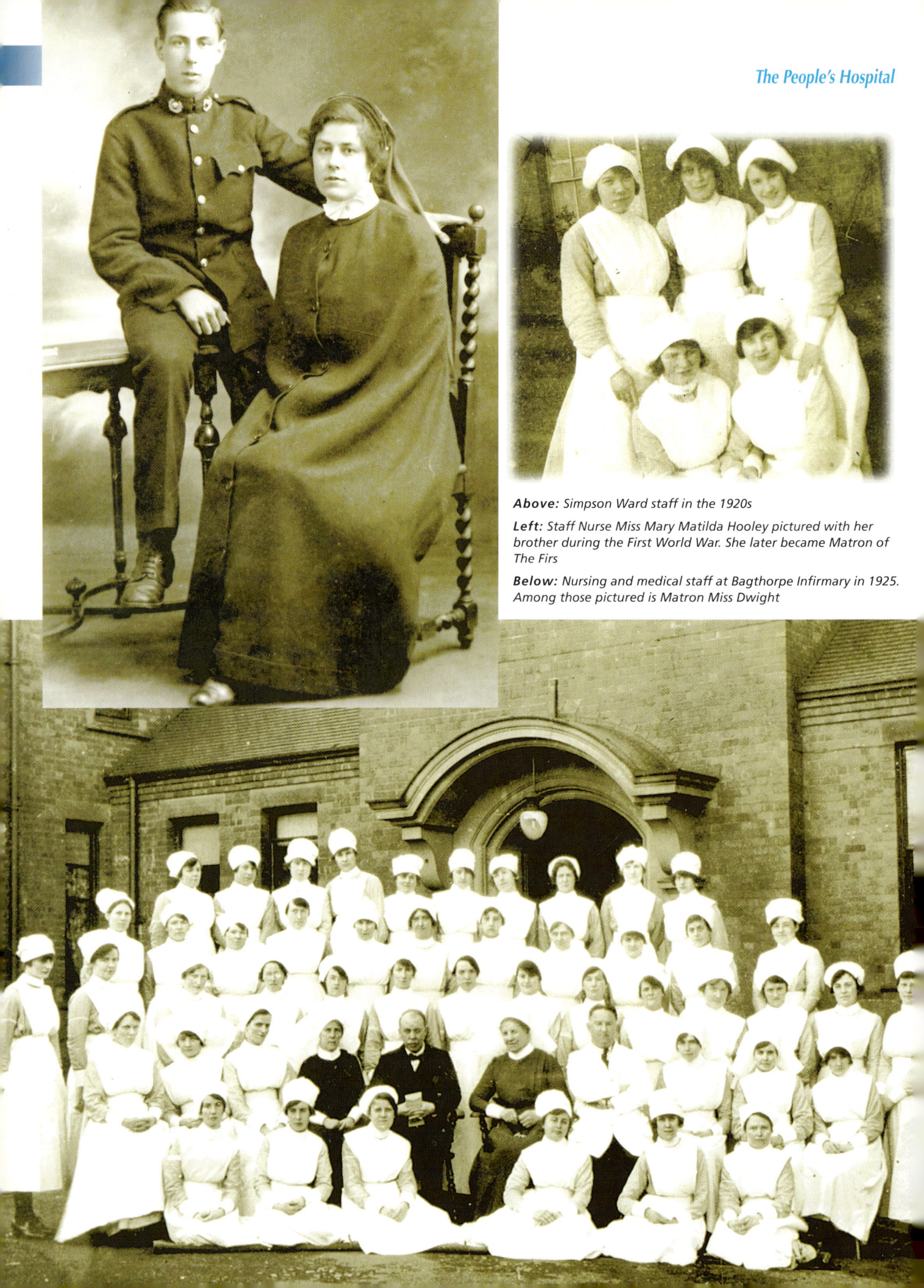

Above: Simpson Ward staff in the 1920s

Left: Staff Nurse Miss Mary Matilda Hooley pictured with her brother during the First World War. She later became Matron of The Firs

Below: Nursing and medical staff at Bagthorpe Infirmary in 1925. Among those pictured is Matron Miss Dwight

The People's Hospital

Conditions were tough in the 30s but it was a far cry from the harsh days of nursing before the First World War. Miss Ivy Gill, of Mapperley, wrote an account in the *Nottinghamshire Guardian* in 1950 of her nursing memories after starting her training at the City Hospital in 1910.

"Hucknall Road was then just a lane and a very lonely one at that with the prison half way along. We scampered down the hill from the prison till we got to the gate and the night porter saw us safely home. Having been interviewed by matron, the home sister took charge and showed me how to put on my uniform. I have never felt such a freak in all my life. Still as time went on, I managed to hide my hair and keep my cap on straight. No preliminary training was given before we went on the wards, which were divided into No 1 (acute cases) and No 2 (chronic cases). My first ward was Edward – a male ward in No 2 with a second year nurse. What a horrid feeling! All the patients were aware you were new and often they asked you to do things for which I was told off severely later. However, you learn as you go along. Sister Meads was the sister on the women's ward, Nightingale Two. The old ladies needed a lot of changing and feeding. Woe betide us if a patient had a red spot on her back. We were taught it was a disgrace to get a bed sore or to lose a case of pneumonia.

"There was no penicillin in those days. It was linseed poultices every four hours and how we were told off if we made them too heavy.

"We had two hours off duty either in the morning or afternoon. If you were on duty in the afternoon, it was either bed bathing or combing heads. The hygiene in those days! My first six months was more like the life of a glorified maid – cleaning baths, taps, and lavatories. Only cleaners did the floors. Floors had to be polished to shine like glass. This caused many a fall, often at the most inconvenient times, during the matron's or doctors' inspection.

"My first night duty was terrifying. I was put on a ward full of old chronic cases, and after doing the round and seeing everyone was comfortable, I sat down. Soon I saw the night sister coming towards me and I could not move. It was my first experience of what was called night nurses' nightmare. It was a lesson to me never to sit down again while on duty.

"Night nurses took their meals into the ward with them. A slice of bread and butter or sardines and maybe an egg. It was all very inadequate unless we added to it. If patients were seriously ill or dying there was no time for a meal.

"The kitchen maid would get up at 5am and make us tea and toast. We often had to start washing patients before 4am and in between midnight and 1am cut bread for the patients' breakfasts. We went off duty at eight in the morning and we were often expected to attend lectures and write essays following the lecture. All lessons and lectures were attended during your off duty period, as it was not part of your working day. A sister, tutor, matron, or assistant matron, and members of the medical staff gave us our lectures."

Miss Gill, who was eventually appointed Sister, recalled the hospital being given over to the military after the outbreak of the First World War in 1914.

"All the patients and ourselves were moved to the St Francis unit mental block. All ward sisters, apart from myself, were required to nurse the wounded soldiers. I was the only sister in charge of the whole female

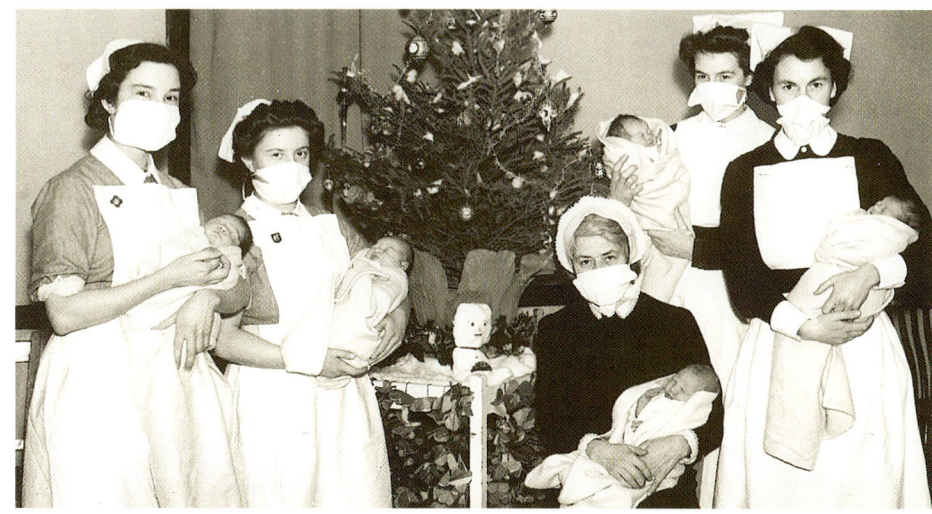

Above: Presentation of newly-born babies at the Firs Maternity Hospital during the Second World War

Right: An example of a nurse's bedroom in Nurses Home Two in the 1950s

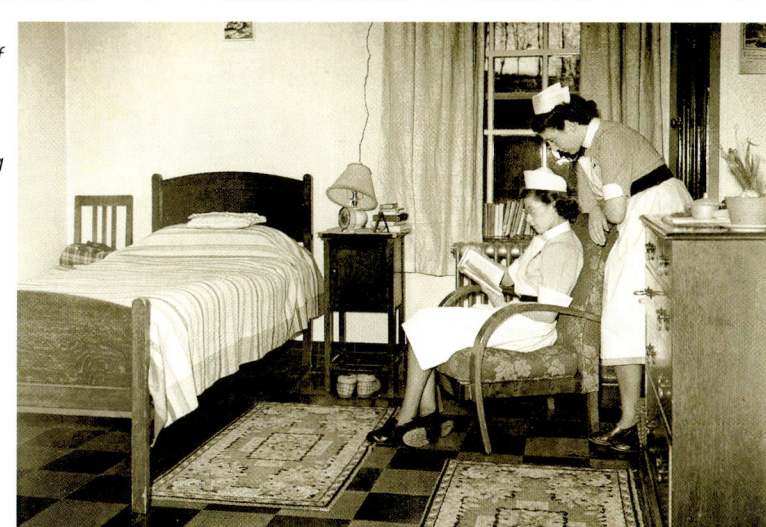

The People's Hospital

side. The uniform we had to wear had to be six inches above the ground. No ankle was allowed to be shown and we always had to wear black shoes and stockings."

Later during the war Sister Gill was posted to France and was mentioned in despatches.

City Hospital midwife Judith Scott has two precious family photographs illustrating the experiences of her grandmother Minnie Barnett (nee Alliss), who was a nurse on a female ward at Bagthorpe Infirmary.

Judith says: "Minnie was born in 1887. She told my mother that many people arriving at the workhouse had to have their hair cut off because they were covered in fleas. She also told her about the high number of deaths during the influenza epidemic. Minnie had influenza herself but recovered." (More people died of the flu in

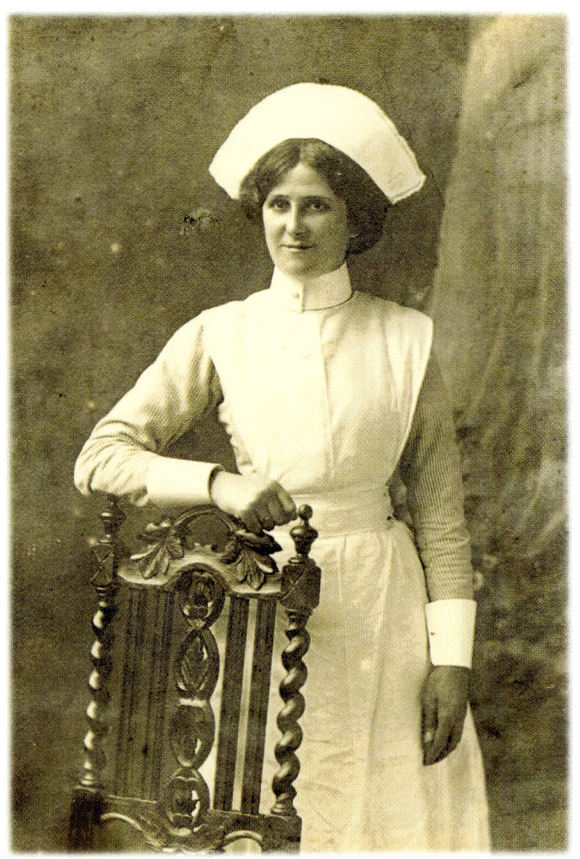

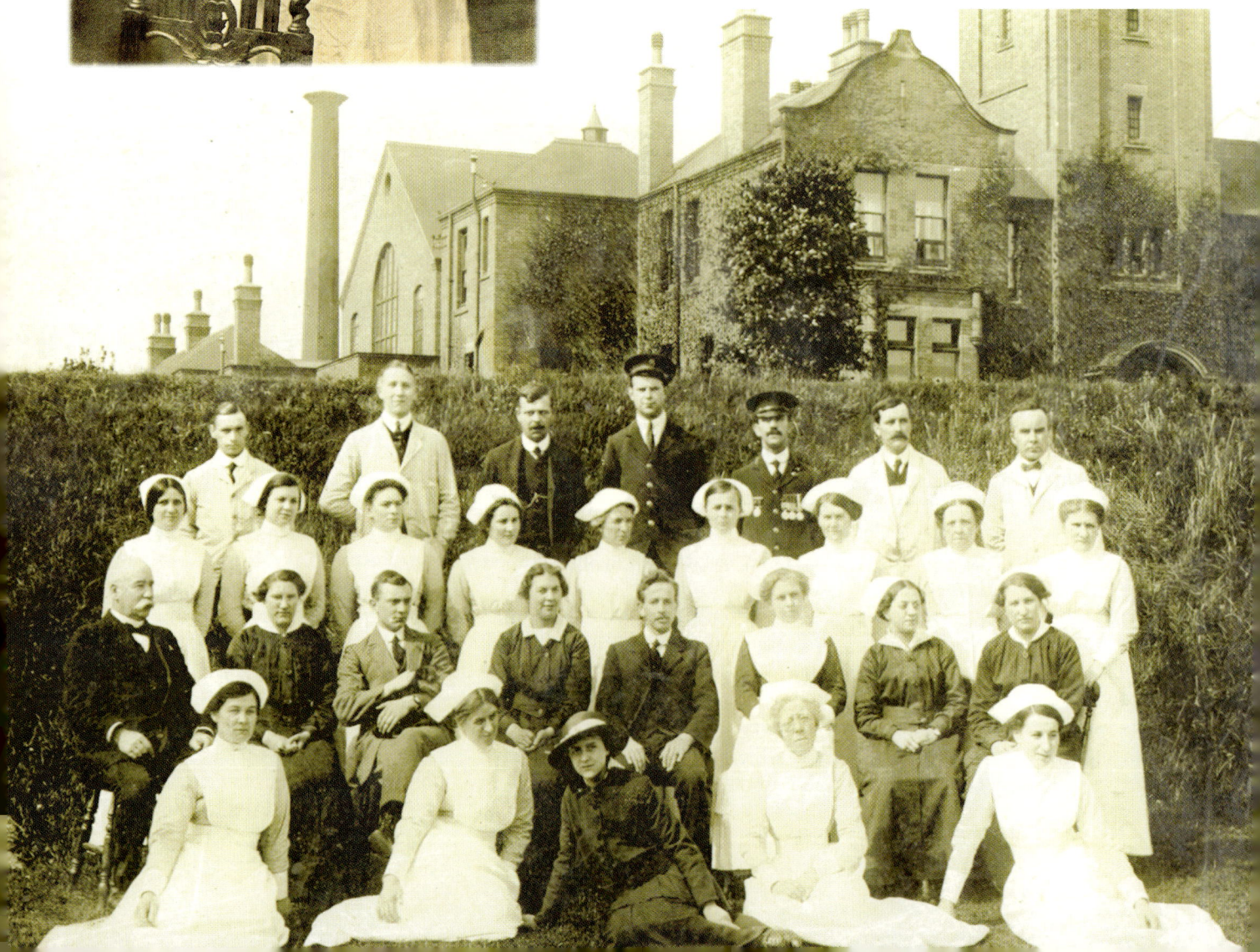

Left: *Minnie Barnett (nee Alliss) in her uniform as a nurse at Bagthorpe Infirmary before the First World War*

Below: *Nursing and other staff at Bagthorpe before the First World War. Nurse Minnie Barnett is pictured on the extreme left (second row from the back). The building at the rear was the living quarters for the workhouse master and matron*

The People's Hospital

1918/19 than the entire First World War).

Mrs Ann Wood, of Aspley Park, treasures certificates belonging to her aunt Miss Mary Matilda Hooley, who was a nurse at the workhouse/infirmary during the First World War. Miss Hooley eventually became Sister Tutor (Midwifery) and later was founder Matron of the Firs Maternity Home, an annexe of the City Hospital.

When Miss Norah Ware started at the City Hospital in 1930 it was compulsory for all nursing staff to live in. Their day started at 6am. Breakfast was at 6.30am and they were on the ward by 7am. Day duty hours lasted from 7am to 8.30pm with a two-hour break given at a moment's notice if it suited the ward sister. All lectures were taken in off-duty time. Night shift was even more rigorous. Two nurses and a 'runner' (so called because she had to dash from one end of the ward to the other) shared 88 beds between them. On night duty it was one night off in 16 and nurses found it virtually impossible to sleep day or night. They were kept awake by the sound of trains shunting on the railway line behind the nurses' home.

Night nurses never left the ward for meals. Each nurse had a basket with her cup, saucer and plates and the food was delivered to the wards. Duties included all ward cleaning (except scrubbing), checking cutlery, crockery and linen, in addition to what would normally be regarded as nursing. In the operating theatres, sterilisers were constantly boiling over and the floors were usually wet.

Nurses had little time or money for a private life outside the hospital. Any leisure hours were often spent on the campus - playing tennis and hockey or watching cricket on the ground between Sherwood Hospital and Valley Road.

One late pass until 11pm was granted each month and there was an elaborate drill to make sure this was not circumvented. Discipline was strict and crimes such as addressing a medical officer or the matron without

Advertisement for the appointment of an assistant matron at Sherwood Hospital in 1952 at a starting salary of £500 a year

being spoken to first, or leaving a ward without rolling down sleeves and putting cuffs on, or being late on duty, usually meant a terrifying interview with matron.

Mrs Agnes Page recalled that her pay in the 1930s was 49 shillings (£2.45p) a month. "It wasn't much but we used to enjoy ourselves all the same. When pay day came round we used to go a little café in Trinity Walk and have sausages and chips and a cup of tea for 1s 6d. Then we might spend 9d going to a see a film at The Mechanics.

"Nursing meant sheer care in those days. We didn't have any antibiotics or incubators. The hours we used to spend sponging patients and holding tiny babies. And of course patients were kept in hospital so much longer then - mums stayed in for 10 days after giving birth."

During the 1930s a nurse in training earned 26 shillings (£1.30p) a month. Even in 1947 the rate for a full sister was only £14, both figures being net after provision of board, lodging, uniform and superannuation.

In 1938 the new Nurses' Home Two was officially opened by Health Minister Walter Elliot. The accommodation included separate rooms for the assistant matron, sisters, home sister's office, 161 nurses' bedrooms, a nurses' dining room, a large lecture room and a demonstration room, a devotional room, studies and writing rooms, bathrooms, shampoo area and light laundry. But one feature - a nurses' smoke room - would have raised a few eyebrows today. Yet during his tour of inspection Mr Elliot said the occasional foible, such as smoking, was not frowned upon. Two further classrooms and tutors' offices were added in the new Nurses' Home Two in 1940. By this time a ward sister at the City Hospital was earning £85 a year.

At this time Matron Alice Rose was finding it difficult to staff the wards. She planned to engage 24 more ward orderlies and in the absence of probationer candidates, eight assistant nurses were engaged for Nightingale and Edward One wards.

Accounts of wartime conditions for City Hospital staff make fascinating reading. In September 1939 permission was given to spend £30 on making the lecture and demonstration rooms in the nurses' home shrapnel-proof. There was an urgent need to create a satisfactory blood transfusion service and Sir Julien Cahn offered a wing of his house at Stanford Hall, near Loughborough as a convalescent home. In 1940 the visiting committee discussed arrangements for evacuating patients in the event of the hospital being badly damaged in an air raid. Later that year, 10 casualties were admitted to the City Hospital after an air raid on Nottingham on the night of August 30/31. A seven-year-old child died seven hours after

The People's Hospital

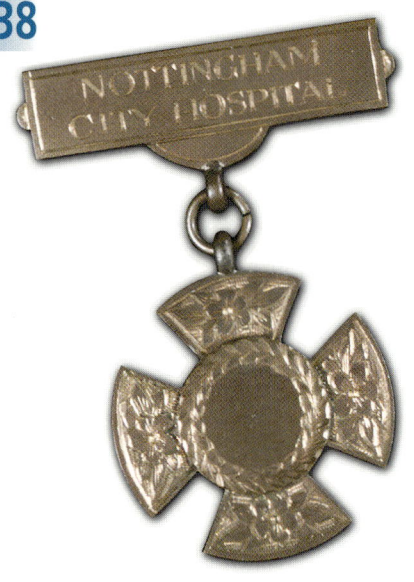

Above: Bronze medal won by Audrey Wade

Below: Presentation of medals to four nurses in 1969. Left to right, Doreen Elston (silver), Marilyn Lomax (gold), Elaine Scott (bronze) and Audrey Wade (bronze)

Bottom: Presentation of the Tennis Trophy by Alderman Ernest A Braddock in Nurses Home Two in 1942

admission. The casualty service and consulting staff were praised for the "expeditious" way they had handled the emergency.

The committee agreed that stretcher-bearers could have a cup of tea while on siren duty at night and matron requested that nurses be allowed to wear strapless aprons during the remainder of the war to save material and minimise laundry wear and tear. At the outbreak of the war, 1,184 beds were in use at the hospital. Bed reductions were recommended by the end of 1944 because of overcrowding on at least eight wards and the unsuitability of some accommodation. Hardened soldiers complained about the cold while being nursed on the veranda of a military medical ward.

By June 1946 the hospital was so short of female nurses that the committee decided to appoint another 20 male nurses. During the same year male nurses were up in arms over pay - their salaries were insufficient to pay for living-in billets of 35s (£1.75) to 37s 6d a week.

Recruitment would remain a persistent problem. (In 1978 one of the hospital's operating theatres was closed because of a shortage of technicians and trained nursing staff.)

When Mrs Margaret Bullen (nee Haugh) started her training at the Nottingham City Hospital in 1948, the matron was Miss Annakin, whom she remembers as strict but fair.

The National Health Service was just four months old and changes were on the way. Nurses no longer had to give up their careers if they wanted to get married and old style uniforms were being phased out. Starched aprons and long sleeves with detachable cuffs were replaced with more practical uniforms but the nurse's cap was retained.

Despite the long hours she believes nurses in those days were more contented than they are now.

"As we had so little time to ourselves most of our socialising was spent on the hospital premises. For example, at Christmas time all the nurses would sing Christmas carols. This was something we all looked forward to especially when we sang on the maternity wards. Another happy time was the Christmas pantomime and we looked forward to the hospital fancy dress party. On these occasions Consultant Gynaecologist Mr Cochrane would dress up as King Farouk and walk into the party pushing a pram carrying a male nurse dressed as a baby. If there was a band he would always take a turn to play as he was an accomplished jazz drummer."

Mrs A McDermott, of Chilwell, who was accepted as a cadet nurse at the City Hospital in 1950, began her training in the linen room.

"Linen was marked with ward names and nurses' uniforms were

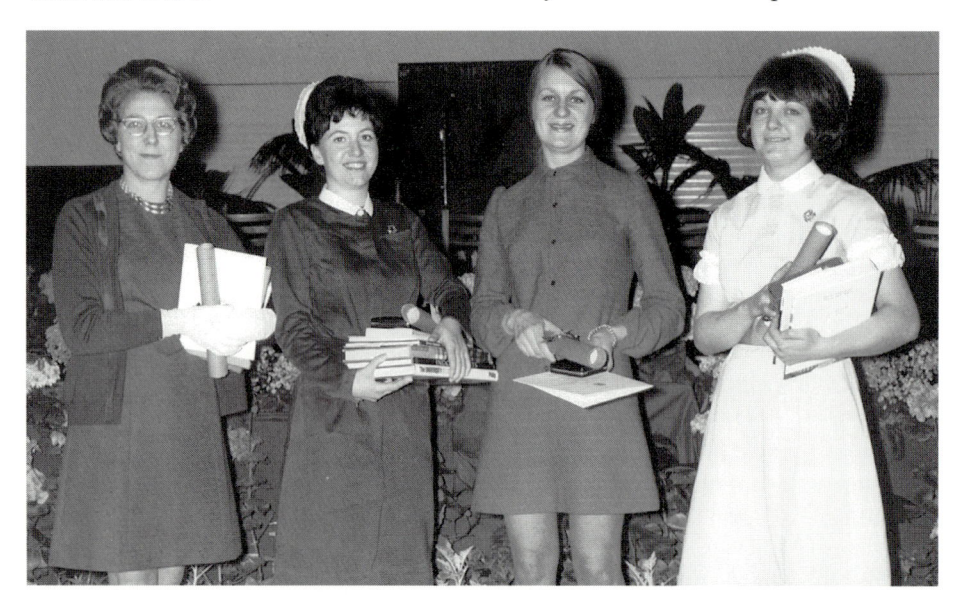

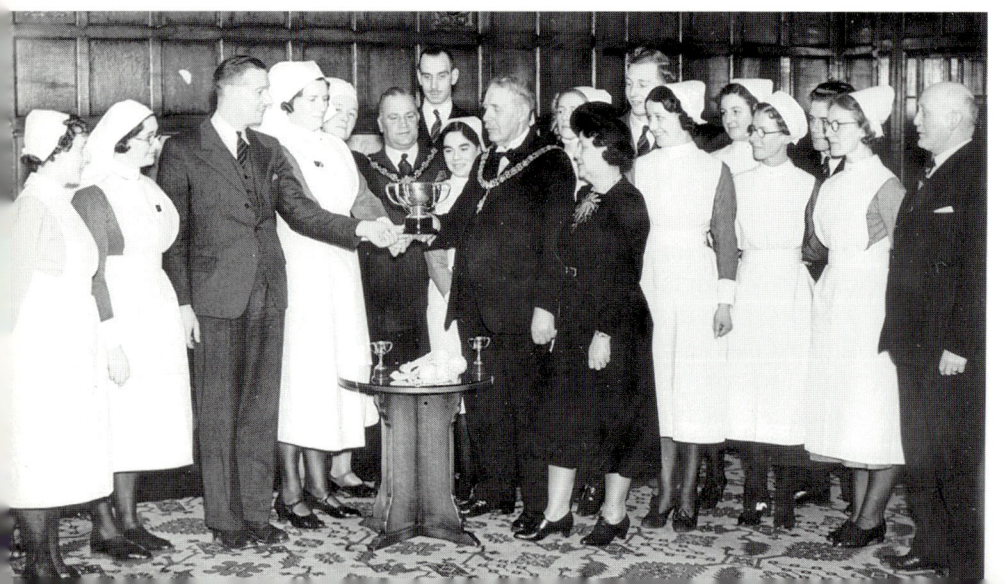

The People's Hospital

altered to fit before being issued. We worked from 9am to 4.30pm for 25s a week. After paying bus fares from home, there wasn't much left for spending money or board at home."

She recalls Matron Miss Annakin taking her Scottie dog on tours of the hospital. "She or her deputy visited every ward, every day and they were always very visible to staff and patients (if only that happened today).

"The Deputy Matron Miss Gerrard had been a sister in the Queen Alexandra's Royal Army Nursing Corps. She wore a green uniform and was known to all staff, nursing and others, as the 'Green Dragon'.

"I worked at The Firs and the Women's Hospital as well as the City Hospital. Most staff lived in; the first two years of training was residential, even if your home was close by. We began at 7am with one day off a week and split shifts. No weekends or Christmas off."

She has fond memories of working with Consultant Gynaecologist John Cochrane on the wards and in the operating theatre. "He was a super person as well as an excellent surgeon. But woe betide anyone who answered his phone calls. Telephone operators would ring three times on the bell for JB's calls and he answered himself. New staff only made the mistake of picking up a 'three bells' once."

The 1960s saw major changes in the social fabric. The age of consent was lowered from 21 to 18; the oral contraceptive pill was introduced; the first heart transplant was performed in 1967 and man landed on the moon in 1969. Nursing adapted to these changes and the 1968 Salmon Report, which introduced new style management, saw the phasing out of the hospital matron.

Sister Audrey Wade recalls the uniform she wore as a nursing cadet at the City Hospital from 1962 to 1964. It comprised a purple and white check dress, white cap, black stockings and black lace-up shoes, a navy blue cardigan and navy blue cloak. The uniform could not be worn outside the hospital grounds.

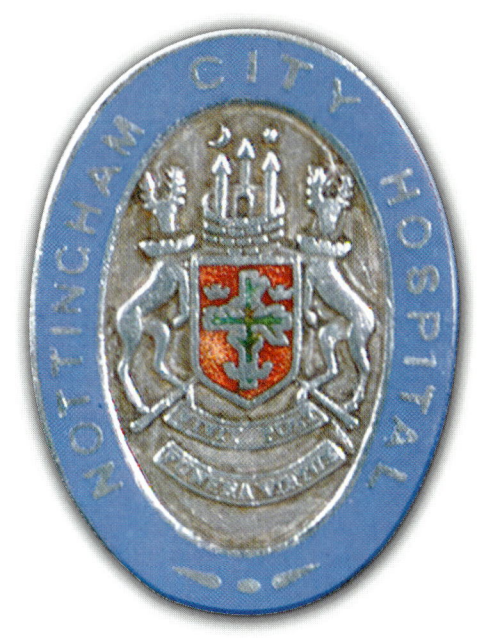

Nottingham City Hospital School of Nursing badge

"I worked on children's wards, pathology reception, the nurses' homes and the admission ward. Cadets were not allowed on adult wards."

She attended Clarendon College one day a week from 1964-67 and was in the first group to do new style training - an eight week introductory course instead of 12 weeks. By then she had a new uniform - lilac and white striped dress, starched white detachable collar, white cap, black stockings and black lace-up shoes and white starched apron. The belt was dark green for first year students, mid blue for second year students and red for third year students.

"Living in the nurses' home was compulsory for the first year of training unless you were married. Age of consent was 21 and your parents signed parental rights over to the matron for the duration of your training. If you wanted to live out after the first year permission from your parents was needed. Matron also had the power to bring you to live in the nurses' home if she felt necessary - and she did on a number of occasions.

"Anyone had access to the matron every morning at 8.30am - no permission was necessary and no appointment; you queued at the door and waited your turn. Matron walked round the hospital once a week - never at the same time or the same day. If she was away the deputy matron took her place.

"Matron Miss Greta Hayre wore a navy blue dress, a lace collar and cuffs and a lace starched cap with a bow under the chin. Deputy matron wore a bottle green dress, white starched cap and no bow under the chin. Known as the 'Green Dragon', she used to stand in the main hospital corridor, observing the passing traffic, looking for nurses inappropriately dressed such as dress too short (the hem had to be 14ins from the floor) or ladders in stockings. Inappropriate behaviour included nurses talking to doctors or porters.

"One of matron's favourite sayings was: 'A hole in your stocking is a hole in your mind.' She also urged us to: 'Drink from the fountain of knowledge every day and you should say to yourself: today I have learnt something new.'"

Audrey has vivid memories of Nurses' Home One. "This is where you slept when on night duty as night duty lasted three months (four nights on, three nights off; every fourth week, five nights on, two nights off). You moved all your belongings into Home One. Sick bay was also in Home One, presided over by home sister. Principal tutor also lived in Home One. She had a flat on the corner and could observe all the comings and goings. One of her favourite sayings was: 'You will never guess what I saw when I looked out of my window last night . . .'

"The dining room in Nurses' Home Two was very hierarchical with large tables seating 12 down the middle of the room for student nurses. Pupil midwives and staff nurses sat at smaller tables against the walls. Sisters had a separate dining room. We had maids to serve us and make sure we sat in the appropriate place. No aprons were to be worn in the dining room.

"At the end of the eight-week introductory course a tea party was held to which your parents were invited. This was hosted by matron and the principal tutor. As a group we were expected to perform in front of this invited audience. We were lucky; in our group was a girl who played the piano very well. The tea party was held in the sitting room of Nurses' Home Two. The covers were put on the armchairs. I remember telling my mother not to put anything on the chair arm as under the cover they were full of holes - cigarette burns or just wear and tear. The covers were only used when visitors came.

"The wards were Nightingale type wards - one big room, beds in two lines, with parquet floors that were kept polished. Some ward sisters insisted on you counting 10 floor blocks between each bed and kicking the bed wheels into a straight line with your heel.

"At that time there was no pre-sterile equipment. All gauze swabs and cotton wool balls were made on the ward by student nurses. This was done during visiting time. There were no curtains between the beds, screens had to be pulled around the ward. Two screens were needed for one bed.

"Pre-sterile equipment was introduced in 1965 beginning with equipment to do ward dressings. We still had to boil everything else in the ward steriliser or send it to be autoclaved. The first defibrillator came in 1966. It was extremely heavy and hard to manoeuvre.

"There was no vehicle access onto Edwards Lane, just a gate for matron. She lived in a hospital house on Edwards Lane, opposite the hospital. Vehicle access was from Hucknall Road, Heathfield Hospital (Gate 1), City Hospital (Gate 2) and Sherwood Hospital (Gate 3). All the gates were locked at 11pm and the porter was on duty at the City Hospital gate to let in ambulances and cars.

"When you lived in the nurses' home meals were provided. Breakfast was cereal, cooked breakfast and toast and tea. Mid morning break - cold toast left from breakfast and tea. Dinner - main course (no choice), plus sweet. It was fish every Friday (never fried) and no chips. Tea was bread and jam, tea and cake. Supper was soup, main course (chips and egg once a week, salmon every Sunday), plus a cold sweet and tea. There was never any coffee.

"We had clean bed linen every week but if you didn't put your dirty bed linen outside your door you didn't have a supply of clean linen. It was green to distinguish it from patient bed linen. You weren't allowed to put anything on the wall of your room. There was no desk. So studying was done sat on the bed (a lot of sleeping was done). Lights were supposed to

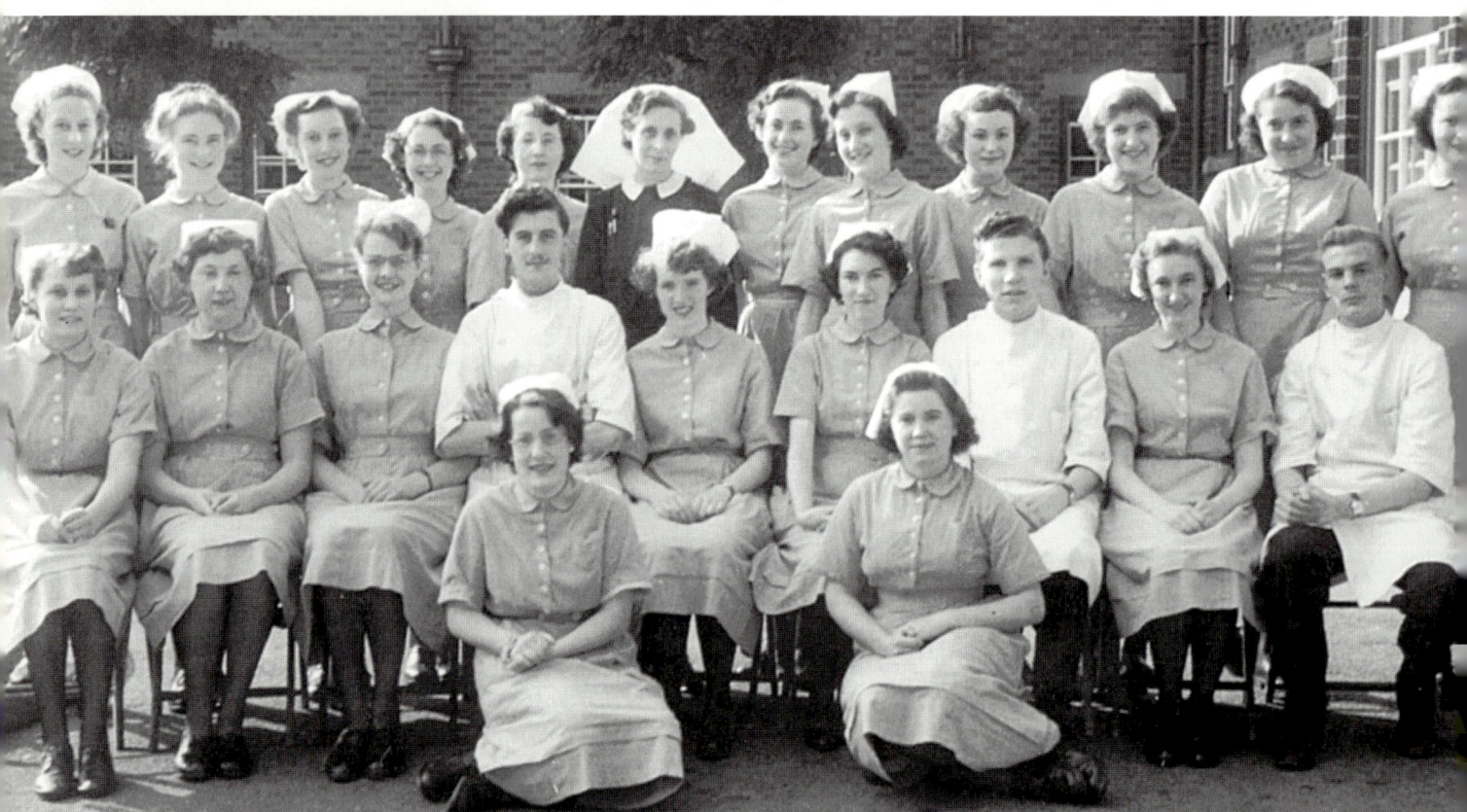

Below: Sister Audrey Wade

Bottom: The Preliminary Training School in October 1951. Among those pictured is Sister Jew, who was responsible for teaching

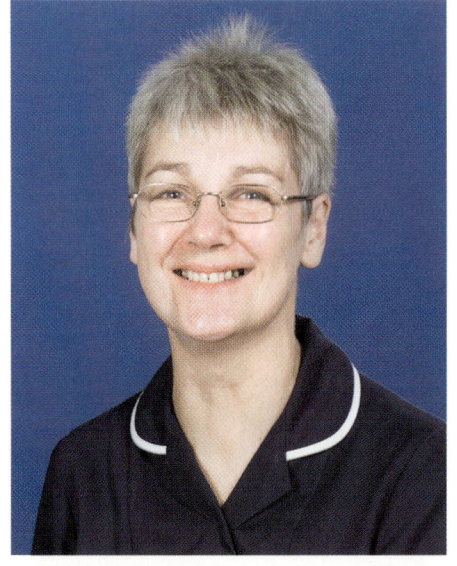

The People's Hospital

be out by 11pm - night sister came round to check and the deputy matron and home sister lived in the nurses' home. In the morning a domestic came round to wake everyone up who was on duty. The way to indicate if you wanted waking was to leave your name card on the door. If you wanted a lie-in you tipped up your name card.

"Shifts were 7.30am to 5pm and 12.30pm to 8.30pm. Night duty was 8.30pm to 7.30am. Sometimes you were required to work a split shift - 7.30am to 1pm, off from 2pm to 5pm, re-start 5pm to 8.30pm. The working week was 44 hours, which was reduced to 40 hours in the late 60s and early 70s. It was then further reduced to 37.5 hours.

"Teaching was all done at the City Hospital. Classrooms were in Home One and Home Two. We had lectures from consultants. Consultant ward rounds were always done with either the ward sister or senior staff nurse and no one else was allowed on the ward. All patients had to be in bed; no one was allowed to talk.

"Visiting was the same on most wards - evening 7pm to 8pm, Thursday afternoon, 3pm to 4pm, Saturday and Sunday, 2pm to 4pm and 7pm to 8pm. No children under the age of 12 and only two visitors per patient. All patients had to be in bed during visiting time. As students it was your job to walk round the ward and make sure the rules were followed. As nurses were known by their surnames with the prefix of status, that is, nurse, staff nurse, you addressed no one - not even your best friend - by their Christian name.

"Sister's office was also the treatment room and in the winter had a coal fire (to be kept going during the night by the night nurse). If a doctor or senior nurse was a patient he/she was nursed in sister's office behind screens and out came the special crockery and a silver teapot! Every ward had a routine which was not flexible or ever questioned. Sister's word was law.

"By the early 70s night sisters stopped wearing aprons because they made a lot of noise when you walked around. The starch made them crackle.

"You were allowed to wear a silver buckle on your belt when you were a State Registered Nurse. Most nurses had them bought by parents or members of family, usually bought from antique shops but new ones could be bought by mail order.

"New uniforms were introduced in the early 70s. It was supposed to be a national uniform but of course some hospitals didn't conform. Navy blue for sisters, pale blue for staff nurses and blue and white check for students. No aprons but caps were still worn."

Training techniques were changing too. Specialist courses for nurses to work in coronary care, the renal unit and neonatal unit, were run at the City Hospital in association with Nottingham School of Nursing. Pupil nurse training for State Enrolled Nurses started in 1964. Formal lectures diminished in importance as slide and sound projectors came into their own. In 1970 the City Hospital School of Nursing was absorbed into the Nottingham School of Nursing in the Queen's Medical Centre, which replaced the six independent schools that had previously existed in the area.

One of the big changes resulting from the 1968 Salmon Report on senior nursing staff structures was the disappearance of figures of authority such as matron. Nurses were largely relieved of non-nursing duties with ward domestics, theatre technicians, nursing auxiliaries and ward clerks to take some of the burden. Specialist nurses were introduced into many areas such as coronary care, intensive care, burns and plastic surgery, special care baby units and the renal unit.

Even taking a patient's temperature changed - from 1972 it was recorded in Centigrade instead of Fahrenheit.

The introduction of the central sterile supplies department brought another big change in nursing practice. Nurses no longer had to boil

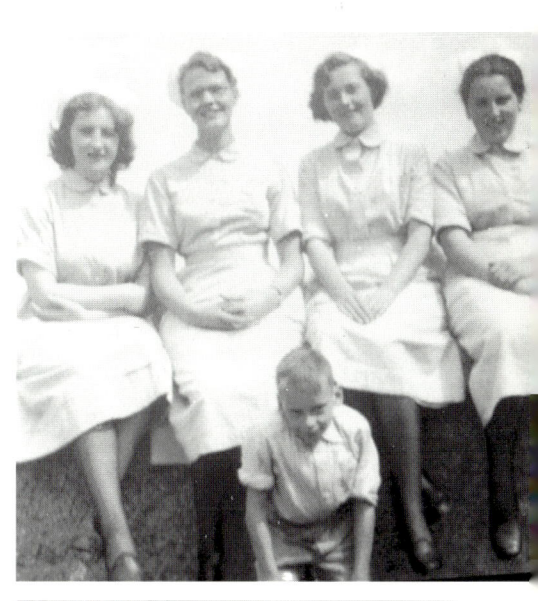

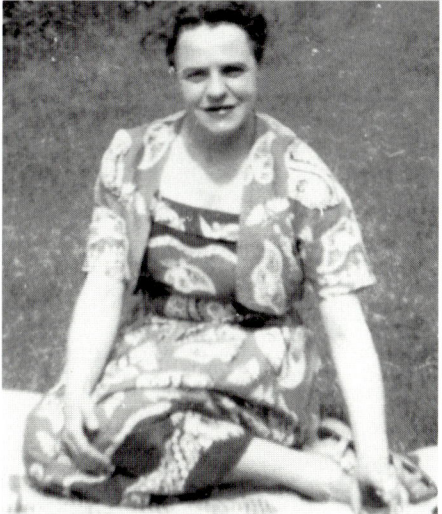

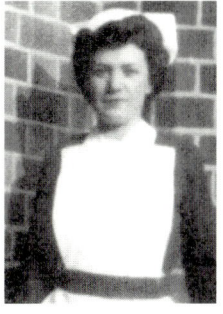

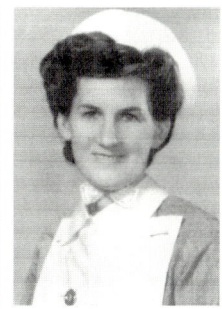

Top: Nursing cadets at the City Hospital in 1951. Pictured left to right are Margaret Briddon, Avis Williamson, Irene Cooper and Valerie Mills with a young patient named Dennis

Centre: Miss Thornton, the Home Sister, pictured on the lawn at the rear of Nurses' Home One

Above left: Sister Gladys Jenkins, who retired around 1975, worked with J B Cochrane on the women's ward

Above right: Norah Ware, who retired around 1975, was Sister in charge of theatres

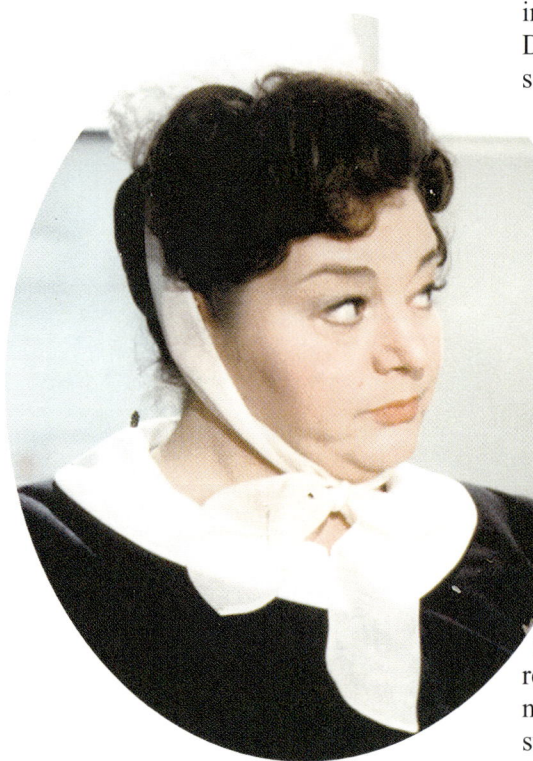

The image of the matron has been personified by the tough, uncompromising figure of Hattie Jacques in the Carry On films

Nightingale Two ward in 1961

instruments, syringes and needles. Disposable items proved a boon, saving nurses from spending hours making cotton wool balls, gauze swabs or checking and patching surgical gloves. Disposable bedpans replaced the stainless steel ones. Changes in medical practice and the early mobilisation of patients meant the routine toilet, bedpan rounds and bed baths were no longer necessary. There were downsides too. A faster turnover of patients gave nurses less time to know their patients. Ward routines changed with great emphasis on individual care plans and each patient had a nominated nurse responsible for their care. Specialist nurses were introduced to advise and support patients with breast cancer, diabetes, leukaemia and genetic conditions.

The opening of a new maternity unit in 1973 brought more changes. Parentcraft classes were held in the ante-natal clinic and fathers were encouraged to stay with the mother in labour. Later a water birthing pool was installed in the labour suite. A family planning service was started with family planning sisters visiting the postnatal wards twice a week. A vasectomy clinic was also introduced on Friday evenings.

The City Hospital's neonatal services were nationally recognised as being at the forefront of medical and nursing care. Former Matron Wendy Parsons recalled: "Parents were encouraged to visit and hold their very small babies. Siblings and grandparents were allowed to visit the unit. Today this is accepted as the norm but not in the 1970s."

Nurse recruitment remained a nagging problem. For a whole year in 1980/81 one of the hospital's 10 operating theatres closed down each week on a rota basis because there were not enough theatre nurses to keep them all going. Nursing Officer in charge Judy Brooksbank organised a cheese and wine party to try and persuade former nurses to come back.

The social scene was changing too. Many nurses no longer lived in nurses' homes, which meant a decline in hospital social activities such as concert parties, drama groups and tennis tournaments.

Retired Sister Janet Hodges

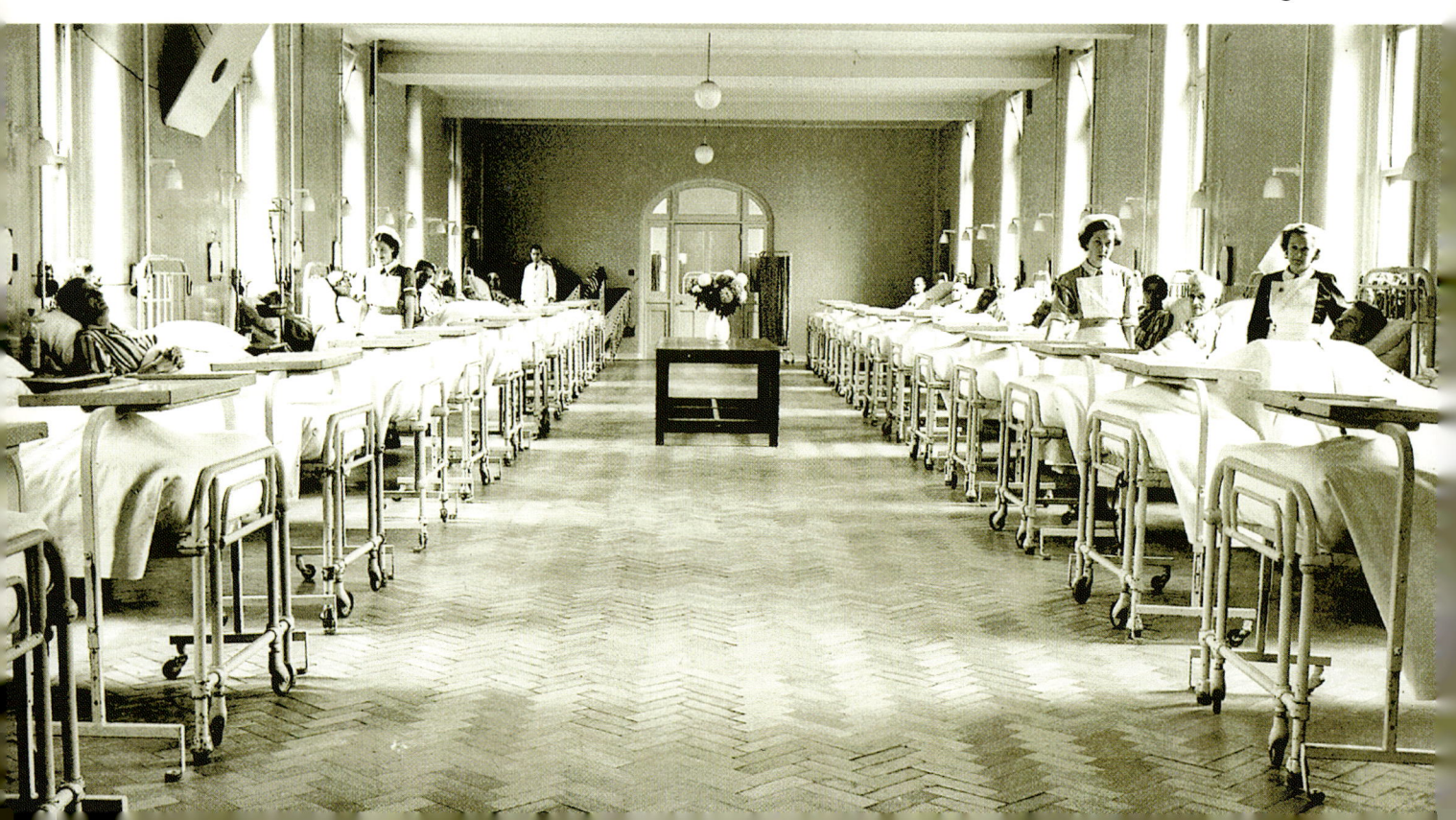

The People's Hospital

recalled: "Patients used to stay in hospital much longer, both medical and surgical cases. Day surgery came into being in the early 1980s, starting with gynaecology. Matron did a round at least twice each week. Her visits were not always welcome especially if the ward was very busy at the time because the sister or the senior staff nurse had to accompany her. These so-called visits were in effect ward inspections because she would always see something amiss, usually in connection with the tidiness of the ward or the appearance of the nurses (such as a nurse not wearing her belt, or having a ladder in her stocking). However they did speak to all the patients and this seemed to give the patients confidence.

"Mixed sex wards were introduced, although this had always been the case with high dependency wards such as coronary care. Most nurses did not want this arrangement for many valid reasons but this is an issue that is still being hotly debated. Many patients are not happy with mixed wards either.

"Visiting times were very much restricted. In the 1960s and 70s one hour each evening and one hour on one afternoon midweek and on Saturdays and Sundays was the norm. Now many wards have open visiting most of the day.

"Consultants' ward rounds were treated like the arrival of royalty, with the procession of his or her team, including senior and junior registrars, house officers, secretaries as well as the ward sister or the senior staff nurse. Unfortunately hardly anyone, least of all the patients, would dare to ask the consultant questions or voice an opinion. Fortunately these days are gone. The wishes and requests of the patient are taken into consideration, procedures are explained and choices are given wherever possible. Patients know their rights today and their expectations are much higher.

"The nurses' dress code has also changed significantly: dresses used to be made of heavy duty cotton, over which were worn starched white aprons and starched caps. This dress code commanded respect from patients and other members of staff. The introduction of man-made fibres allowed a more casual appearance. Gradually it became accepted in society for men to be equally competent as nurses as women. Also during the last 20 years it has become the norm to use first names for both staff and patients alike. Sometimes one has to ask if all such changes are for the better!"

Miss Ellen Treweek started work at Nottingham City Hospital in 1947, a year before the NHS was officially inaugurated. She initially worked as a nurse teacher and rose to the post of Deputy Matron before retiring in 1967.

She said: "A matron was never above rolling her sleeves up and getting stuck in when she found a problem. It's no good telling someone to do something unless you knew how to do it yourself. She didn't grumble, she helped, she understood and she co-ordinated. But patients also knew she was the person responsible for their overall care. They liked to see the matron as she treated them like another human being.

"I remember a little man in a brown suit who was doing a time and motion study at the hospital. This bureaucrat was telling us we should only spend 10 minutes with each patient. I asked him what he meant. You may only need 10 minutes with one patient but with another you may need half an hour. He couldn't understand that; so I ordered him out."

When Miss Treweek worked at the City Hospital, nurses, not cleaners, were responsible for keeping the hospital clean. In an age before antibiotics and high-tech cleaning equipment, they used the disinfectants lysol and carbolic - and plenty of elbow grease.

The image of the matron has been personified by the tough, uncompromising figure of Hattie Jacques in the Carry On films. But

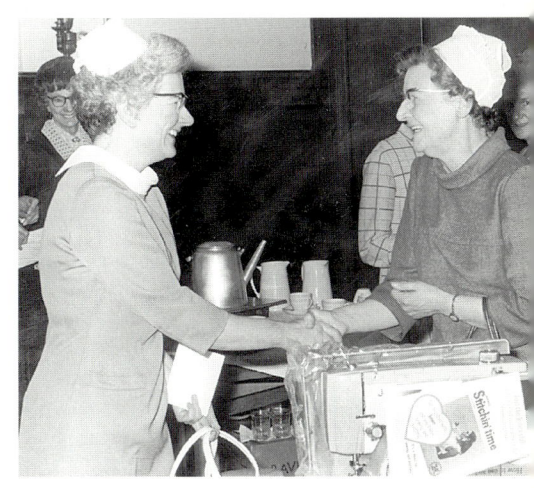

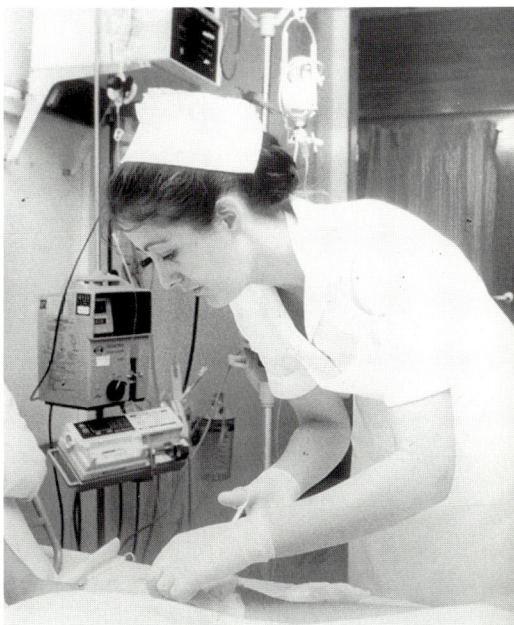

Top: Deputy Matron Miss J M Evans presents Miss Ellen Treweek with a sewing machine to mark her retirement in 1970 after 22 years' service

Above centre: State enrolled nurse Julie Ledger nursing a burns patients in 1988

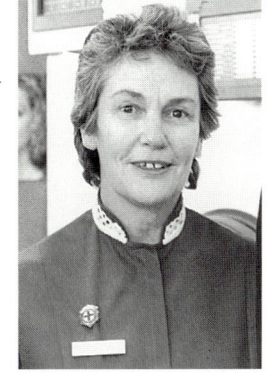

Above right: Wendy Parsons in 1986 when matron was back on her rounds at Nottingham City Hospital after a 18-year break

Miss Treweek claims that image was far from the truth. She said: "The Matron was the person at the top and although she didn't deal with the medical staff, they worked together as

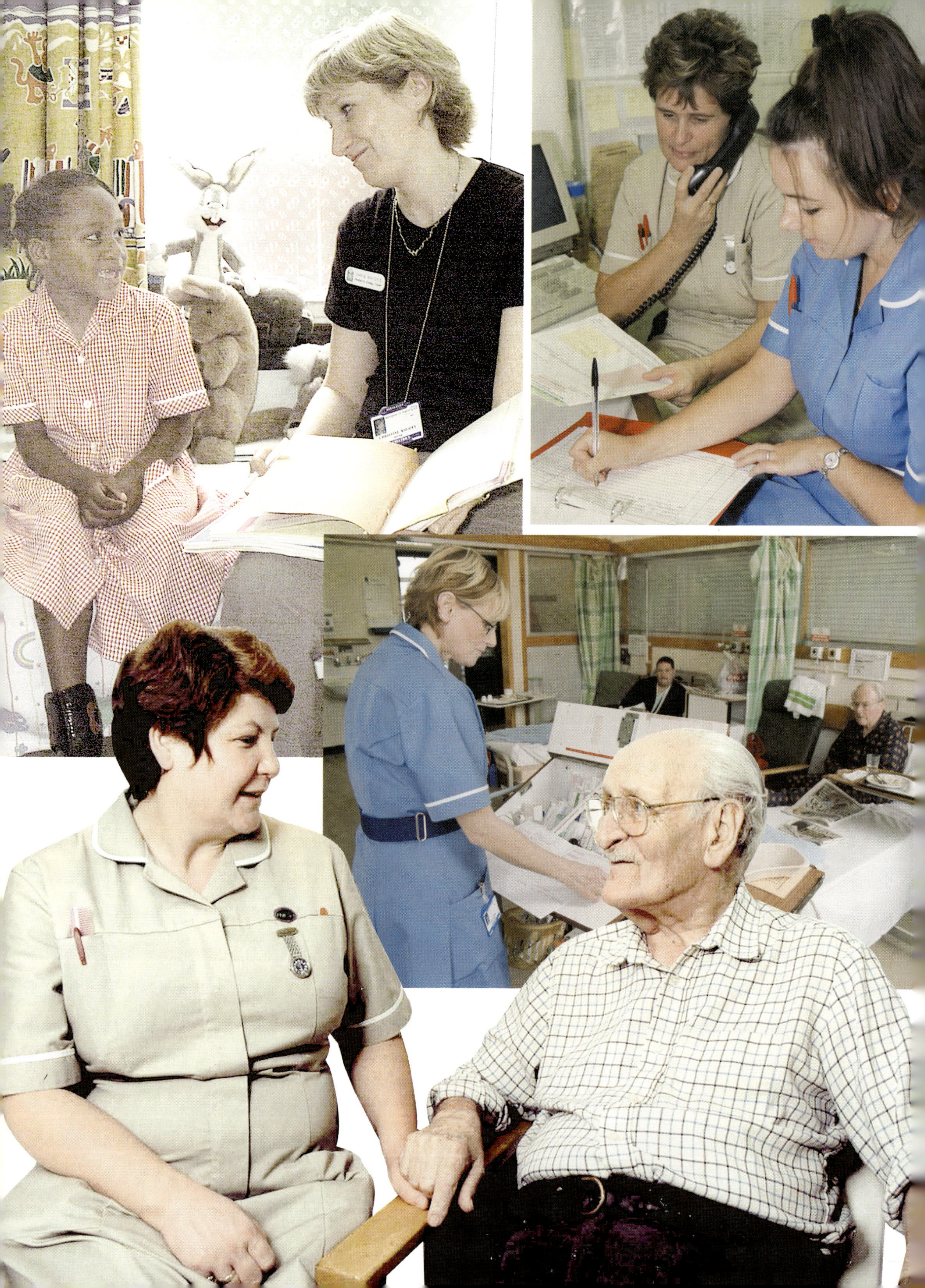

The People's Hospital

a team. It was about respect. We respected each other because everyone knew each other's value. matron was a mother figure in the hospital."

By 1986 matron was doing her rounds again at Nottingham City Hospital - after an 18-year break. Interviewed at the time Wendy Parsons said: "The reaction is overwhelming. People know who a matron is." Before her appointment as Matron her previous post was Director of Nursing Services and she was known as Mrs P." But as she said: "It just didn't have the same ring."

Mrs Parsons came to Nottingham in 1973, specialising in midwifery until nursing was reorganised in 1982 and she had to apply for her old job. She didn't get the post but was given responsibility for the acute services and care of the elderly. She recalled: "It turned out to be the best thing that ever happened. I think I had done midwifery for too long."

She started nursing in 1955 when matron was still a forbidding starched figure who ruled the wards. Wendy prefers to think of the modern image as much more human.

She believed the biggest problem facing staff on the 60-acre site was communication. And her decision to appear regularly on the wards was one step towards breaking down those barriers.

Now Nottingham City Hospital has not one, but a string of matrons. They were introduced to look after the interests of patients and staff on a group of wards, making sure the quality of services is raised and that these high standards are maintained.

Today they are called clinical nurse managers, providing support to their nursing colleagues, making sure the wards are clean, that patients are treated with respect and courtesy and, if there's a problem, they have the authority to sort it out as quickly and efficiently as they can.

Clinical Nurse Manager Sharon Saunders, who works in the surgical division, says: "This is a great opportunity to make a difference to the care our patients receive. I understand the day-to-day pressures of working on the wards but I now have time to stand back and look objectively at what we do and how we do it and to suggest changes which I think would make a difference. Patients and their relatives are welcome to ask for our help at any time."

Another modern matron is Clinical Nurse Manager Jane Roe, who has been working with a team of colleagues from many different parts of the hospital to plan the replacement of all the beds.

And the hospital began the new millennium in winning style. Pioneering work by staff in children's services clinched a batch of top national honours. Urology nurse Christine Rhodes brought the *Nursing Standard* Paediatric Nurse of the Year Award back to Nottingham, following in the footsteps of the City Hospital's cleft lip and palate nurse specialist Vanessa Martin who had won the award in 2000. Vanessa was also named overall Nurse of the Year in 2000.

So the nursing spirit, so vital in the first 100 years, is burning as brightly as ever as Nottingham City Hospital enters a demanding and exciting new era.

Main picture: Multi-disciplinary team in 2002
Inset: Staff nurse using a Tympanic thermometer
Opposite page: Nurses in action including award-winning Christine Rhodes pictured top left

4

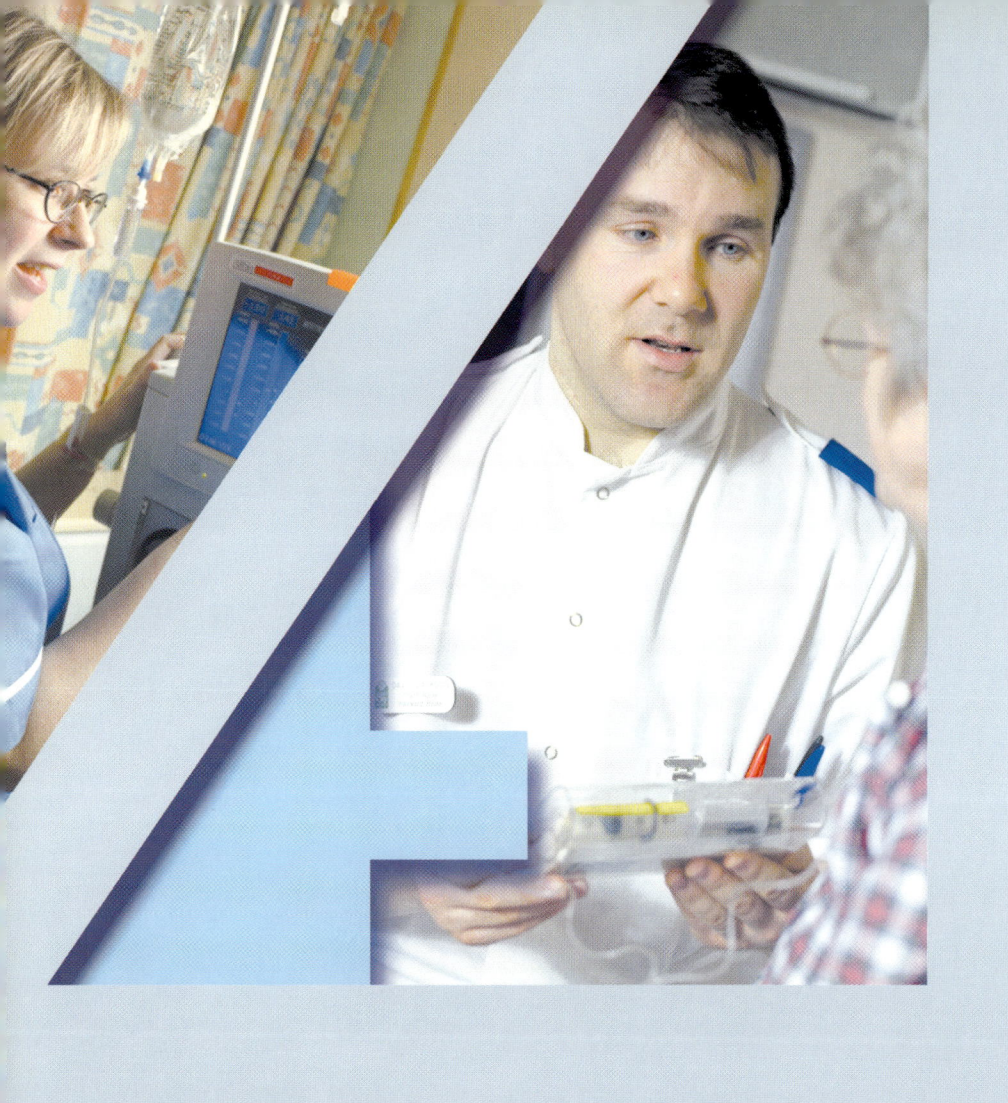

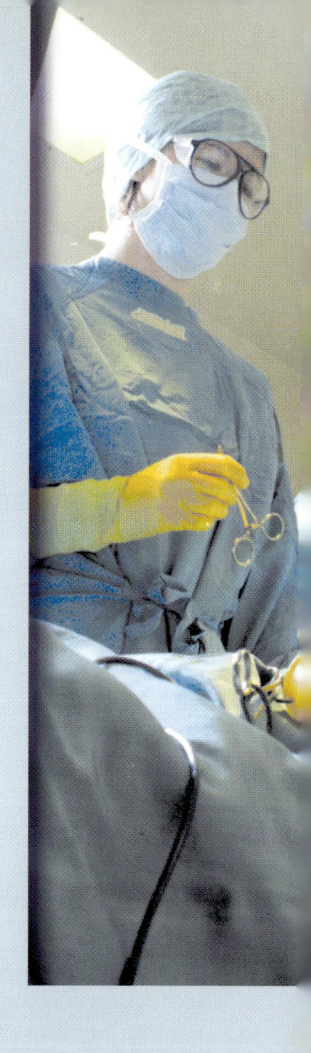

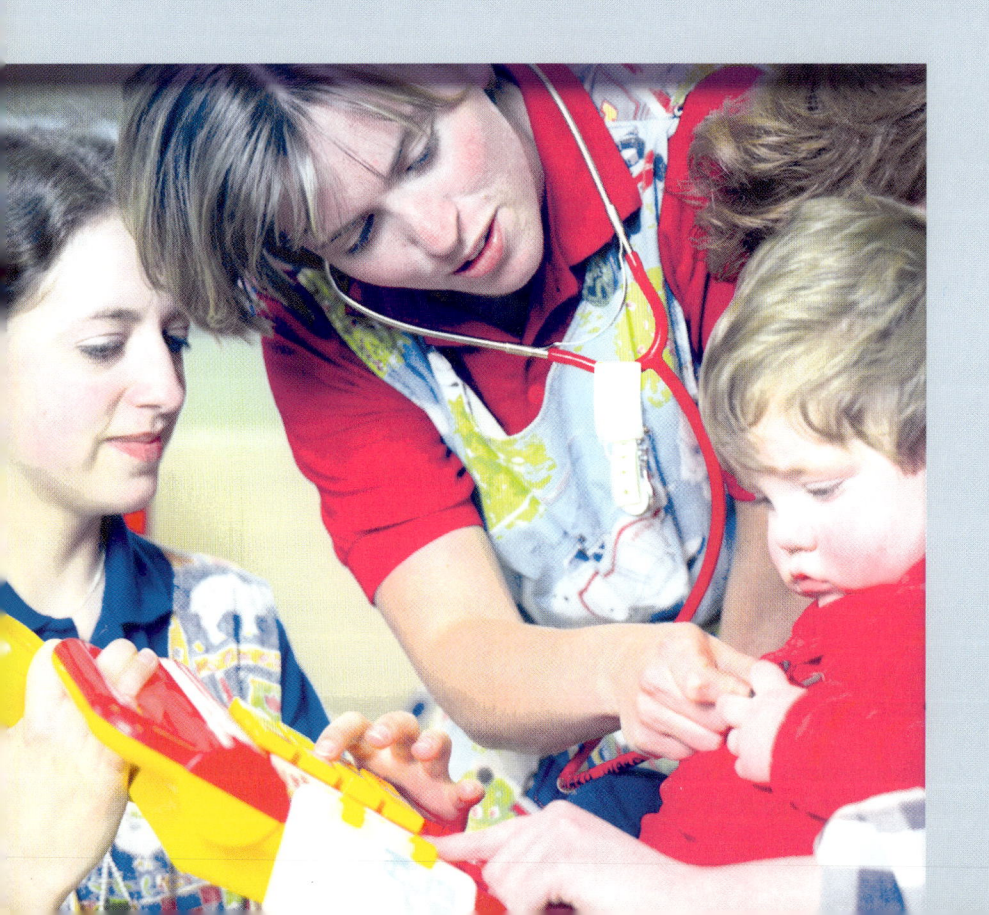

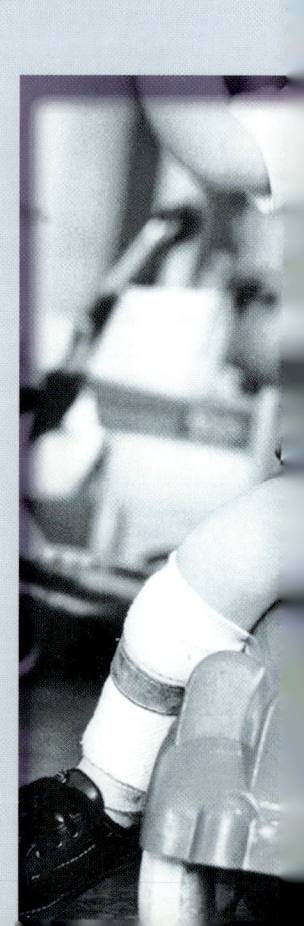

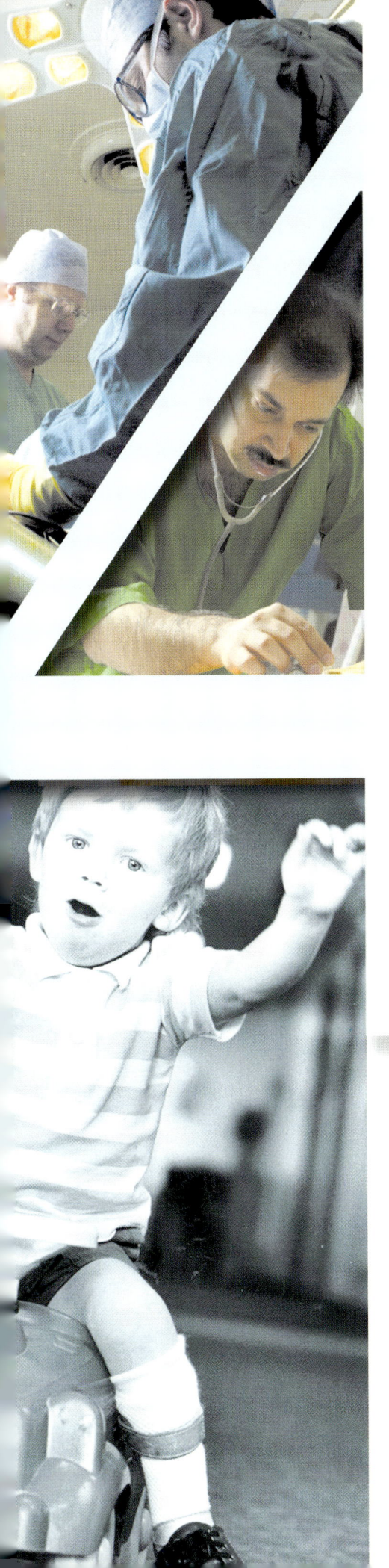

The emergence of specialist services

A thriving centre of excellence

BY the 1970s the City Hospital was on the move. It had shrugged off its humble roots and had brought together an able team of consultants and key personnel with the drive to forge ahead as a major teaching hospital. By the end of the millennium the hospital would be renowned locally and nationally as a centre of excellence in many areas, including kidney transplantation, maternity and neonatal care, breast screening, stroke care, cancer treatment, genetics, heart surgery and bone marrow transplantation.

Nottingham City Hospital's current service directory runs to 78 pages, reflecting the breadth of services now provided - and new developments are continually coming on stream. So this section, selected and edited from a wide range of sources, outlines how some of the specialist services developed through the eyes and personal experiences of many people who have contributed to the hospital's history.

Department of radiology

By Donald Rose

THE first X-rays were taken at City Hospital by Dr Rigby in the early 1920s. At that time the films took a week to develop. By 1931 the number of X-ray examinations had risen to 498 in one year.

When Mr L S Hall was appointed the first Superintendent Radiographer in 1957, the staff comprised himself, a nursing sister, three radiographers, a dark room technician and two clerks. The work at that time was mostly basic radiography with barium sessions and a few kidney examinations. Dr Donald Munroe, an anaesthetist from the thoracic unit, carried out cardiac catherisations and a few bronchograms.

In 1959 radiology moved into a new department, opposite the theatres in the old outpatients department. This had four X-ray rooms and the workload really took off. The number of X-ray examinations rose from 12,000 in 1961 to 40,000 in 1970, the workload doubling every 8.5 years. During the late 1960s percuteneous angiography (X-rays of blood vessels and blood vessels within organs) was introduced and the new imaging techniques of ultrasound and nuclear medicine started to become available to radiologists. Dr Alun Morris pioneered an integrated radiology department at the City Hospital with the introduction of a gamma camera in 1970 and an ultrasound machine in 1971, together with a third consultant radiologist.

A major expansion into purpose-built accommodation on the southern side of the main corridor took place in 1975/76 and when a second

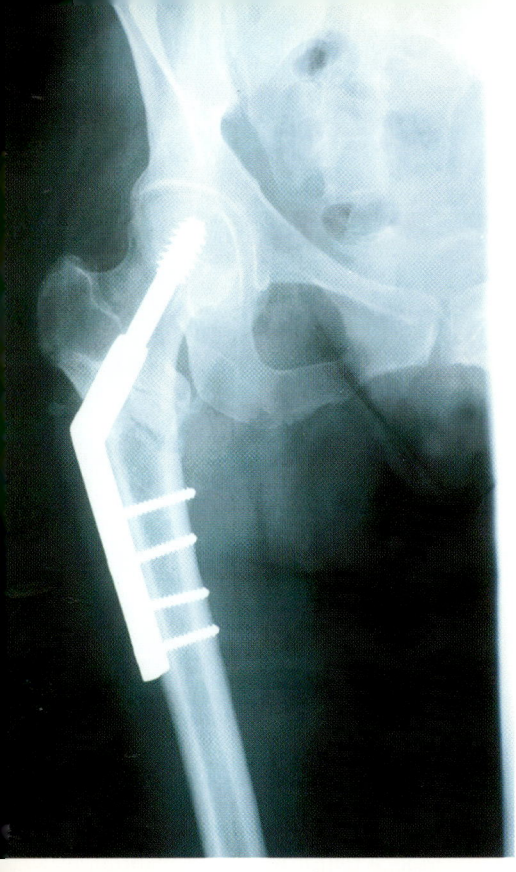

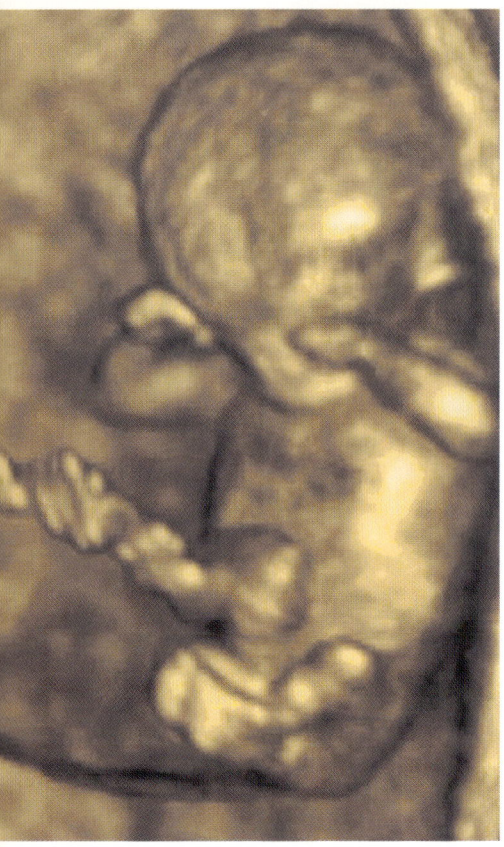

The People's Hospital

ultrasound machine was installed in 1977, the department had 17 rooms and five consultant radiologists, all dedicated to the City Hospital but also providing a radiology service to Newark Hospital.

Radiology was entirely a diagnostic specialty until the late 1970s when therapeutic techniques such as cyst aspiration, removal of retained gallstones via drain tracts, and embolisation (blockage) of bleeding arteries under radiological guidance were introduced in the department. These were the early days of interventional radiology, which included the drainage of blocked kidneys and keyhole disintegration of kidney stones by the early 1980s. Ultrasound also proved to be an extremely valuable imaging tool.

Computed tomography (CT), a sophisticated X-ray technique which demonstrates internal structures in great detail, was invented by Nottinghamshire man Sir Godfrey Hounsfield in 1973. In 1984, a CT scanner was installed at the Queen's Medical Centre, and City Hospital radiologists investigated their patients there in the evenings until 1988 when a CT scanner was installed at the City in a purpose-built suite adjacent to the pathology department. This was paid for by the local population after three years of fundraising.

A purpose-built MRI (magnetic resonance imaging) suite was built in 1994 as a Private Finance Initiative by Lister Bestcare and run by them using NHS consultants. Radiology of the breast is undertaken in a separate department - the Helen Garrod breast screening unit, established in 1979 after years of fundraising.

In 1987 the department installed a computerised reporting system to allow requests for and reports of examinations to be sent electronically. Other practical improvements in recent years have been the digitisation of images (computed radiography) and the widespread use of daylight processing facilities that are quicker, cleaner and more accessible than the old dark rooms which were used for film processing.

Today the department comprises 18 X-ray rooms, five ultrasound rooms (plus three in antenatal clinic) and a nuclear medicine section which contains two gamma cameras, three bone densitometers and radiopharmacy. The radiology team performed 160,000 examinations in the year 2001. Interventional procedures, which can be complex and time consuming, rose from 800 in 1991 to 2,500 in 2001.

Teaching is undertaken at all levels of the department. The number of radiologists at the City Hospital has more than doubled in the past 20 years and there are now many more in training. The department has 44 radiographers of various grades, four nurses, 28 clerical and administration staff, 42 trainee radiographer assistants and radiographer helpers.

Thoracic surgery and the start of intensive care services

By Robert Barclay

THORACIC surgery was one of the earliest specialist services at the City Hospital. Harley Street consultant Lawrence O'Shaughnessy held regular surgical sessions from 1936, operating on many patients with pulmonary tuberculosis. Regarded by many as the father of modern thoracic and cardio-vascular surgery, he was killed in France in 1940. Mr George Mason from Newcastle-on-Tyne took his place. Mr William Buckley was appointed the first full-time Thoracic Surgeon in 1947 and was joined by a second consultant in 1952. Between them they covered a large area extending as far as Grimsby and Lincoln.

I was appointed Senior Registrar in April 1949, working at the City Hospital, the Ransom Sanitorium and other hospitals in the area. I had previously worked at Harefield

Top: *X-ray of hip following operation using pins and screws*

Above: *Scanned image of baby in womb*

The People's Hospital

Hospital, where some cardiac surgery was being done. Mitral valve surgery was just beginning to be recognised by the cardiologists. I was very keen to do more cardiac surgery. In 1950 Mr Buckley and I went to Guy's Hospital to see the eminent surgeon Sir Russell Brock, who was doing mitral valve surgery. He encouraged us and we came back to Nottingham and started performing the operation.

After I was appointed full-time Consultant Thoracic Surgeon in July 1952, the need for an intensive care unit to give post-operative respiratory support became evident. Following another fact-finding visit to Guy's, we dedicated part of the male thoracic ward to post-operative intensive care and offered to take patients requiring respiratory support from other parts of the hospital and other hospitals. This was the start of intensive care in Nottingham.

But our efforts to establish cardiac surgery in Nottingham suffered a number of setbacks. Both Leicester and Sheffield were keen to set up 'open heart' units, but in approving this, the Regional Board did not want a third unit in Nottingham as well. This had to wait until coronary artery surgery was widely developed. By that time I had retired.

Cardio-thoracic surgery

By David Richens

THERE had always been the desire to develop cardiac surgery in Nottingham because of the size of the city and the fact that it contained two large acute teaching hospitals. There was already a thriving thoracic surgery unit with close links with two other providers in the Trent region at Leicester and Sheffield which each had a cardiac surgery unit. It was considered necessary to let Leicester and Sheffield grow to their maximum capacity before opening a third unit in the Trent region in Nottingham.

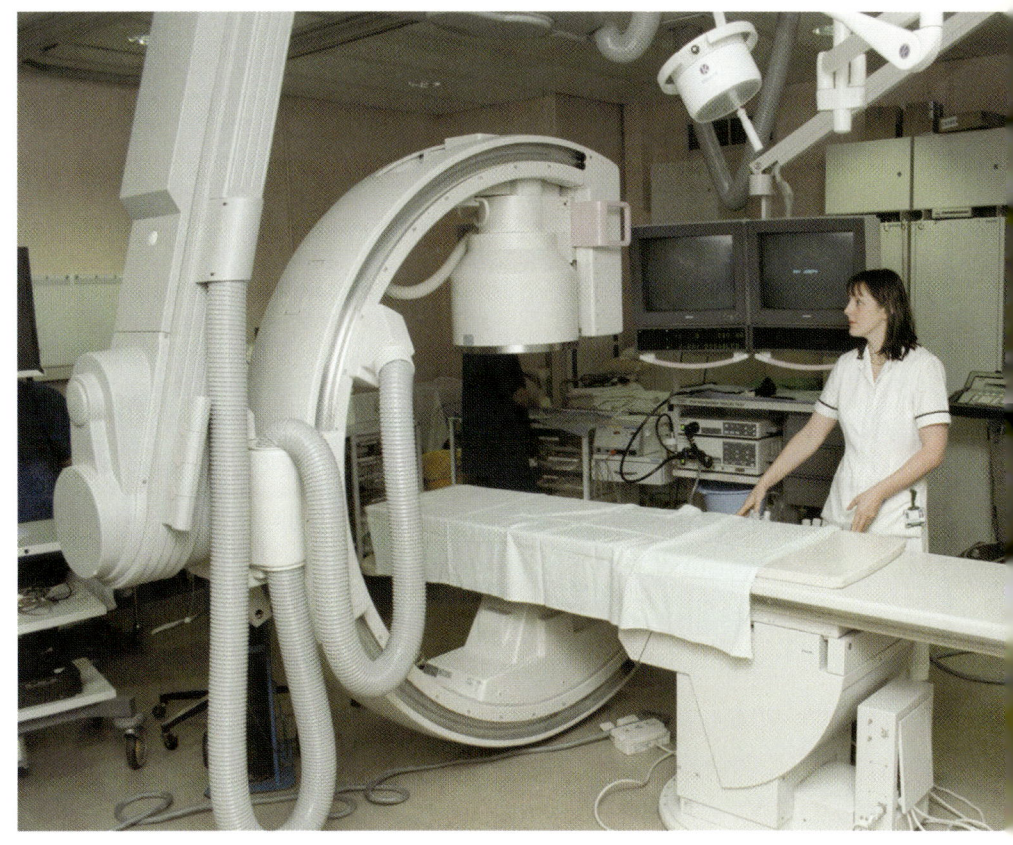

In 1994, Nottingham City Hospital decided to go ahead with the development of a cardiac surgery programme. Two consultant cardiac surgeons and two consultant cardiac anaesthetists, together with a full complement of theatre, intensive care and ward staff were employed between 1994 and 1995.

The first case was performed in September 1995 and since that time, more than 3,000 operations have been carried out. The unit provides adult cardiac surgical care for the full range of operations with the exception of cardiac transplantation. Milestones in the development of this programme have been the appointment of a third surgeon and anaesthetist in 2000, and the publication of the Department of Health's League Tables for results of cardiac surgery, which place Nottingham City Hospital top of the league with the lowest mortality rate in the country. The unit is now looking to grow further with the promise of a large new building in the hospital, which would integrate cardiology and cardiac surgery.

A digital X-ray camera

Operating theatres

By Robert Coultas, Judy Brooksbank and Mike Bromige

BEFORE 1973 there were twin theatres off the main corridor and one theatre near to wards B1 and B2 (now James ward). These served all the surgical specialties including maternity. The Firs Maternity Unit on Mansfield Road, Sherwood had its own operating theatre.

In late 1972 the central sterile supplies department (CSSD) opened and Judy Beaver (soon to become Judy Brooksbank) was appointed Theatre Manager.

A new six theatre block was brought into use gradually from April, 1973. This had a post-operative recovery area for patients to be looked after by specially trained theatre staff before they returned to the wards. The small theatre close to the plastic surgery wards was closed but the twin theatres remained and eventually became a dedicated urological surgery unit.

The new maternity unit opened with two theatres staffed from the main unit which were used for neonatal surgery and obstetric emergencies. The old unit closed and the Firs Maternity Hospital followed soon afterwards.

Below: Consultant Respiratory Physician Dr John Macfarlane

Bottom: The Mayor of Gedling's Charity raised £10,795 which paid for four new electronic beds in the Beeston ward stroke unit at the hospital. Councillor Dennis Walker (Mayor 1999-2000) is pictured testing one of the new beds while talking to stroke patient Marjorie Langsdale

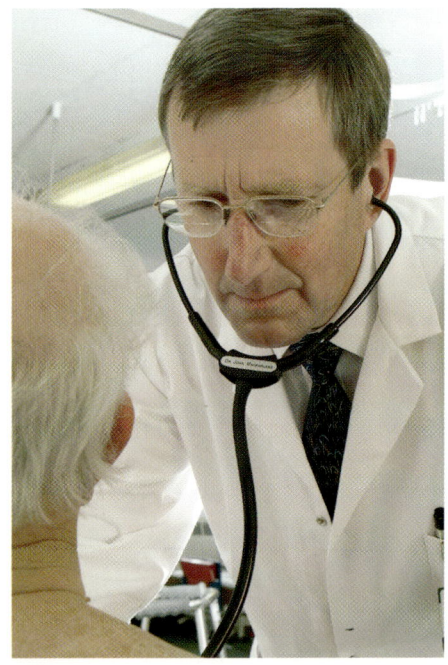

A burns unit with a small theatre, which had provision for general anaesthesia, was opened near to the entrance to the plastic surgery wards B1 and B2. This subsequently moved to the new H block with plastic surgery and the small theatre became, in the new unit, a plastic surgery theatre plus a burns dressing area.

The theatres were gradually modernised over the years to keep pace with changing health and safety legislation and the requirements of more complex surgery and anaesthesia. For example, a laminar airflow unit was installed for joint replacement surgery.

In the early 1990s a day surgery unit was opened in a vacated ward on top of the maternity unit, and a few years later plans were put in place to create more theatres to cope with the increasing amount of day surgery, orthopaedic surgery and the decision to begin cardiac surgery.

A twin theatre day surgery unit was built on a separate site adjacent to the maternity unit and two new operating theatres were squeezed into a space adjoining the main theatres. One of these had a second laminar flow unit for orthopaedic cases. At the same time the recovery and reception areas were redesigned and enlarged.

Throughout this entire time staff training and development were a high priority and the City Hospital became committed to the National Award in Operating Theatre Practice. Judy Brooksbank retired in 2000.

Chest diseases in Nottingham

by Dr Dewi Davies

IN 1948 the NHS took responsibility for running chest clinics and sanatoria treating patients with tuberculosis from the local authorities. There was a heavy caseload but this gradually changed as tuberculosis declined and staff entering new posts underwent wider training.

In 1955 Nottinghamshire had 588 beds for chest diseases (the majority at Newstead and Ransom Sanitoria) but there were also beds in five other hospitals. Nearly all were occupied by patients with tuberculosis. There were more than 700 cases a year in Nottinghamshire and hospital stays were long. By 1966 the number of beds had reduced to 299 and 85 per cent of the patients had non-tuberculosis diseases. Newstead closed in 1969.

At that time the outpatient chest service in Nottingham was run from Forest Dean, a large house on Gregory Boulevard, and the inpatient facilities were based at Ransom Hospital near Mansfield. Medical staff were keen to avoid this isolation and to integrate with general medicine. A few beds were made available for the chest physicians in the thoracic surgical wards at the City Hospital in the early 1970s. In 1975 Ransom Hospital closed and Oxton and Gedling wards, which were no longer needed by maternity, were used for medical patients. These were run by the two chest physicians (myself and Dr Deri Roderick-Smith) and Dr David Banks, who took part in the general medical take as well as dealing with an increasing number of patients with respiratory diseases. By

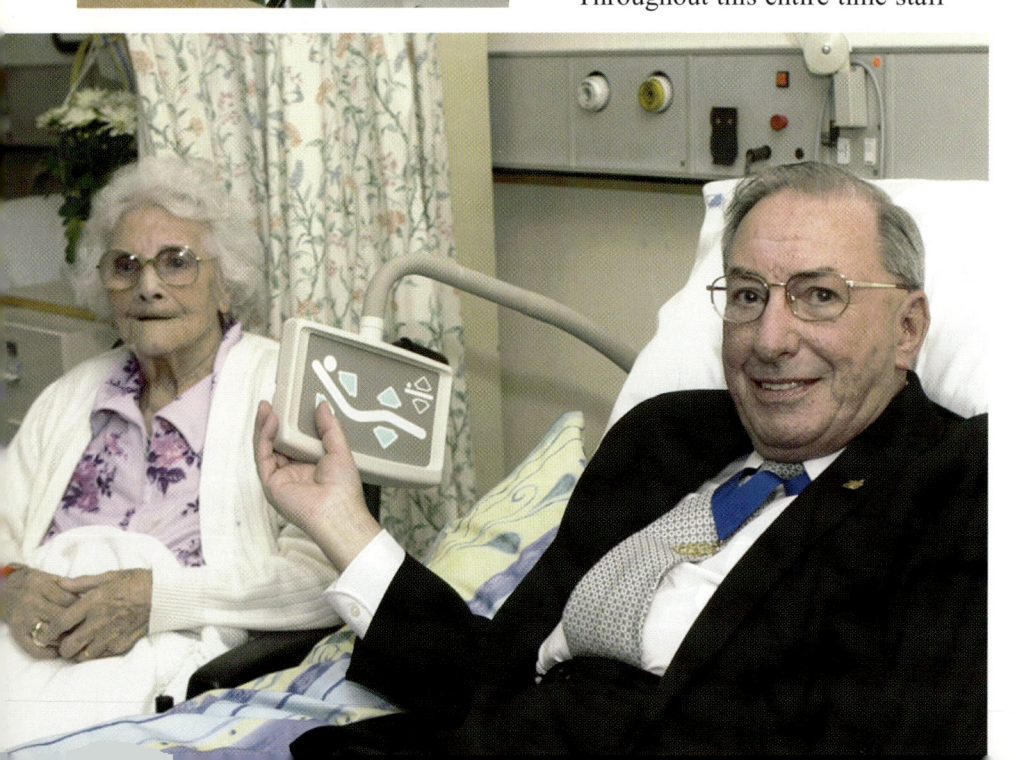

The People's Hospital

then six beds at Heathfield Hospital were sufficient for patients with tuberculosis. In 1977 the outpatient clinic at Forest Dean closed and the outpatient chest service then operated from the main outpatient department at the City Hospital. At last integration of the chest service into the body of general medicine was complete.

Staffing was very inadequate with only two consultant physicians. They also provided support for the University Hospital because there was no specialist chest physician on the staff and they ran an outpatient clinic in Newark.

Relief came in 1984 when Dr Anne Tattersfield from Southampton was appointed Professor of Respiratory Medicine and a specialist chest physician started at University Hospital in the following year.

Respiratory medicine
By Professor Anne Tattersfield

WHEN I came to Nottingham in 1984, there were between 65 and 91 students at the City Hospital. The Medical School intake is now 250 in each academic year. Respiratory medicine started from scratch in 1984 with money from the NHS and university for a chair, senior lecturer and secretary. The group has grown progressively with support from the university and funding from research bodies. We now have three professors, two senior lecturers and a lecturer, plus secretaries and several technicians, research fellows and research assistants: 30-35 people in total.

Our main research area has been in asthma but we are also carrying out research into cystic fibrosis, cryptogenic fibrosing alveolitis, chronic obstructive pulmonary disease and a rare lung disease called LAM. Our integrated approach has worked well and the group collaborates widely within Nottingham and outside from as far afield as Harvard in America and Jimma in Ethiopia.

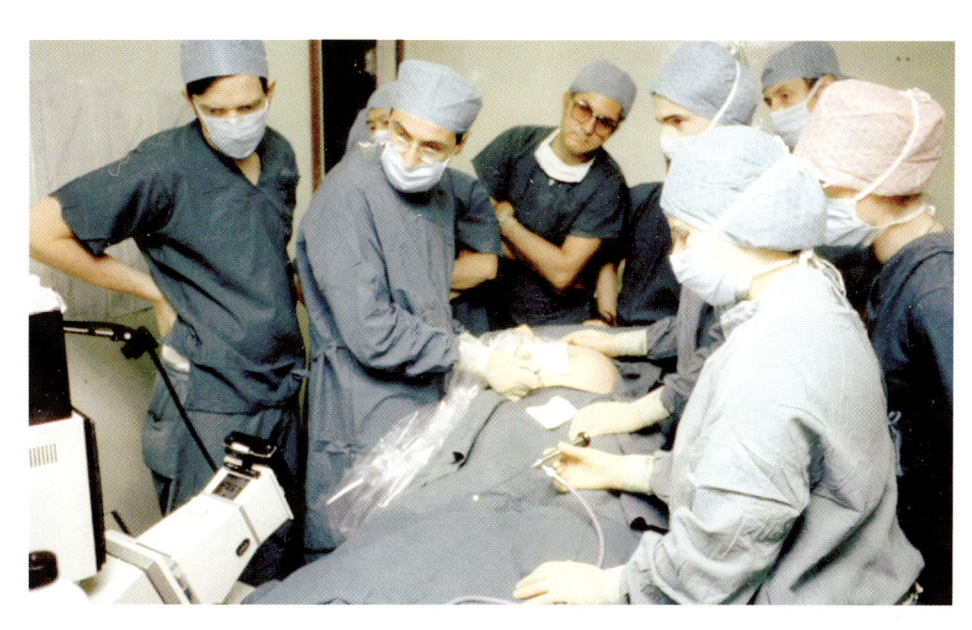

On the clinical side we have played a major role in developing the adult cystic fibrosis service. In 1984 there were 15 adults with CF in Nottingham and the average life expectancy was 15-20 years. In 2002 we have 100 adult patients on the books and their life expectancy is 35-40 years.

From a standing start 25 years ago, Nottingham is now internationally recognised as an area of excellence for respiratory medicine.

Stroke research
by Professor Philip Bath

THE stroke research unit, now called the Division of Stroke Medicine, was set up at Nottingham City Hospital in 1982, initially with funding from a local charity - the Nottingham Fights Stroke Association. The unit at that time was headed by Dr (now Professor) Nadina Lincoln. The research emphasis was on rehabilitation after stroke and the unit justly achieved national and international status. A key project showed that rehabilitation in a stroke unit led to improved outcome; this trial along with others from the UK and elsewhere led to the introduction of stroke units around the world.

In 1992 the Stroke Association (then the Chest, Heart and Stroke

Keyhole surgery being performed at the hospital

Association) funded the UK's first Chair in Stroke Medicine based in the stroke research unit. The foundation Chair was held by Professor Peter Fentem who had previously been Dean to the Medical School. The unit expanded during his tenure and extra funding, agreed in 1996, allowed a senior lecturer and lecturer to be appointed. The research emphasis remained on rehabilitation with the addition of studies into risk factors, notably exercise, Professor Fentem's interest.

Professor Fentem retired in 1997 and Professor Philip Bath commenced in 1998. His research interests of acute pathophysiology, treatment and secondary prevention have added to the division's repertory. The unit was visited by the Duke of Kent in 1992 and the Queen in 2000.

Cardiology
By Dr Keith Morris

THE first steps towards dedicated, specialised care for patients with heart attacks at the City Hospital were taken in the late 1960s. A few beds on a general medical ward, equipped with specialist monitoring equipment, became the first coronary care unit. When the old maternity unit closed in the early 1970s, the obstetrics ward was turned into a specialist coronary care unit and the old delivery ward became the base for inserting temporary cardiac pacemakers. The unit was supervised by Dr David Banks who had joined Professor Michael Langman's therapeutics department. Dr Banks, a former member of the university department of medicine, continued to be closely involved with all the heart attack research which took place in Nottingham over the years.

One of the unit's proud boasts is that none of the senior nursing staff has ever left to do anything unrelated to cardiology - reflecting the unit's great friendship and teamwork.

Lynne Dale, who initially trained on the unit, teaches doctors and nurses the art of resuscitation and the unit runs successful training courses for coronary care nurses, masterminded by Jenny Fox.

In the 1960s/70s the ECG department was established in the old annexe buildings. Senior Technician was Mrs Eileen Mullins, a real enthusiast who was later appointed to the National Council and became heavily involved in the training of cardiac technicians.

She recalled: "When I began work as an ECG technician in 1961 there was just one ECG machine which was very large and heavy in comparison to today's machines. It was only portable on a trolley. I used to receive request cards from consultants to record ECGs on patients in the wards. This entailed moving the bed to the nearest power point before recording. After about a year a battery-operated ECG machine was purchased, which made life easier."

Jan Prewitt, who joined the cardiac department in 1974, added: "A typical tracing from the early ECG machines was about 20ft long. Abrasive jelly was rubbed into the patient's skin, on their limbs and their chest. Metal plates were attached to the limbs and suction cups were attached to the chest. Unfortunately in warm weather the jelly became runny and the electrodes would slide about all over the patient's chest.

"The early defibrillators were huge pieces of equipment. Some were mounted onto large wooden cabinets which were painted red with the words 'Danger - high voltage' emblazoned across the doors. They were called the 'Red Devils'."

Gradually the department took on more and more investigations and the equipment became more complex. When the respiratory unit was established they wanted their own testing department, so this was split from the main department by Sue Revill, who went on to obtain a PhD.

Today the highly specialised ECG department, supervised by Martin Giles, provides technical services for all the modern developments in cardiology, including the assessment of abnormal heart rhythms, management of pacemakers and implanted cardiac defibrillators. It also provides technical expertise in the cardiac laboratory, where angiography and angioplasty procedures take place and technicians now run the echocardiographic and exercise testing services.

Cardiac catheterisation was being carried out at the City Hospital in the late 1960s by Dr Monroe, an anaesthetist and Dr Robert Duff, the cardiologist, but most patients who required surgical intervention, had to travel to Leicester.

Dr Keith Morris, who succeeded Dr Duff in 1985, had already established a cardiac catheter service at University Hospital and repeated the process at the City Hospital. This led to a great increase in workload and eventually the department of cardiothoracic surgery was established.

Other consultants have been appointed with specialist expertise in electrophysiology and angioplasty. The City Hospital now offers a full range of services in cardiac surgery and cardiology, including a service for adult patients with congenital heart disease.

A protoype ECG machine

Health care of the elderly

By Dr Angela Trueman

THE many changes in care of elderly patients during the past 50 years have been reflected in the development of services at the City Hospital. Dr William Morton was appointed Consultant in Geriatric Medicine in 1948 shortly after geriatric medicine had been recognised as a speciality. The department was based in the old Sherwood Hospital which had been the old workhouse (Bagthorpe).

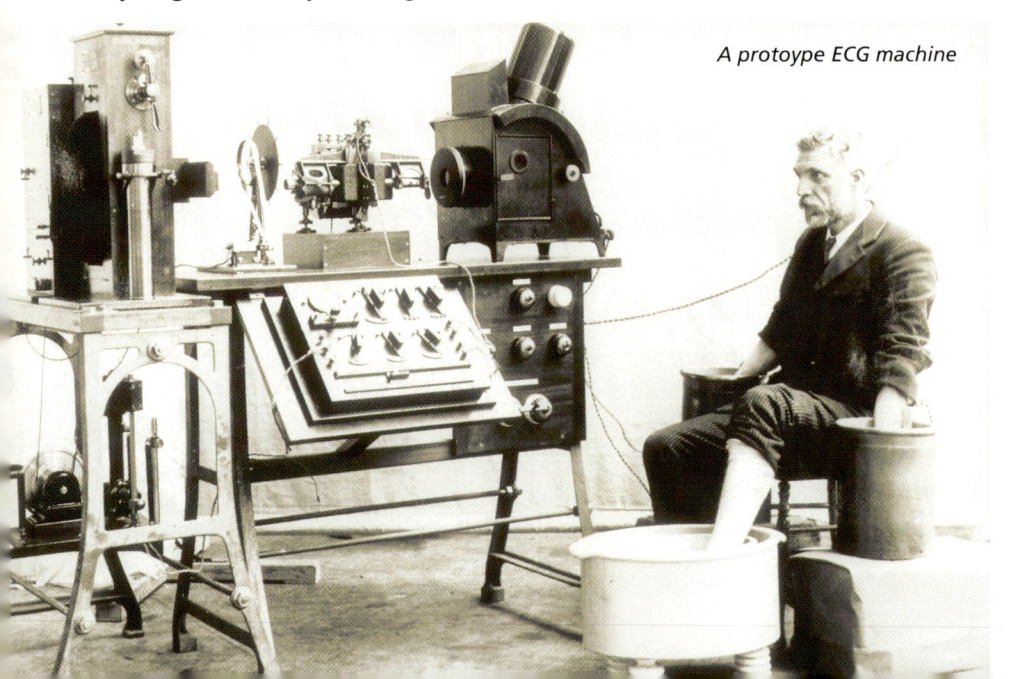

The People's Hospital

There were many beds crowded on three floors in six wings. During the 1960s and 1970s new wards were added and geriatricians were appointed who, not only looked after the 440 beds in the Sherwood wing, but had to supervise the care of patients in hospitals in Newark (Hawtonville), Highbury Hospital, Basford Hospital, Ellerslie House (the young chronic sick unit), other peripheral units and also St Francis Hospital (where there were psychogeriatric patients).

In 1977 the Academic Unit of Health Care of the Elderly was formed and Tom Airie was appointed Professor of Health Care of the Elderly. His background was in psychogeriatric medicine and he further developed links between psychiatry and medicine. The department increased in size and many trainees pursued academic careers in furthering geriatric medicine. For example Dr Graham Mulley developed his reputation in research on the problems of daily living before moving on to become a Professor of Geriatric Medicine in Leeds; Dr Horan, an SHO in the department, became Professor of Geriatric Medicine in Manchester; Dr D Barer, a Registrar in the department, became Professor of Geriatric Medicine in Newcastle.

The 1980s saw the closure of the old wards in the Sherwood wing and the building of new facilities. The academic unit moved to the University Hospital, the stroke unit transferred from the old General Hospital to the City Hospital and Professor Fentem was appointed as Professor of Stroke Medicine. During the 1990s geriatric medicine at the City Hospital integrated with general medicine and the geriatricians have worked as general physicians looking after patients of all age groups but still with a responsibility for care of the elderly. With the publication of the National Service Framework for Older People there will be an increasing need to take on the responsibilities of intermediate care in community settings, developing the functions of the Day Hospital and increasing research and teaching into the needs of an increasingly older population.

Department of gastroenterology

By Dr Richard Long

RIGID endoscopy of the stomach, lungs and colon has been performed by surgeons and, to a lesser extent, physicians for many decades. The fibre optic endoscope, developed in the 1960s, allowed a bending tube to see round corners and to relay an image to the eye of the endoscopist.

The technique of looking into the stomach in this way was developed by Professor Michael Langman in the 1970s with Tom Balfour quickly doing more extensive fibre optic colonoscopy (imaging of the lower bowel). Tom Balfour then went on to perform imaging of the bile ducts and pancreatic ducts; he started to remove gallstone via sphincterotomy (short surgical incisions performed by a knife down the endoscope) and to alleviate jaundice in malignant obstructions with stents. In the late 1980s, video endoscopy became common whereby the image can be viewed on a television screen. Other techniques such as laser surgery and the development of more advanced stents allowed the technique to have a therapeutic role rather than diagnostic as initially envisaged.

A new endoscopy centre opened at Nottingham City Hospital in summer 2001.

Department of therapeutics

By Professor Michael Langman and Dr David Banks

IN 1972 the Boots Company gave £100,000 to endow a chair in therapeutics and Professor Michael Langman was appointed. The number

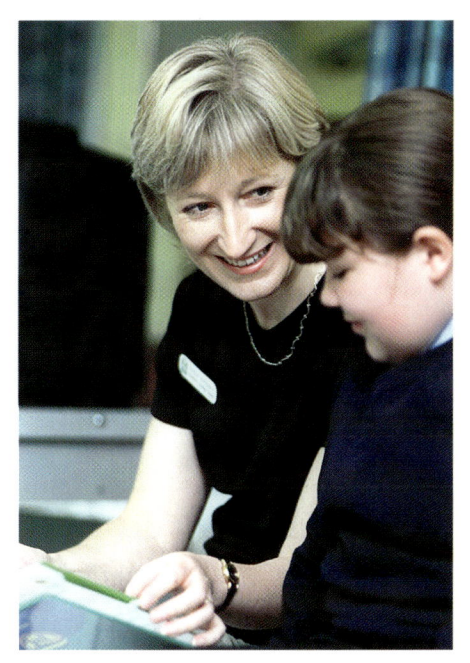

Christine Rhodes, a Paediatric Urology Sister, who was nominated for Nurse of the Year after being named Child Health Nurse of the Year in 2001. She is pictured with long-term patient Emma Barratt whom Christine has been treating since she was six months old

of medical students was expected to increase rapidly. So the department of therapeutics was sited at the City Hospital as support for the hospital's academic role.

The department started in a medical ward converted at a cost of around £30,000. The first staff were Dr David Banks as part-time Senior Lecturer and part-time Consultant Physician, and Chief Technician Alan Bramall. They were soon joined by Duncan Bell, now Professor in Sunderland.

Research was based in gastroenterology and cardiology but not only in drug action. The first lecturers were Malcolm McIllmurray, now a Consultant Oncologist in Lancaster and David Henry, now Professor of Clinical Pharmacology in Newcastle, New South Wales, followed by Rodney Burnham, now Consultant Physician in Romford. The core department was small, close-knit and worked well.

There was a strong partnership between academe and the hospital, working closely in clinical trials, research and patient care.

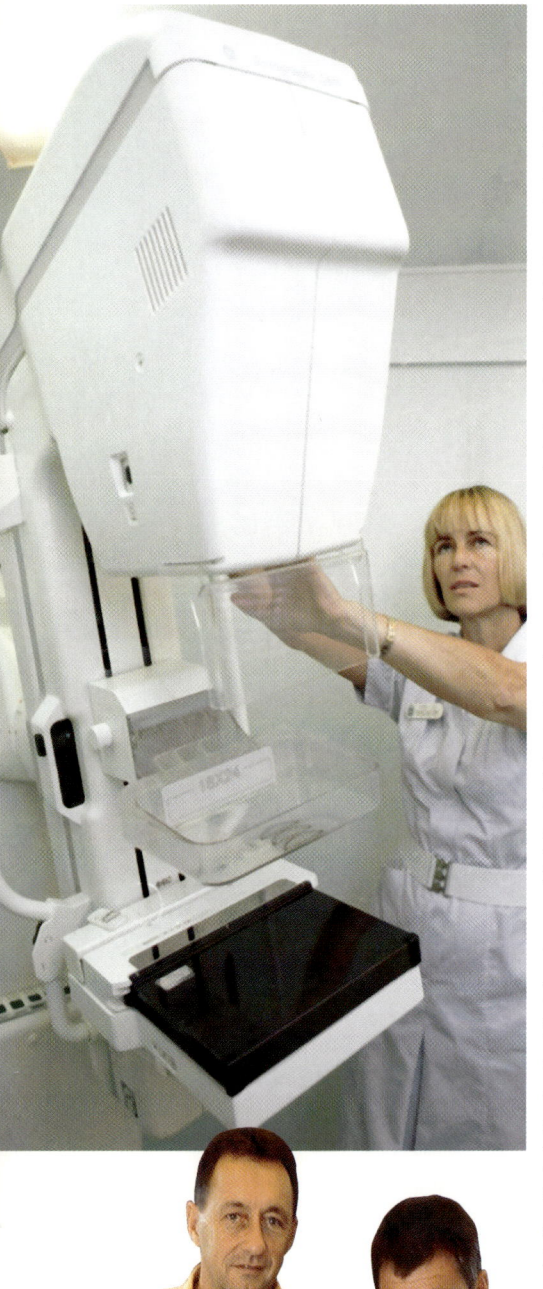

In 1979 the department produced an antibiotics policy to help rationalise drug usage in the Nottingham hospitals. A multi-author book on medical treatment was also published in the same year. This was later translated into both Italian and Japanese. In addition drug cards were produced by the department and the Pharmacist Peter Golightly to guide staff in the correct use of drugs. This was before the revamped National Formulary - now the mainstay of all prescribing - was readily available.

Urology

By Patrick Bates and Michael Bishop

UROLOGICAL surgery started to separate from general surgery in the early and mid 1970s. This was largely the result of a single operation - transurethral resection of the prostate - and the development of much better endoscopic instruments and fibre optics for medical use by Professor Harold Hopkins of Reading University.

The City Hospital initiative was led by Matt Gray, a general surgeon who had become a full-time Urologist. A former chairman of the medical committee, he was extraordinarily energetic and determined. He was also an eccentric. In his earlier days he had taken part in a motor race around the City Hospital campus with another general surgeon, Johnny Masterman.

Patrick Bates, who was appointed the first Urologist in Nottingham in early 1973 at the General Hospital, later joined Mr Gray and, together they formed the new department of urology in the old operating block in 1977.

This became a model for virtually all urology departments which have been established since then, providing operating facilities, an outpatient department, day case surgery and secretarial services on one site.

Sister Doria Pear became a tower of strength organising the nursing unit, followed by Gillian Swannell. They provided a welcoming and happy atmosphere to the very busy day case and outpatient activities associated with urology.

Another of Mr Gray's innovations was persuading a patient to provide the first dialysis machine for Nottingham before there were any renal physicians in the town. The first patient he treated on this machine made a full recovery and was present for Mr Gray's retirement party in 1978.

This machine led to Mr Bates receiving an unusual request - he was phoned by the owner of a nearby zoo to ask if they could dialyse one of his lions! Mr Bates recalled: "Being quick on the uptake I wanted to have the diagnosis confirmed by a measurement of the blood urea (which our path lab agreed to do). So I stipulated that he would have to take the blood, and let us know the normal level for lions. The phone discussion went back and forth until about 2am when the owner had to admit he could not find a vet who would take the specimen."

After Mr Gray retired in 1978, his successor was Mr Mike Dunn. Mr Michael Bishop was appointed in 1981. In 1993 the department successfully set up a £750,000 appeal for a lithotripter, which received generous support from patients, industry and medical staff. The machine has made the unit a leading centre for the treatment of stone disease.

Above left: *Breast screening equipment*

Left: *A golf day at the Sherwood Forest Golf Club raised over £3,000 for the Millennium Millions Appeal at Nottingham City Hospital. Handing over the cheque in 2002 were organisers Mike Braithwaite (left back) and Kevin Cooper. Receiving the cheque were Consultant Radiologist Dr Robin Wilson and hospital Business Manager Dawn Anderson. They're pictured with a model of the new Nottingham Breast Institute*

The People's Hospital

There are now six urologists at the hospital and there are plans for a new department.

Breast care services
by Dr Robin Wilson and Professor Roger Blamey

PROFESSOR Roger Blamey (Surgeon) and Dr (later Professor) Christopher Elston (Pathologist) were appointed at the City Hospital in the same year, both with a strong interest in breast disease. They established a breast clinic at the City Hospital, when previously there had been none in Nottingham and referrals to the clinic steadily grew. Dr Myles Benton (Radiotherapist) and Dr Eric Roebuck (one of the pioneers of mammography) joined the team and Dr David Morgan took the place of Dr Myles Benton when he retired. The clinic has become one of the largest in the country and has a staff of international experts in all fields of breast cancer.

Research work was carried out by a number of research fellows supported by Tenovus. The research is such that more papers are produced on breast cancer from the City Hospital than from any other single institute in the United Kingdom and this research is world-leading in several aspects (prognosis, pathology, screening, hormonal therapy, tumour markers). Very large research grants have been received over the years from the MRC and from the European Commission.

The unit now diagnoses over 6,000 women a year with breast symptoms. This results in the treatment of more than 600 new patients a year with breast cancer. Any further treatment that is required is carried out by the single unit. It is the major teaching unit for breast cancer in the UK, with over 70% of all staff engaged in the national screening programme having attended the Nottingham courses. Dr Robin Wilson, Radiologist (widely recognised internationally as an expert in breast cancer screening) is the Clinical Director of the unit.

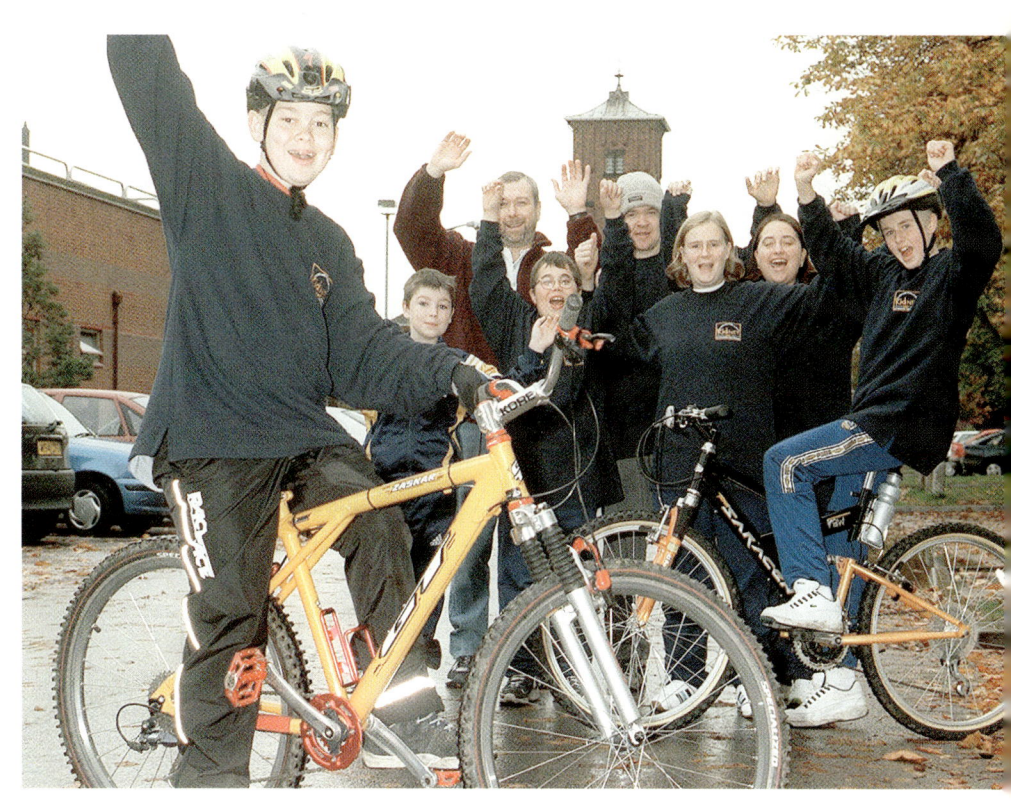

The Nottingham International Breast Cancer meetings are held biennially and attended by close to 1,000 delegates from some 20-25 countries.

Members of the unit have achieved recognition in a number of national and international honorary posts and are in receipt of honorary degrees and fellowships and frequently present research work or are called upon to lecture internationally.

The renal unit
By Dr Richard Burden and Professor Roger Blamey

THE unit was founded in the early 1970s by Dr Martin Knapp. The first dialysis patients were treated in a small room at the end of one of the surgical wards on the North Corridor (Lister ward) but when the maternity block opened in 1975, part of the old maternity department was adapted for renal patients.

The number of patients on dialysis began to grow and in 1980 a fully equipped dialysis unit was opened in the H Block. For some time this unit

Young cyclists setting off in 1999 on a coast-to-coast bike ride to raise money for facilities for teenagers in the Kidney ward

was only open for part of the week but as the number of patients grew even keeping it open every day from early morning to late at night wasn't enough and a satellite dialysis unit was built in the grounds of King's Mill Hospital in Sutton-in Ashfield, with staff employed by the City Hospital. Meanwhile the converted maternity unit wards with just six beds had become too small. A portable building provided a clinic for transplant patients but the waiting area was so small that people often queued outside. When it was hot they were joined by the transplant sister at a makeshift desk (but she always managed to find room inside when it rained).

Peritoneal dialysis was introduced in 1980, offering an home-based alternative treatment, but more space was needed for training and was provided adjacent to Nightingale One. In 1993 a new building was opened next to the dialysis unit with wards as well as clinic space, offices and seminar rooms. For the first time all renal patients could be looked after at the same site in first class accommodation. Unfortunately this is now nearly bursting at the seams and plans are underway for yet more beds and another satellite unit - possibly at Queen's Medical Centre.

In 1973, 350 dialysis treatments were completed. Now twice that number take place in a single week. We currently have 427 patients on dialysis. There are two reasons for the continually increasing numbers. Routine treatment for kidney disease is relatively new (I remember very clearly seeing a young man die from kidney failure in 1969 just a few weeks before the hospital where I worked acquired its first dialysis machine) and it used to be that because of very limited facilities in this country, only the young patients were treated. Now almost everyone is treated. Secondly, the treatment works - and some of our patients have been on treatment for many years, including two of the very first patients who started dialysis in Nottingham in 1972. Treatment was very different then and there was only room at the City Hospital for temporary dialysis, so patients had to travel to the regional centre in Sheffield. Each dialysis took 12 to 15 hours, compared with four hours now.

There have also been many improvements in kidney transplants since the first one in Nottingham was carried out by Mr (later Professor) Roger Blamey in February 1974. In the following calendar year a further 10 transplants were carried out and since then the rate of transplantation has steadily increased. Patients now stay in hospital for about a week rather than two or three, and there have been major advances in the drugs needed to combat rejection. Because the waiting list continues to grow, kidneys are often donated by members of the patient's family - the operation carried out by 'keyhole' surgery, pioneered in this country by City Hospital surgeons. Transplantation is the best treatment for many patients as it can enable people to return to a normal life, and this includes being able to have children, which is unusual for people on dialysis treatment.

Over the years many research projects have been completed by renal unit staff. Research was carried out by a series of research fellows working in the Professorial Unit of Surgery. Peter Wenham and Graeme Cooksey did one of the first studies in the world on cytology and needle biopsy in the management of acute rejection. Studies by doctors Foster, Dennis and Beckingham were among the first to study chronic rejection and Dr Christine Evans did an early study of lymphocyte traffic.

Another major study looked at the reasons why kidneys are sometimes rejected after transplantation and the introduction of different treatments has helped to improve the chances of long term success. Other work has concentrated on reducing the risks of complications occurring in the bones of dialysis and transplant patients. Several projects have concentrated on preventing people getting kidney failure through better treatment of high blood pressure and diabetes.

The staff team has grown to more than 100 nurses, including 12 sisters. There are six secretaries, six clerical staff, four technicians, three dieticians, two social workers, four consultants and eight junior doctors.

Above left: *Chris Bark, (right), manager of the oncology and palliative care social work team, talks to a colleague*
Above right: *Professor Roger Blamey*
Left: *Nine consultant histopathologists produce more than 70,000 tissue samples a year from which nearly 100,000 slides are individually screened using a microscope*

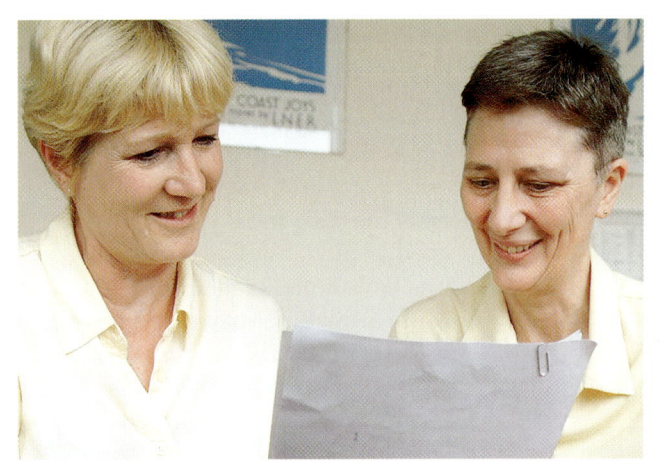

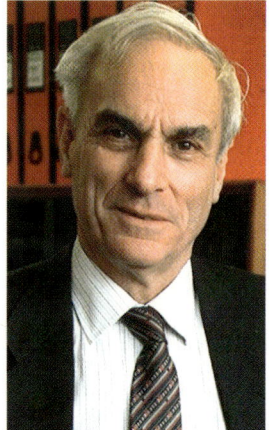

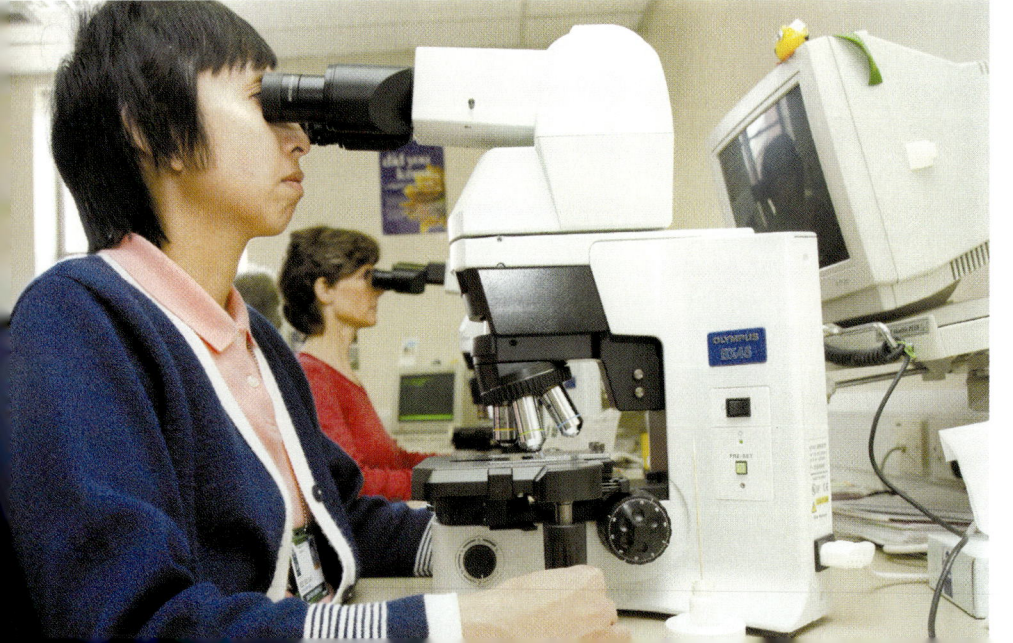

Histopathology

By Professor Roger Cotton and Professor Chris Elston

WHEN Dr (later Professor) Roger Cotton arrived to take up his post as Consultant Histopathologist in 1963, the City Hospital department provided a service to most of the hospitals in the Nottingham No 2 Hospital Management Committee.

The histology workload was about 3,000 specimens a year. This grew progressively over the years, reaching 16,000 by 1990 when Professor Cotton retired.

Professor Cotton recalled: "The range of techniques provided in histology was rather basic but the technical staff were excellent and very responsive to my plans to widen and modernise the service urgently. Of note was the absence of frozen sections for immediate (20 minute) reporting of fresh surgical specimens - a necessity for surgeons wanting a diagnosis on things like breast lumps before embarking on radical surgery. This service was instituted before the end of 1963."

Microbiology services were taken over by the Public Health Laboratory Service in Shakespeare Street, Nottingham, following the retirement of Dr Tony Johns. Dr Eric Mitchell was in charge and he speedily set up a satellite laboratory in the City Hospital department, introducing a wide range of sophisticated techniques together with a personal consultative service for individual case problems. Dr Mitchell became a very important driving force in the modernisation of the City Hospital, not confined to microbiological matters.

A cytology service was urgently needed, particularly for cervical smear testing. By late August 1963 an embryonic service was up and running. This was initially confined to requests from gynaecology and obstetric clinics, but was rapidly expanded as technical staff were trained and space, equipment and money were secured. The service was extended to GPs in the early part of 1964.

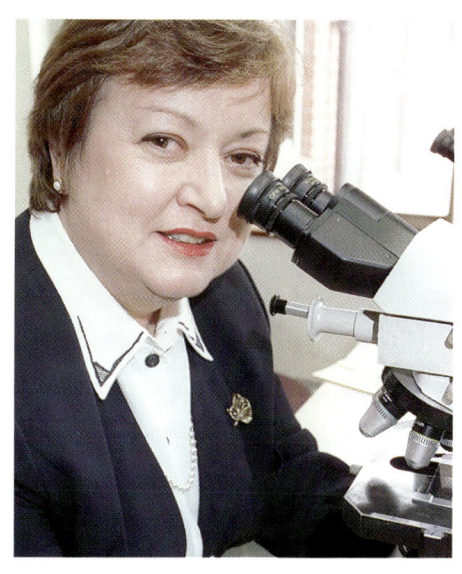

Dr Jane Johnson of the department of histopathology looking at a smear test through a microscope

There clearly was insufficient senior medical staffing for pathology and by the end of 1964 Dr Stephen Jones joined Dr Cotton as a second consultant. By the early 1980s six full-time posts were filled in histopathology/cytology to manage the workload which had increased by 500% since 1963.

Chris Elston came to the department of histopathology in March, 1974 as the fourth consultant, joining Roger Cotton, Stephen Jones and Jenny Dyson. Within a year Dr Dyson left for London and was replaced in 1975 by Dr David Ansell.

The department (along with the rest of pathology) was housed in wholly inadequate accommodation converted from the previous plastic surgery ward and operating theatres until 1985 when staff moved into a new, purpose-built department - later formally opened by the Duchess of Gloucester.

There are now 11 consultants (including two part-time, two academic) in a total of more than 50 medical, scientific and secretarial personnel. Because the hospital is an integral part of the University of Nottingham Medical School and a designated Cancer Centre, histopathology has evolved from a small district general hospital type department into a specialist teaching hospital department with an international reputation.

Professor Elston said: "Credit for much of this expansion is due to the foresight and energy in the early days of Roger Cotton and Stephen Jones. It is interesting that despite the fact that the current building is less than 20 years old we have already outgrown it and further development will be necessary."

Three of the consultant staff - Roger Cotton, Christopher Elston and Jane Johnson - have chaired the medical staff committee. Professor Cotton's tenure in the early 1970s coincided with a marked expansion of the hospital as a result of the need for clinical teaching in the new Medical School. Professor Cotton was also responsible for the decision to site a new Post Graduate Education Centre on the City campus in the face of considerable opposition.

Professor Elston was Unit General Manager from 1987 to 1990 and Jane Johnson was Chairman of the Hospital Medical Committee in the late 1990s.

Oncology department

By Dr David Morgan

PLANS were first developed in the mid 1980s to move the oncology department from its old site at the General Hospital to a new building at the City Hospital. At the time it was agreed that the Cancer Research Campaign would be involved and would fund a new academic presence in oncology. Jim Carmichael was appointed to the chair and took up his post in 1992. The department, which includes the academic and NHS department, moved in October 1993.

Two of our ward names were retained from the General Hospital. Fraser ward is named after Dr William Fraser, Nottingham's first Consultant Oncologist, and Gervis

Pearson ward takes its name from Lt Col Gervis Pearson, who was Chairman of the Monthly Board when the General Hospital became part of the NHS in 1948. A third ward in the new oncology building was named after Robert George Hogarth, founder of the radiotherapy department at the General Hospital.

There had always been strong links between the oncologists and many of the departments at the City Hospital and these have been developed since the move. Links with Queen's Medical Centre have also been strengthened and the two hospitals work closely together as part of the Nottingham Cancer Centre.

One of the first cancer multi-disciplinary teams was set up in the late 1980s when Professor Roger Blamey, Professo Chris Elston and Dr David Morgan established a protocol to review the management of all newly-diagnosed breast patients.

The department serves a resident population of 1.1 million and currently sees around 3,000 new patients each year, providing a comprehensive range of non-surgical oncology services to the East Midlands. The development of the Nottingham Cancer Centre provides opportunities for cancer services to be developed over the next five years. In 1950 the number of patients registered with oncology was around 2,000.

Ten years ago the department moved into purpose-built accommodation at the City Hospital and since then has seen some expansion in radiotherapy facilities with more planned over the next three years. There are strong links in cancer care between the two major trusts in Nottingham that forms a seamless cancer care service for residents in Nottingham. There is a planned expansion in cancer care services at Queen's Medical Centre and The King's Mill Centre specifically in chemotherapy services. This has meant that the number of consultants has also increased over the last five years.

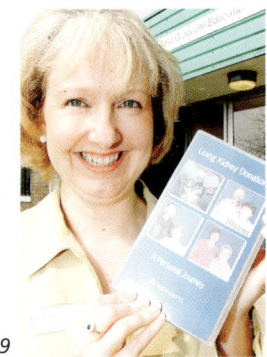

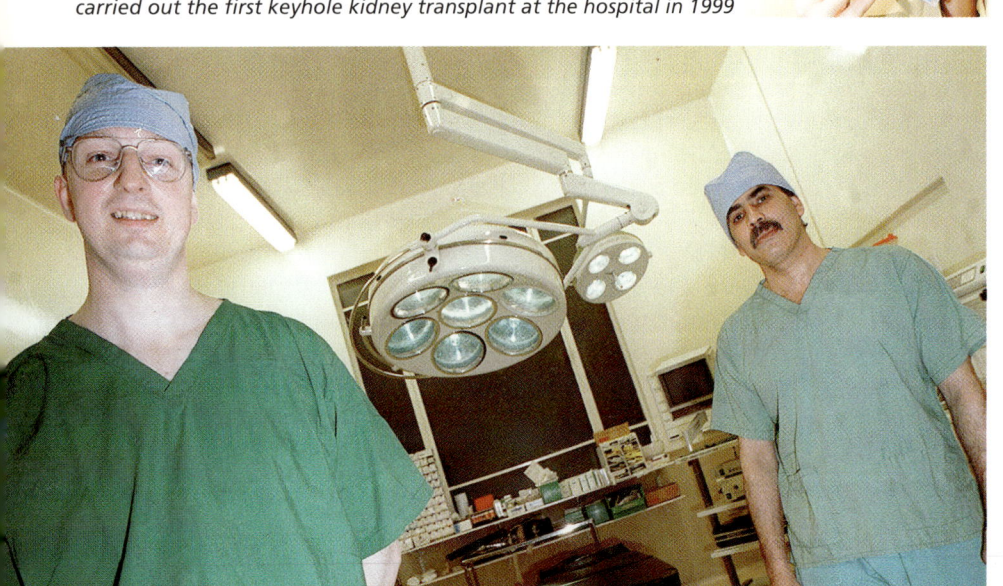

Haematology services

By Professor Nigel Russell

CLINICAL haematology developed as a separate speciality from general medicine following the appointment of John Fletcher as Consultant Physician with an interest in clinical haematology in 1971. Dr Fletcher worked closely with the laboratory haematologists to develop a combined clinical and laboratory service with beds on Patience One and Patience Two wards. He had a special interest in lymphoma and developed a clinical trials collaborative group with other centres in Birmingham and Leeds which developed into the Central Lymphoma Group and piloted many clinical trials in the treatment of lymphoma patients. Dr (later Professor) Fletcher, also had a strong research programme in haematology in the Medical Research Centre.

Following the appointment of Dr Nigel Russell, Consultant Haematologist/Senior Lecturer in Haematology in 1985, a bone marrow transplant programme was developed for both autologous and allogeneic transplants. The original bone Marrow transplant unit was on Patience One ward with just two beds funded by the Leukaemia Research Fund. The unit moved in 1994 to Hogarth ward with 18 beds, including six beds for transplantation. In 2002 the BMT unit moved again to two new wards comprising 26 beds, including 12 isolation beds for patients undergoing bone marrow transplants. During this period of time the numbers of transplants performed annually has risen from six in 1986 to 96 in 2001.

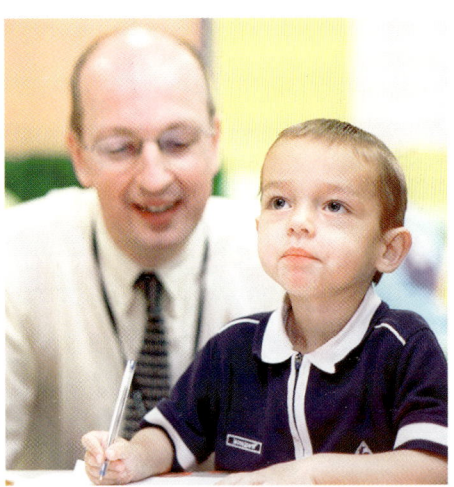

Above: Thomas Bird - one of the youngest patients to have a kidney transplant. The kidney was donated by his father Jason. Here Thomas is with Keith Rigg, Consultant Transplant Surgeon who was part of the team which carried out the operation in 2001
Below: Consultant Surgeons Keith Rigg and Magdi Shehata who carried out the first keyhole kidney transplant at the hospital in 1999

Right: Renal Transplant Sister Anne Frankton with a copy of video about living kidney donation

The People's Hospital

Professor Roger Cotton (centre right) shakes hands with Laurie Bourne, former Senior Chief Medical Laboratory Scientist, during the professor's retirement reception at the Post Graduate Education Centre in 1990

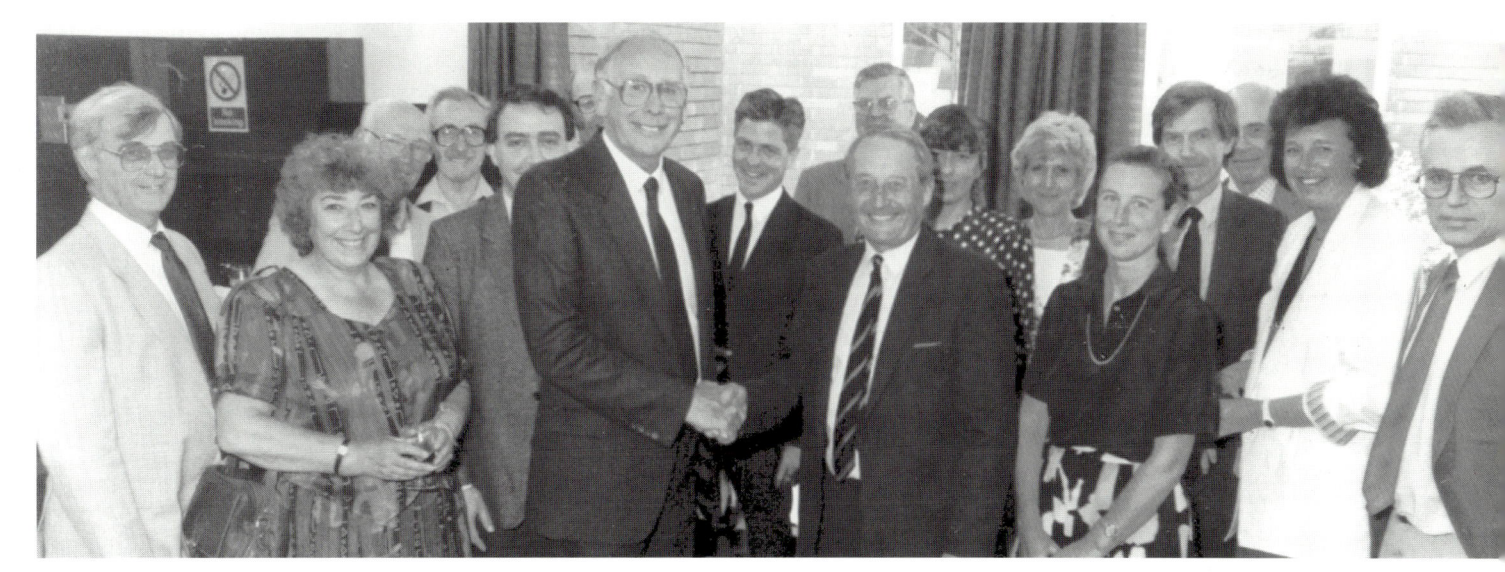

At the same time the haematology department has grown with Dr Andrew Haynes replacing Professor Fletcher as lead consultant for lymphoma, and more recently with the appointment of Dr Jenny Byrne and Dr Andrew McMillan to strengthen the clinical team. It is now recognised as one of the cutting edge centres for the treatment of patients with haematological malignancies in the UK.

Bone marrow transplantation

By Professor John Fletcher

BONE marrow transplantation is one of the City Hospital's success stories. The unit has a national and international reputation as a result of pioneering work, particularly in the use of the patient's own stem cells for the treatment of leukaemia, myeloma and lymphoma. It started in 1986 when a grant from the Leukaemia Research Fund was used to convert three side wards on Patience One ward into two isolation rooms. In the first year six transplants were carried out by Nigel Russell, the newly appointed senior who is now Professor of Haematology. Over subsequent years the numbers steadily increased, particularly after the move into the new Hogarth ward with six isolation rooms. Now nearly 100 transplants are carried out each year. The number of patients being cured of life-threatening diseases is increasing as is the range of diseases that can be treated. The result is that patients are now coming to the hospital from all over the East Midlands, and a few from as far away as Scotland.

Many aspects have contributed to this success. Firstly, the hospital has provided appropriate facilities and levels of staffing particularly on Hogarth ward. Secondly the clinical work has been integrated with a programme of research and development carried out for the first years in the David Evans Research Centre, and more recently in the Clinical Sciences Building. Thirdly, there has been a unique collaboration between Nottingham City Hospital and the Leukaemia Research Fund to set up the Nottinghamshire Leukaemia Appeal. This appeal has raised more than £1.5m since its launch in 1994. This money has provided research grants, the purchase of state-of-the-art equipment and allowed the appointment of key research and clinical staff. These three factors have put Nottingham City Hospital 'ahead of the game'.

What of the future? The transplant unit has now moved into two new wards as a temporary arrangement until a purpose-built unit becomes available in 2005. The new unit is going to cost more than £8 million and will provide some of the very best facilities in the country. There is no doubt that with this backing bone marrow transplantaton will continue to expand, providing a world-class service for the patients and bringing prestige to Nottingham City Hospital.

Pharmaceutical service (1970 to 2002)

By John Gilby and Shelagh French

IN 1971 the dispensary opened in the main outpatient department to provide a more convenient service to patients and the following year the resident pharmacist service was introduced. At that time pharmacists lived on site (Heathfield House flat) and were members of the junior doctors' mess. They helped ensure the pharmacy service operated 24 hours a day, seven days a week.

In 1973 the drug information service was developed and the following year a decision was taken to cease manufacturing standard intravenous fluids on site and to switch to commercial sources. Previously the hospital had been self sufficient for all saline and dextrose infusions.

Between 1974 and 1977 a service

providing bespoke intravenous feeding solutions for neonates was developed. Again this operated seven days a week.

The 1980s saw continued expansion of the clinical service to the wards and in 1982 a post graduate diploma was introduced in association with the University of Nottingham. Some 25 pharmacists have now completed the diploma while based at the City Hospital.

When the renal/oncology block opened in 1993, a satellite pharmacy was included, providing a cytotoxic manufacturing service and dispensing service to cancer wards. The workload has more than doubled in the last 10 years with more than 22,000 cancer injections being prepared in the pharmacy each year.

More than 40 clinical trials are currently being carried out in this one specialty.

Pharmacy staffing has grown significantly over the last 25 years - from 30 whole time equivalents in 1977 to 76 whole time equivalents in 2002. Many innovations have been introduced. Pharmacists are now specifically attached to the hospital's clinical directorate teams (16 in all). A teacher-practitioner post works jointly with the City Hospital and the university and a clinical pharmacist works jointly with Gedling Primary Care Trust.

Drug costs have increased from £2.2m in 1988 to £11.5m in 2002. The majority is spent on antibiotics and drugs used to treat kidney disease, cancer and leukaemia.

Infectious diseases
By Professor Roger Finch

IN 1979, Dr Roger Finch was appointed as Physician within the newly-established academic department of microbiology. The latter was initially housed in the Bagthorpe Building (currently clinical chemistry) before transferring to Queen's Medical Centre in 1978.

He set about developing the infection services by setting up a satellite diagnostic microbiology laboratory which complemented that at Queen's Medical Centre. The infection control service was also formalised and supported by infection control nurse and link nurse arrangements throughout the hospital. Patients admitted to the City Hospital requiring specialist care were looked after in the side rooms of the medical wards, since the Heathfield wards were no longer suitable for managing acutely ill infected persons. 1991 saw the opening of Nightingale Two as the infectious disease ward with 13 beds, seven of which had single room en suite facilities and an air control system to protect against the spread of airborne infections.

The combined clinic and laboratory approach to the management of infectious disease gradually expanded to cater for an increase in the requirements for in-patient care, cross-specialty consultation and outpatient referrals. The latter included community infections and

Left: *In October 2001, six-month-old Romanian baby Cristina Cocor had life-changing surgery at the City Hospital's regional centre for children born with a cleft lip or palate. Pictures show Cristina before the operation and (inset) a year later*

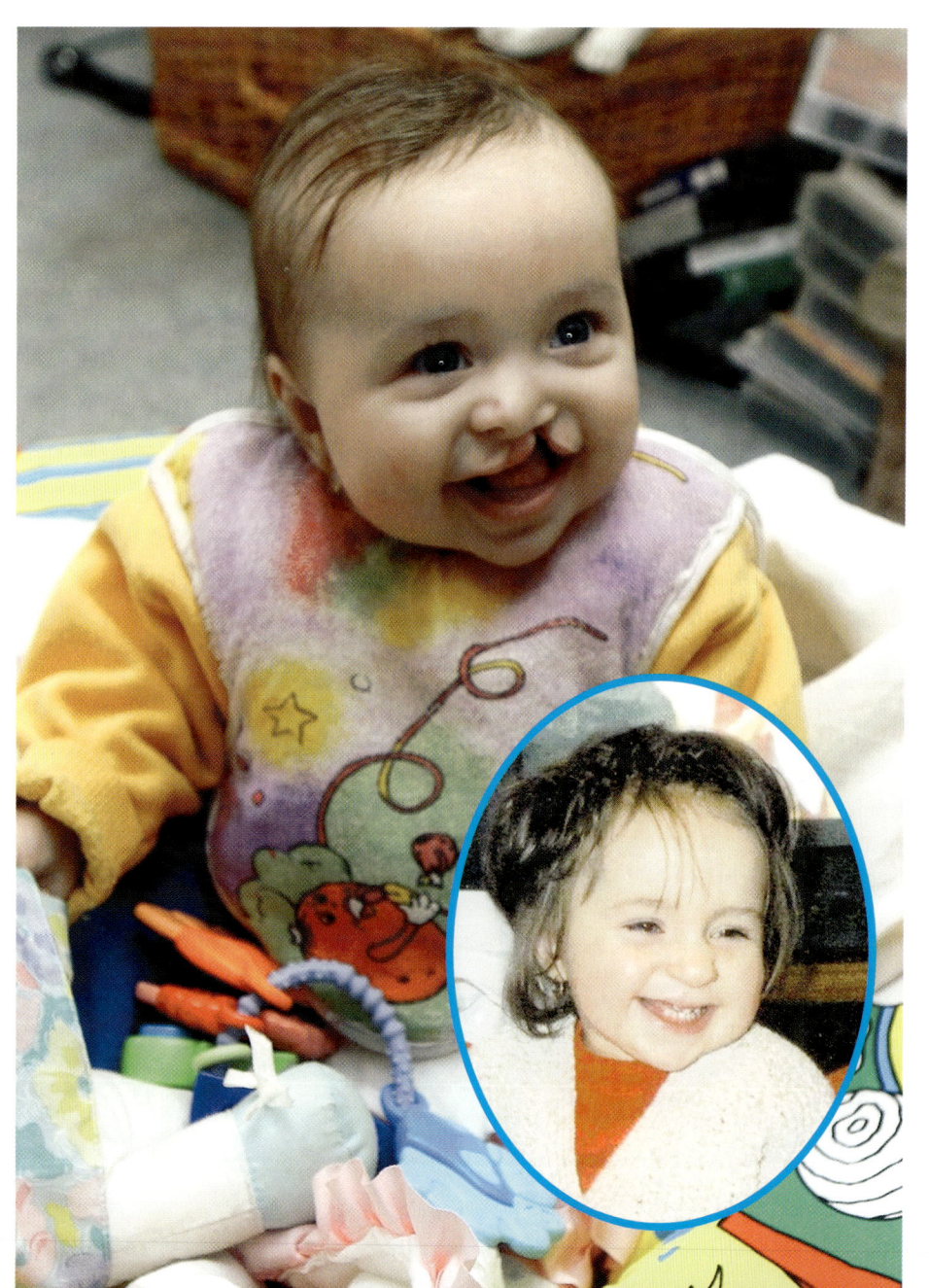

The People's Hospital

imported diseases as well as the emerging problems of HIV and hepatitis C virus infections. Dr Finch (subsequently Professor Finch, 1991) sustained the service single-handed for many years. He was joined by Dr Brian Thompson, Senior Lecturer in Infectious Diseases in 1996, and on the retirement of Dr David Banks in 1999, Dr Prith Venkatesan was appointed Consultant Physician with a specialist interest in infectious diseases.

The workloads of the satellite microbiology laboratory steadily increased and Dr Fiona Donald was appointed as Consultant Microbiologist in 1989. As the laboratory activities further expanded, additional appointments were made. Dr Tim Boswell, currently Infection Control Doctor, and Dr Shiu Soo further strengthened the staff arrangements. The infection control service has undergone a major expansion in recent years in response to local and national concerns over the growing impact of hospital-acquired infection. It is now considered one of the major quality checks for hospital service provision and as such, is supported by a staff of six infection control nurses and a pharmacist responsible for supporting antibiotic prescribing policies.

Specialist training in infectious diseases and medical microbiology is an active component of post graduate education training at the City Hospital. Indeed, the hospital unit was one of the first to appoint a trainee in the new national scheme that provides a joint training programme in infectious disease and medical microbiology. This reflects national developments in the staffing of infection services which rely heavily on laboratory investigation complementing sound clinical expertise. The manner in which the services developed at the City Hospital has been adopted as a model for many other infection units and academic centres in the UK and beyond.

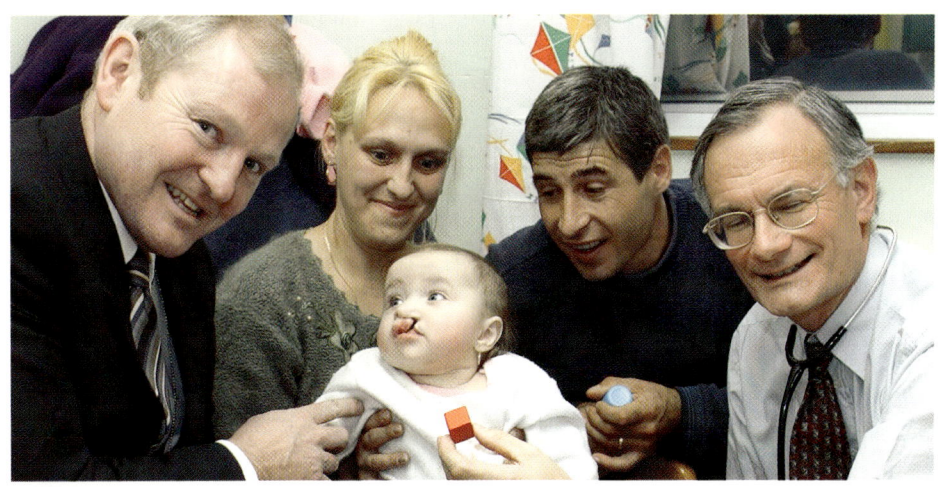

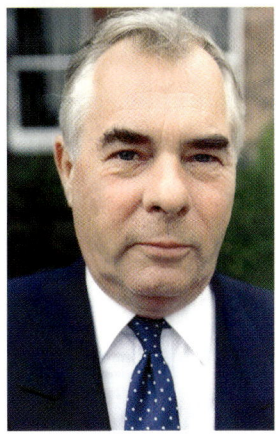

Above: Baby Cristina Cocor who underwent cleft palate surgery at the hospital is pictured with her parents Gabi and Vasile during a meeting with Surgeon Mark Henley (left) and Consultant Paediatrician David Curnock (right)

Left: Chairman of Nottingham City Hospital Trust Norman Deakin cut the ribbon to open the Nightingale ward for infectious diseases in 1991

Plastic surgery

By Paul Swift

SOON after the Second World War, plastic and reconstructive surgery began to be recognised as a specialty in its own right. But until 1955 patients requiring plastic surgery in the Nottinghamshire and Derbyshire areas had to travel to hospitals in Sheffield and Leicester. This changed when David Wynn-Williams was appointed Consultant Plastic Surgeon to cover Nottingham, Derby, Mansfield and Grantham. His central unit, which included burns, was in B Block in the City Hospital. There were 12 female and 12 male beds on B1 ward (now James ward) and 12 children's beds on B2 ward (now the Charnley Suite).

David Wynn-Williams retired in 1971 and was replaced by Lance Sully. The B Block accommodation became inadequate, particularly for complex cases, where many consultants may be involved. For example, surgeons in accident and emergency departments, metabolic physicians, plastic surgeons, renal physicians and anaesthetists who often have to provide adequate analgesia or even general anaesthesia for painful dressings.

A temporary burns service was set up in 1979 in a small prefabricated unit with a minor operating theatre but this too proved to be inadequate to deal with all the cases, particularly severe burns patients requiring long stay hospital care.

A new plastic surgery unit and self contained burns unit was completed in 1981/82, as part of a new three-storey development (H Block) containing facilities for paediatrics and renal dialysis. The maxillo-facial team was originally led by Tom Battersby.

The plastic, dental and reconstructive department has come a long way since its humble beginnings. It is now housed in its own self contained unit. The burns unit that once accommodated 12 patients in a temporary ward now has a bed capacity of 21 in a state-of-the-art ward with a purpose-built burns and plastic surgery operating theatre. The wards on the first floor have a combined paediatric/adult bed capacity of 51. From just one consultant in 1955, the department has grown to five consultants - and efforts are under way to recruit two more.

The department covers a full range of plastic surgery and burns work for adults and children, specialising in burns and microsurgery. The hospital is also the regional centre for the care of children born with a cleft lip or palate.

Rheumatology
By Dr Tony Swannell

THE rheumatology service was provided single-handedly by Consultant Dr Sam James in the 1960s. It was then known as physical medicine and he supervised outpatient services at the City and General Hospitals and had access to medical inpatient beds at the City Hospital. Dr James also established The Cedars medical rehabilitation unit, which soon had a national reputation. In the 1970s, when the first medical students were starting their clinical course, a second consultant was appointed.

Professor Angus Wallace pictured in 2000 with an artificial shoulder joint

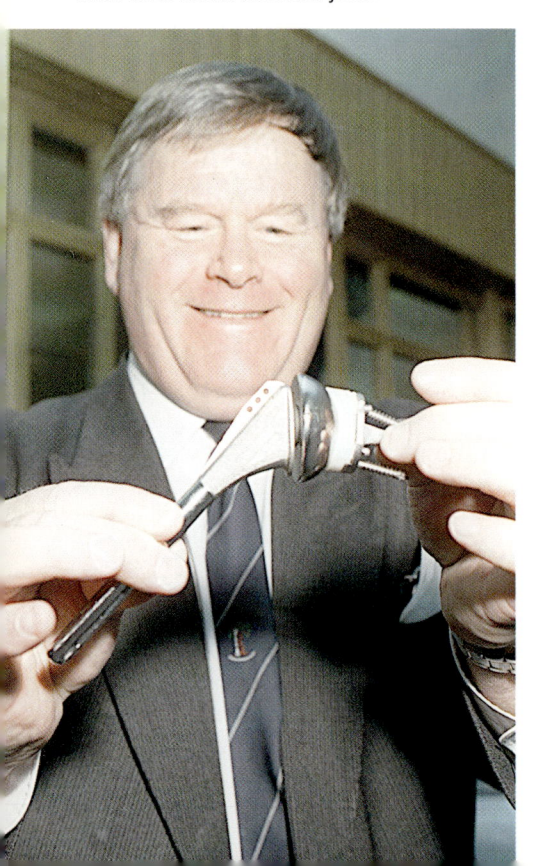

Outpatient services were extended to Ilkeston Community Hospital and paediatric rheumatology consultations were provided at Nottingham Children's Hospital. The inpatient beds, which were scattered across Nottingham, were centralised at the City Hospital to improve patient care and a senior registrar appointed. Rheumatology played a very active part in undergraduate and post graduate education. Also at that time consultants were often asked to see patients at home at the request of their GP - an educational experience for the consultant and GP alike.

The 1980s saw the separation of rheumatology from rehabilitation at national level and gradually separate specialists in rehabilitation were appointed. In 1995 Nottingham City Hospital and the university created and appointed a senior lecturer post in rheumatology, funded by the Arthritis and Rheumatism Council. Inpatient care for rheumatology patients was also improved with the opening of James ward at the City Hospital. This ward was subsequently given over to orthopaedics but still caters for patients with locomoter type problems.

In the 1990s outpatient services were extended to Newark Hospital and great efforts were made to improve the service to patients at the City Hospital. A rheumatology nurse practitioner was appointed, providing easy access for patient problems. The policy of 'shared care' with the GP for patients receiving dangerous drugs for their arthritis was started. This allowed less frequent hospital visits and improved GP knowledge of the drugs used. A third NHS consultant was appointed in 1995 who took on a commitment for general medicine.

Now there are four NHS consultants, a professor of rheumatology with research fellows and technicians, a senior registrar and junior staff providing a full service at the City Hospital and outpatient clinics at the Queen's Medical Centre and Newark. Dr James would be proud to see the present rheumatology service.

Occupational therapy
By Pauline Johnston

THE occupational therapy service, established in the mid-1950s, was originally housed in what is now the Chapel on the North Corridor. The early emphasis was on improving patients' physical and psychological well-being. A training flat was created in the former X-ray department at the eastern end of the corridor with the aim of helping patients to return home.

In the mid-1960s the medical support to the occupational therapy department was provided by Dr James Macfie until the establishment of the department of physical medicine and the arrival of Dr Sam James.

At the same time a temporary rehabilitation unit specialising in older people was built at Sherwood Hospital, now the South Corridor. This was later replaced but the building still stands, having subsequently been used as a day hospital and by the department of human resources.

The rehabilitation unit at Sherwood Hospital developed as a multidisciplinary unit and was one of the first units to employ helpers who worked jointly across the professions of occupational therapy and physiotherapy.

The service moved from the North Corridor to a new department, opened in 1987 by Princess Margaret.

Today occupational therapists work in a range of locations on and off the City Hospital site providing a service to a much wider range of patients and using a wider range of interventions.

In 1993 Pauline Johnston, who is now Clinical Director of the Paramedical Services directorate, was awarded the MBE for her services to occupational therapy locally and nationally.

The People's Hospital

Orthopaedics
By David Lowe

ORTHOPAEDIC surgery has made tremendous strides since the Second World War. Soon after the formation of the National Health Service, TB, polio and rickets slowly disappeared, partly as a result of improved social conditions.

Nottingham's first Consultant Orthopaedic Surgeon was Noel Birkett, who was appointed in 1947. He operated from the General Hospital and the City Hospital until 1970. Dedicated to the care of his patients, he never wore a watch because he paid little regard to time and always refused to stick to a rigid schedule.

Meanwhile a new age had dawned in orthopaedics. Sir John Charnley's contribution to total hip replacement was perhaps the most important advance in surgery since the war. By 1977 the operation had become a standard procedure and the survival of Harlow Wood as an orthopaedic hospital in the 1980s rested on the success of hip replacement. The knee, being a more complicated joint, was more difficult to replace. Progress was slow at first but gradually it became a more common operation at Harlow Wood. Arthroscopy, leading to precise diagnosis of injuries to the knee, was also introduced.

Nottingham and Harlow Wood were linked together to form an organisation with a national and international reputation. This was largely the result of more consultants being appointed with outstanding ability, including Professor Angus Wallace, who succeeded William Waugh as Professor of Orthopaedic and Accident Surgery.

When Harlow Wood closed in 1995, Professor Wallace moved his world renowned shoulder and elbow surgery to Nottingham City Hospital and almost £1m was invested in two new theatres. Professor Wallace, whose lifesaving operation aboard a British Airways jumbo jet at 35,000ft made world-wide news, worked alongside colleagues Simon Frostick and Lars Neumann on the initiative. Another orthopaedic consultant joined the team when a third operating theatre opened later that year.

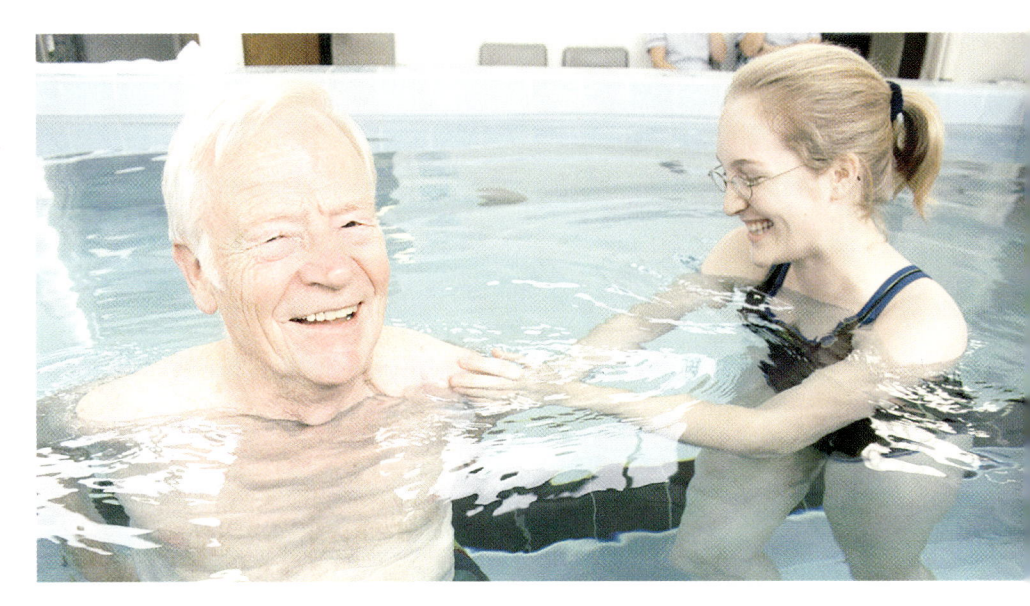

The three specialist wards have a total of 57 beds and the surgeons are supported by physiotherapists, occupational therapists and allied paramedical staff. This includes use of a hydrotherapy pool and there is also a combined clinic, where physiotherapists and occupational therapists assist with referrals to orthopaedic outpatients.

Hucknall Orthopaedic Clinic, a satellite outpatients centre visited by City Hospital consultants, is celebrating its 75th anniversary in 2003.

Nottingham School of Physiotherapy
By Alan Scowcroft

THE establishment of a physiotherapy school in Nottingham in the 1960s was due very largely to the efforts of two superintendent physiotherapists, Elisabeth Trussell at Nottingham Orthopaedic Clinic, and Margaret McMain at Harlow Wood Orthopaedic Hospital, supported by

A physiotherapist working in 2001 with a patient in the hydrotherapy pool

Mr J P Campbell, Consultant Orthopaedic Surgeon. Their persistence was rewarded in 1958 when the hospital authorities met them at the General Hospital in Nottingham to consider a report prepared by another local physiotherapist, John Henry Smith (Mr Smith was one of the first members appointed by the Secretary of State to a proposed State Registration Board for physiotherapists).

But it was not until 1962 that the Sheffield Regional Health Board put forward plans for the establishment of a school in Orchard House, on the City Hospital site. These were not acceptable to the Chartered Society of Physiotherapy, the professional association responsible for the education and training of physiotherapists in the UK. But later that year a second proposal was approved: the conversion of a three-storey reception centre on the Sherwood Hospital campus, with the addition of a single storey annexe.

Work started on the site in 1964 and was completed by August the following year, at a cost of £30,000, with £11,000 allocated to equip and furnish the building. All was complete by September, when 17 students started. And on October 11, the school was officially opened by Group Captain Douglas Bader.

Although located on the Sherwood/City Hospital site it was, in effect, a regional training school. The students gained their clinical experience at first in local hospitals, at the Queen's Medical Centre once it had been opened by the Queen, and thereafter in specialist units in Mansfield, Leicestershire and South Derbyshire.

The main building was over 100 years old at that time. In its early days it had served as a reception centre for the less fortunate members of society, who could have a night's lodging, 'paid for' the following morning by a session of chopping firewood for lighting the coal fires around the hospitals.

In 1993 the school became part of the University of Nottingham, changing its title to the Division of Physiotherapy Education, and offering a three-year BSc with honours course in physiotherapy. And in November 1998 it moved into the new Clinical Sciences Building on the City Hospital site. The old buildings were demolished and a purpose-built day nursery for the children of hospital staff now stands on the site.

Obstetrics and gynaecology

By Lesley Baker

IN 1965 the obstetric unit was situated at the far end of the hospital on three wards. There were three delivery rooms, an ante-natal and a post-natal ward and a neonatal unit. Patients who needed Caesarean sections or other surgical procedures had to be rushed down the long corridor through the centre of the hospital to the theatres, which in those days were situated in the present urological theatres or even further afield near the pathology department.

The gynaecological wards were in C Block, one ward being entirely used for the treatment and care of patients with septic abortions. After 1967, following the legalisation of abortion, the use of this ward altered. Later the gynaecological beds moved to a modernised ward. Victoria Two, and then Lister Two, Edward One and Two. At one stage we had three gynaecological wards.

Initially there were only three consultants, Mr Cochrane, Mr Barkla and myself. The clinical assistant was Dr Ken Emsley, who with Mr Cochrane and I, covered the Firs Maternity Home.

The new medical school arrived in Nottingham in the early 1970s and many changes occurred. A university department of obstetrics and gynaecology was established by Professor Malcolm Symonds, initially at the City Hospital and then at the Queen's Medical Centre. A new maternity unit with proper neonatal facilities and self-contained operating theatres was opened in 1972. The newer consultants appointed after this were Mr Tyack, Mr Bruce, Mr Bain and Miss Jequier, as well as Professor Symonds, senior and junior lecturers.

In the 1960s and early 70s, only 60% of women in Nottingham had their babies in hospital and a flying squad service was provided to support the domiciliary midwifery service. The team that went out comprised a consultant obstetrician or registrar, anaesthetist, midwife and usually a medical student. I remember going out with the squad one cold January night at 2am to the Hyson Green area. We went into the house and arranged for the patient to be brought to the hospital by ambulance for further care. Her ante-natal co-operation card had been left in the home and I went back to get it. When I came out I found that both the midwife in her car and the ambulance containing the patient had left, leaving me standing alone on the pavement. When they got back to the City Hospital, Sister Katie Kirby, the night sister in charge, said: "What have you done with Miss Baker?" I was rescued shortly afterwards.

The opening of the new units at the City and the Queen's led to a 90% hospital delivery rate and the flying squad gradually diminished. This was replaced during the 90s by paramedics and the emergency ambulance service.

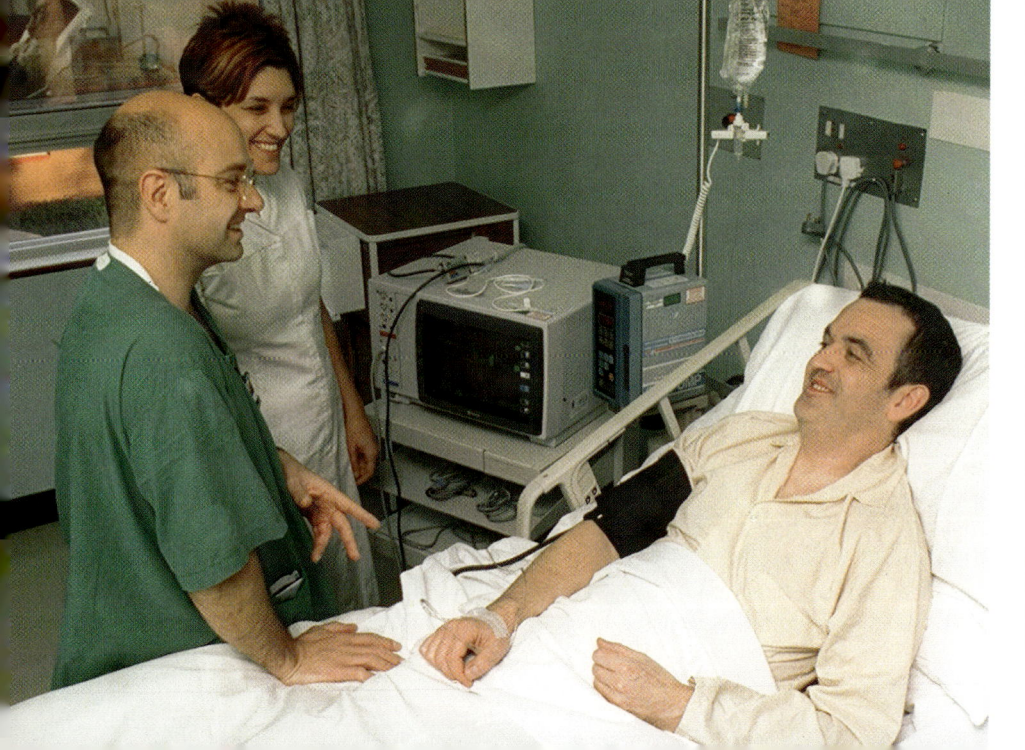

Left: *Charge Nurse Owen Jones and Staff Nurse Maria Higginson seen in 2000 carrying out routine monitoring of a patient in the burns unit*

The People's Hospital

A third new maternity unit was opened in 1994 at the City Hospital, comprising a neonatal unit, a university department of obstetrics and gynaecology and an innovative Patient Hotel, used by new mums as well as patients from other parts of the hospital. Obstetrics itself has changed.

The normal midwifery is now only done by midwives. Scanning has altered ante-natal care and the patient stay in hospital has been much reduced over the years from 10 days down to six hours for a normal delivery.

In the last decade, further changes have occurred. The oncology unit has been moved from The Ropewalk to Nottingham City Hospital and it is now the regional centre. A day case surgical unit was built near the new maternity unit. Many gynaecological surgical procedures are now carried out on a day case basis. In the old days, most gynaecologists were general obstetricians and gynaecologists but there has been increasing specialisation. The fertility clinic, initially mainly run by Mr Tyack, myself and Mr Liu, has now transferred to the Queen's Medical Centre.

The autonomy of midwives has increased, particularly in the labour ward and antenatal clinics, and domiciliary midwives come in and deliver their own patients.

With the reduction of junior doctors' hours, the advent of Calman training, clinical governance revalidation and protocols, life for consultants has changed. The main medical changes that occurred in gynaecology during my 30 years were the introduction of the colposcope and hysteroscope, scanning in the ante-natal clinics and the legalisation of termination of pregnancy. There has been a gradual reduction of maternal mortality and morbidity during these years and much of this has been due to the great improvement in anaesthetic services.

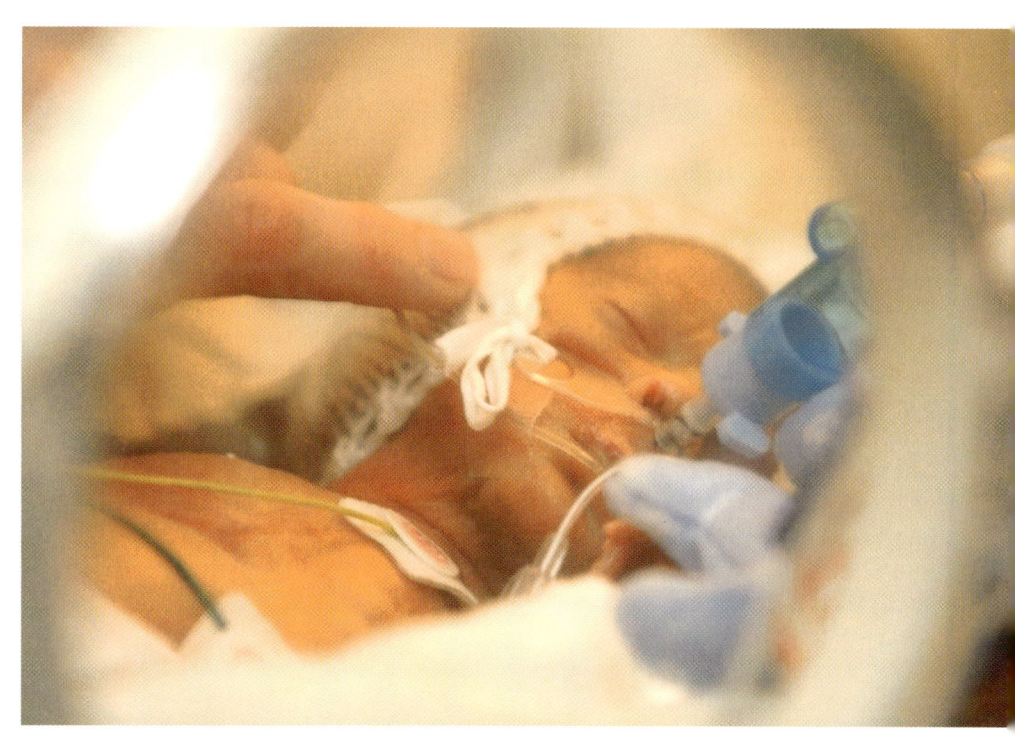

A baby in intensive care

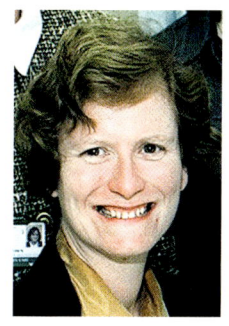

Right: Dr Lucy Kean, Consultant Obstetrician

Paediatric services

By Professor Nick Rutter, Dr Joan Hiller and Dr Alan Watson

THE City Hospital has a long tradition of caring for babies and children and long-stay beds existed from the 1950s, mainly for children with rheumatic fever and TB meningitis. By the end of the 1960s specialist acute paediatric beds were added.

John Fitzsimmons joined Pat Page about 1965 and concentrated initially on developing the neonatal service which was right at the other end of the hospital. Joan Hiller was appointed in 1971 and John left the Children's Hospital, where he shared paediatric and neonatal work with Dr Nick Rutter, a registrar and two senior house officers. Margaret Mayell was appointed Paediatric Surgeon in 1972 and by this time Joan Hiller had developed an interest in cystic fibrosis, setting up a specialist service with a dietician, physiotherapist and social worker. She also held peripheral clinics all over mid-Trent.

The appointment of a series of fellows funded by the Cystic Fibrosis Trust allowed the service to develop with the establishment of an adult clinic, taking part in research studies with Dr Tony Milner relating to very young children with asthma and various drug trials. In addition, she ran clinics for children with diabetes and phenylketonuria (a rare inherited disease in which the body cannot break down one protein component found in many foods) with Chris Jarvis, the senior dietician. Dr Alan Smyth took over from her when she retired.

Children with infectious diseases were admitted to Heathfield Hospital under the care of Dr Don. In the early 1980s when the new H Block opened, better isolation facilities were available, along with wards for general paediatrics, general surgery, plastic surgery and a separate baby unit.

John Fitzsimmons developed an interest in clinical genetics and he set up a department. As clinical genetics expanded, David Curnock took over his paediatric work and Ian Young took on the clinical genetics work upon his retirement. The services they set up continue to thrive.

The children's services have rapidly adapted to the changing needs of children and families, particularly with the emphasis on keeping children out of hospital as much as possible. Children's specialist nurses and facilities have been developed and Linby ward was created as a children's high dependency unit. The baby section of Papplewick ward was joined with the main ward and the space used to provide important parent accommodation.

The paediatric renal unit was created in 1985 and quickly became a regional referral centre, providing all types of dialysis and kidney transplantation for children throughout the Trent region and parts of East Anglia. Initially the unit was housed on Millard ward and in 1992 Lambley ward became the children's nephrology unit with the creation of dedicated dialysis facilities for children. Millard ward will shortly house the regional cleft lip and palate service and the sub-regional cystic fibrosis unit is on Papplewick ward.

In 1989 the Children and Young People's Clinic was built as a national demonstration site, offering a large play area, facilities for teenagers and excellent consultant room facilities. The Child Development Centre, which was originally attached to the old outpatients' building, joined the Children's Centre, run by the Community Unit on the City Hospital campus.

Over the last 100 years children's care has undergone tremendous changes and the whole ethos of short-term admission and assessment units for children with support in the community is a far cry from the long hospital stays and segregation from their parents that prevailed in the last century.

Neonatal service

By Professor Nick Rutter and Dr Joan Hiller

THE 'new' maternity unit opened in 1972, replacing the old one near to the present coronary care unit. John Fitzsimmons and Joan Hiller were joined by two academic paediatricians, David Hull (Foundation Professor of Child Health) and Tony Milner (Senior Lecturer), who came to Nottingham from Great Ormond Street in 1973. The senior nurse was Paula Hale who trained in Nottingham. The unit flourished and throughout the 1970s and 80s it developed a national reputation for innovative practice, particularly in the field of neonatal nursing. Paula founded a national organisation, the Neonatal Nurses' Association, and ran it for many years.

The neonatal service is a recognised centre for the delivery of care to babies, attracting visitors from all

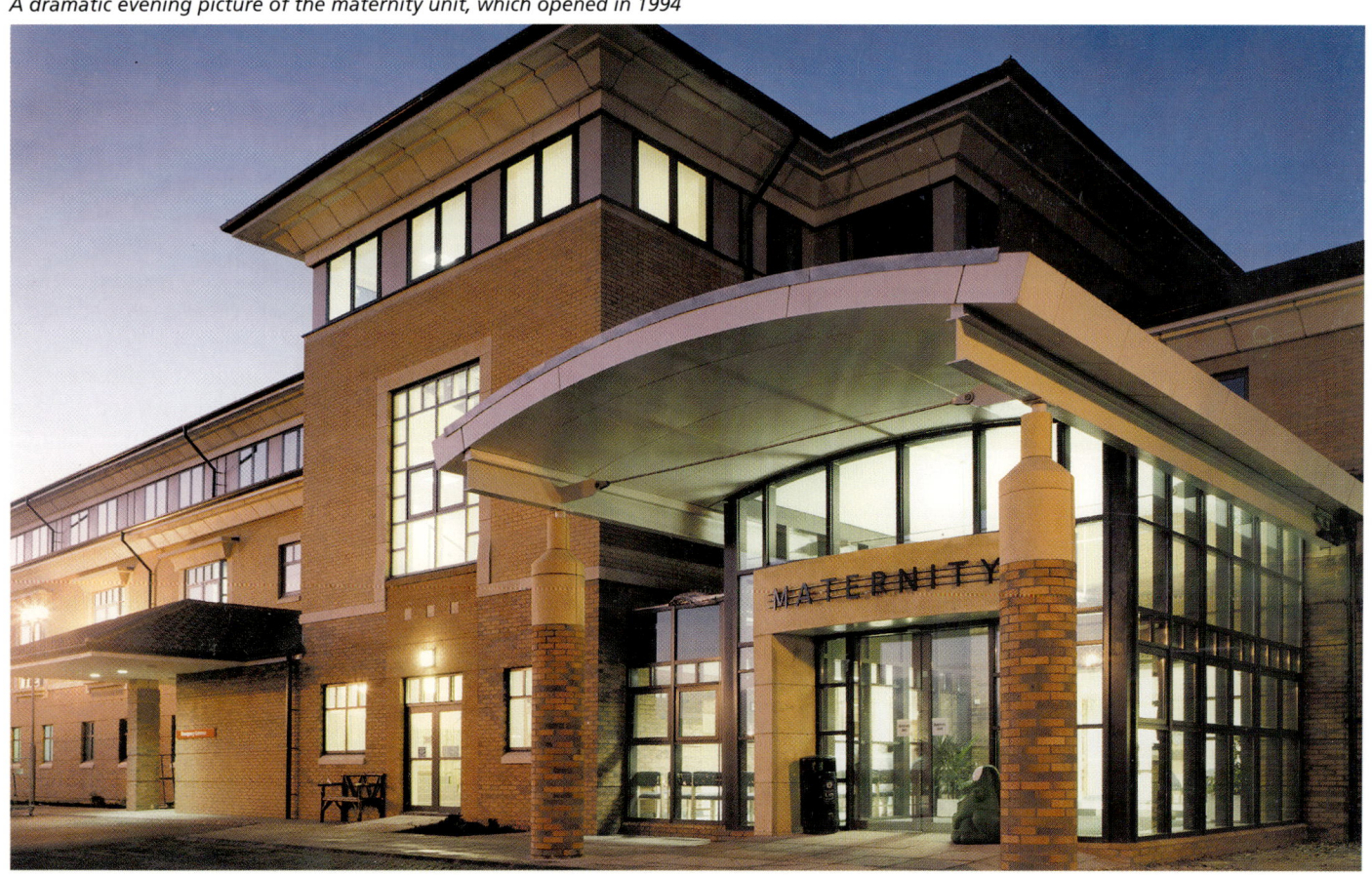

A dramatic evening picture of the maternity unit, which opened in 1994

The People's Hospital

over the UK and abroad. The unit pioneered a family-centred approach to neonatal care which has since been adopted nationally. The intensive care unit, housed in the City Hospital maternity unit which opened in 1994, is recognised as one of the country's leading facilities. The service has also developed an international reputation for its research.

The Academic Department of Child Health was launched in 1972, in readiness for the first Nottingham medical students who came to paediatrics in their fourth year (1974). Although most paediatric teaching was at the old Children's Hospital (which became Nottingham Health Authority HQ in 1979), the City Hospital started to take paediatric students in the 1980s. It currently takes 40 students each year.

The department was based at the City Hospital from 1973 to 1978. It moved to the newly-built Queen's Medical Centre in 1978.

Genetics

By Professor Sandy Raeburn

SPECIALIST clinical genetics developed in Nottingham during the early 1970s under the leadership of Dr John Fitzsimmons, an experienced paediatrician. With his wife Beth, he developed a family-focussed clinical genetic counselling service located in a small department within H Block. This department became a national model for a clinical genetic centre.

The clinical cytogenetic laboratory service was developed under the leadership of Dr Pat Cooke from May, 1974. She headed a team of scientists who carried out 259 cytogenetic tests in that year. The current service under Dr Tony Parkin performed 4,819 tests in 2001/2, most with great complexity and wider case mix. In 1987, molecular testing started, first with Dr Roger Quaife and since 1989, Dr Gareth Cross. In 1991 this molecular team was the first to apply in clinical practice the new knowledge of the gene which causes the Fragile X syndrome. Dr and Mrs Fitzsimmons retired in 1989. Coincidentally Dr Pat Cooke left to become Trent Regional Scientific Officer. Dr Tony Parkin headed the cytogenetics service from February 1990. Professor Sandy Raeburn was appointed in 1990 to link clinical and laboratory services in Nottingham and to provide academic insights. Penny Guilbert became Clinical Services Manager.

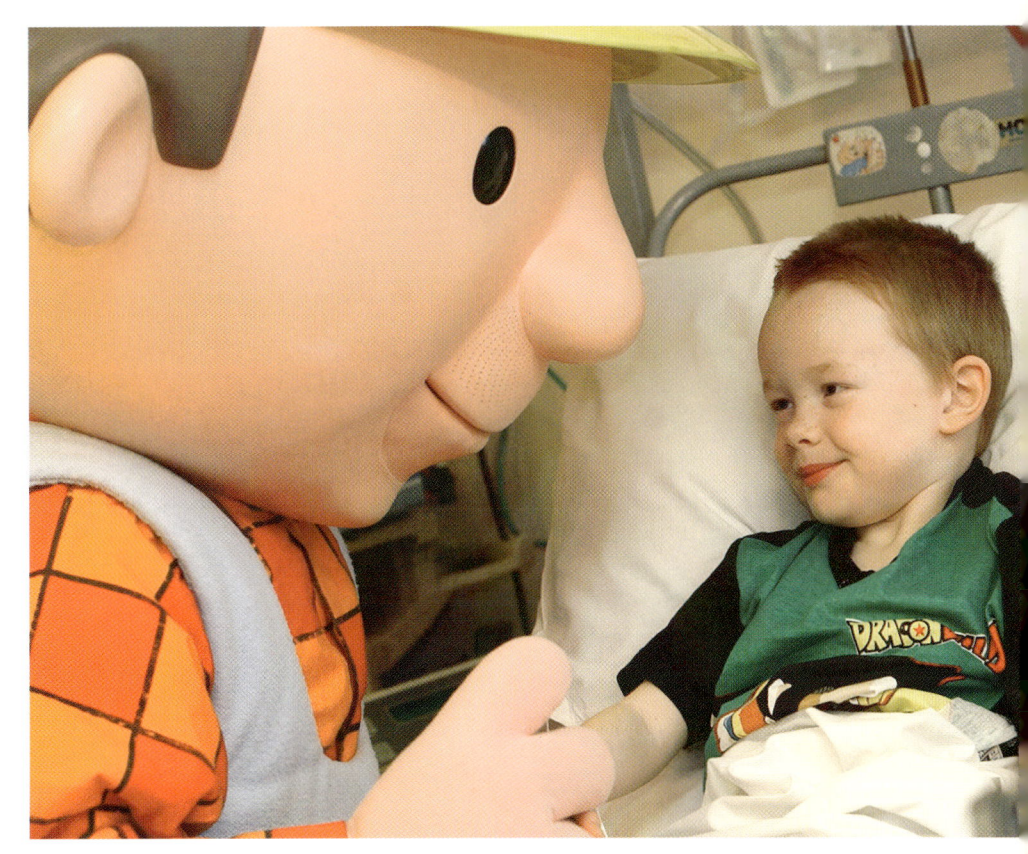

Since 1990, genetic services have been integrated as an independent directorate within the hospital. Unfortunately plans for creating suitable accommodation to house all genetic services together (and also to facilitate links between the University and the City Hospital) have not moved on so rapidly. The dedicated centre for medical genetics, which was John Fitzsimmons' vision, based on the genetic advances of the 1950s to 1980s, has not yet been achieved. However, the university has developed programmes of human genetic research rapidly. There is now an Institute of Genetics, currently under the leadership of Professor David Brook, which has an international standing. With a reputation for providing patient-led, family-focused, genetic services and with genetic research rated at the highest level internationally, Nottingham is well placed to carry genetics into the next 100 years.

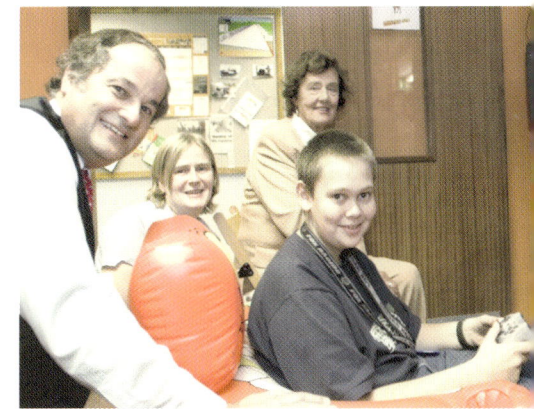

Top: Bob the Builder visited the City Hospital's Lambley ward to cheer up children who weren't able to see his show at the Nottingham Ice Arena. He is pictured saying 'hello' to six-year-old Terry Harrison who was in hospital for a major operation in 2002

Above: Dr Alan Watson, hospital youth worker Donna Hilton, Elizabeth Ward OBE and Tom Winlow (17) at the launch of the new youth room in Lambley ward in 2001

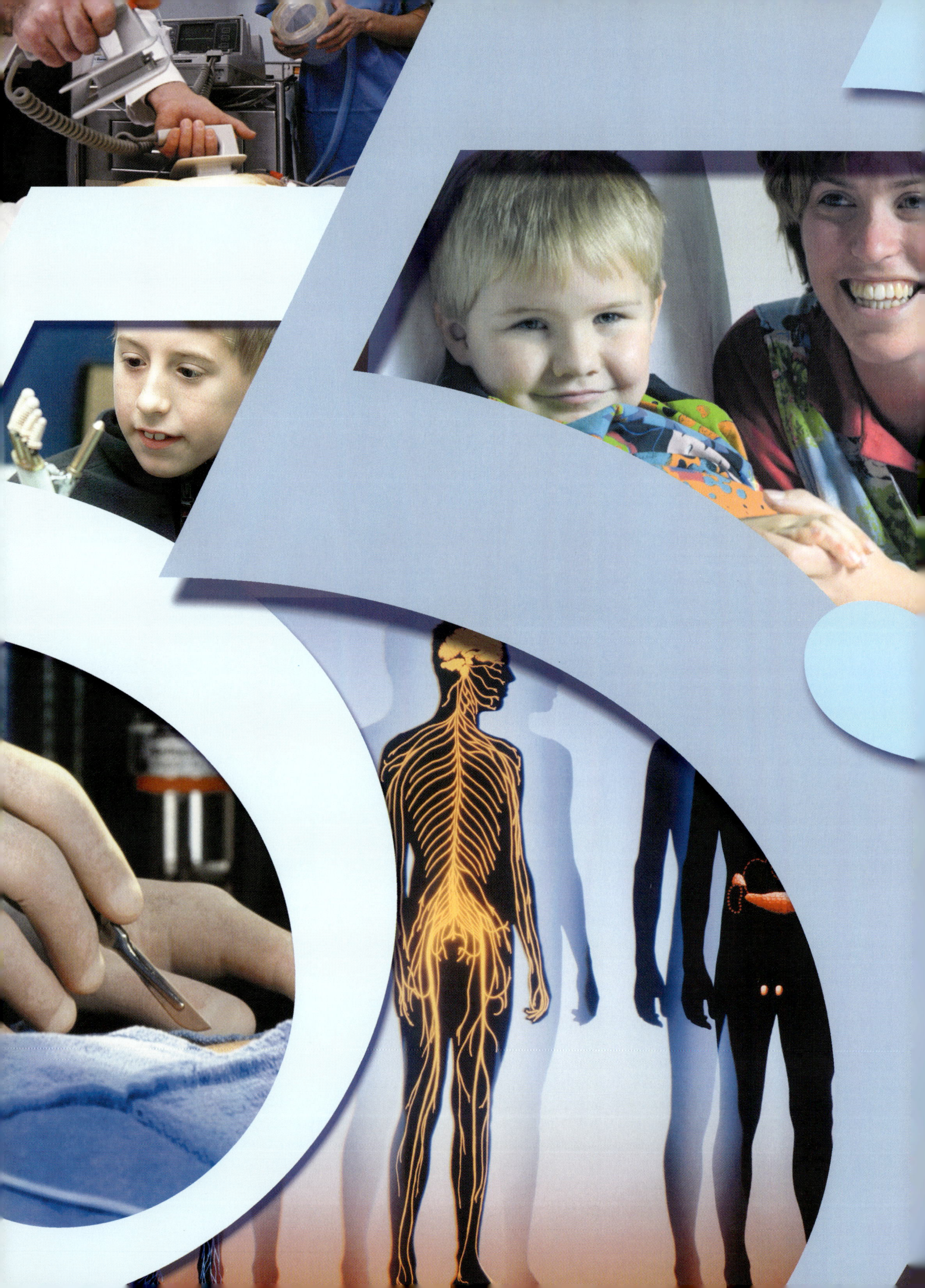

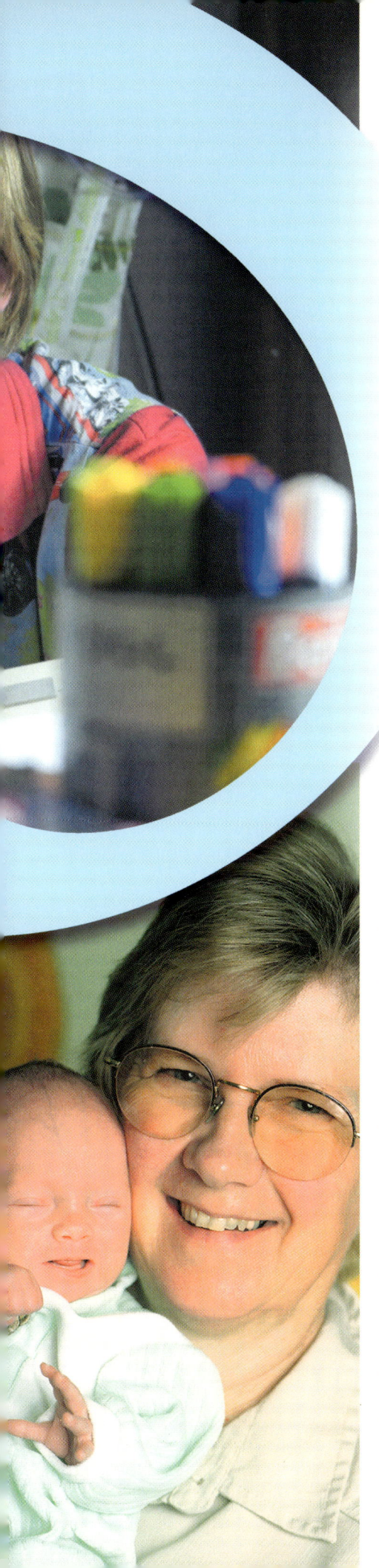

Two decades of development

Looking ahead with optimism

LEECHES were making a come back at Nottingham City Hospital in 1982 and Sister Elizabeth Melbourne was worried about the age of the beds in Patience Two ward.

The first story came from the *Evening Post* explaining how an old treatment was proving invaluable in the after-care of patients who had undergone microsurgery. The second story from the *Financial Times* suggested the City Hospital contained a microcosm of the economic problems confronting Britain's National Health Service at that time.

The hospital's annual budget was then £20m. Yet, said the report, it was constantly hampered by a shortage of funds and staff were under increasing strain as vacancies were frozen in line with the Government's aim of reducing manpower.

At that time the hospital had 908 beds and the Trent region was the most medically deprived in the country in terms of facilities, medical staffing and general health indicators. Since 1976 the Government had been paying the region extra money to try and reduce these inequalities.

It was a crucial time in the development of health care in Nottingham. As part of NHS reorganisation, the new Nottingham health district had come into existence on April 1, 1974. Hundreds of beds remained empty at Queen's Medical Centre because there was no money to run services in unopened wards. The City Hospital's teaching status had profound implications for both the hospital and the district. Medical students were then costing, on average, £100,000 each to train and although the district received extra funds for the additional costs it did not feel it was enough.

Nottinghamshire Area Health Authority, which was abolished on April 1 when an entire tier of NHS administration was removed, had warned in 1981 that without much-needed capital investment in the next 10 years many departments at the City Hospital would continue to operate in "inadequate facilities for years to come, to the detriment of the service in general."

This chapter will show how the hospital responded to that challenge.

But first the fascinating story of the leeches. John Gilby, who retired in 2002 as Director of Service Development, was then the hospital's Principal Pharmacist and "unofficial leech-keeper." He told the *Evening Post* how the blood-sucking worms, which had been used in treatment from the Middle Ages, could now make the difference between a skin graft failing or succeeding. The leeches, he explained, were starved before being introduced to patients to clear up tissue after microsurgery operations. The suckers removed clotted blood which affected the flow of fresh blood to newly-grafted skin.

And the lively leeches, costing £2.50 each, were so keen to get at blood clots that they were sliding out of their tank while off duty. Mr Gilby said the hospital was looking for a more secure receptacle for them.

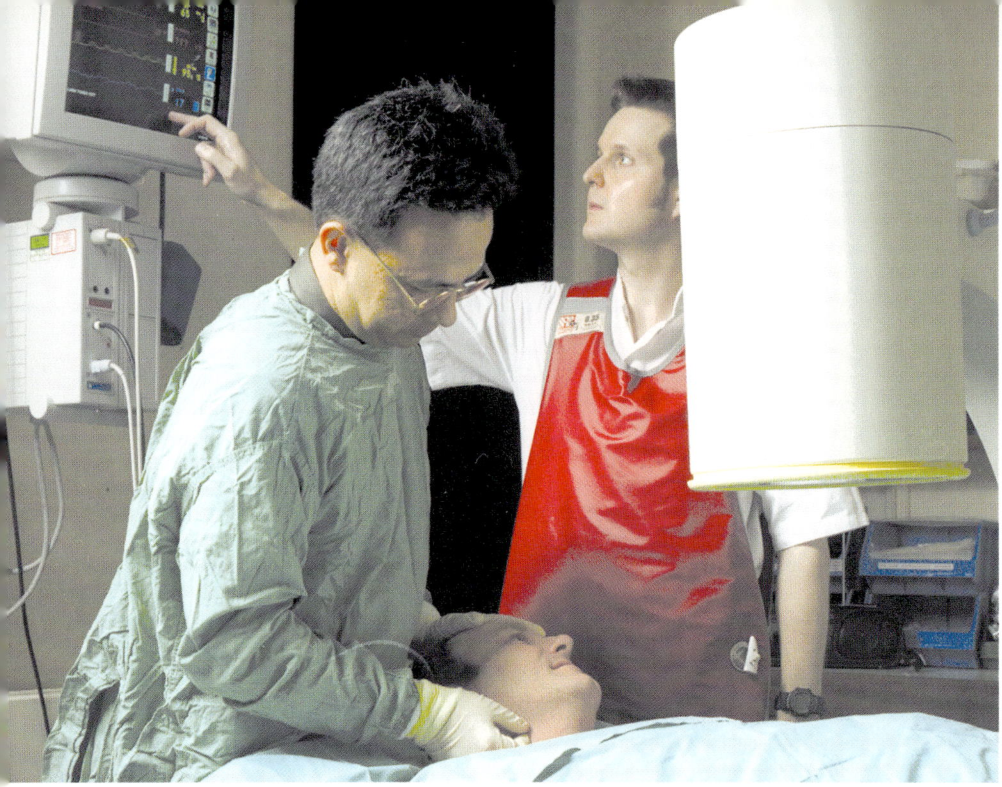
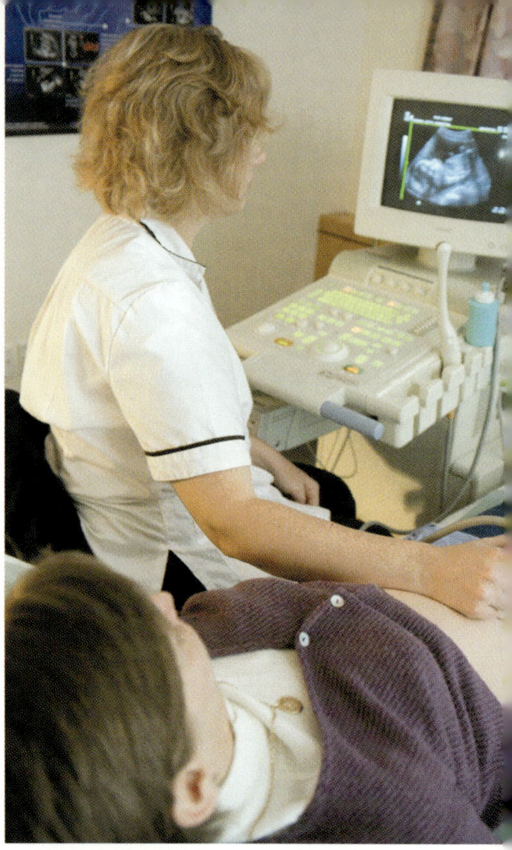
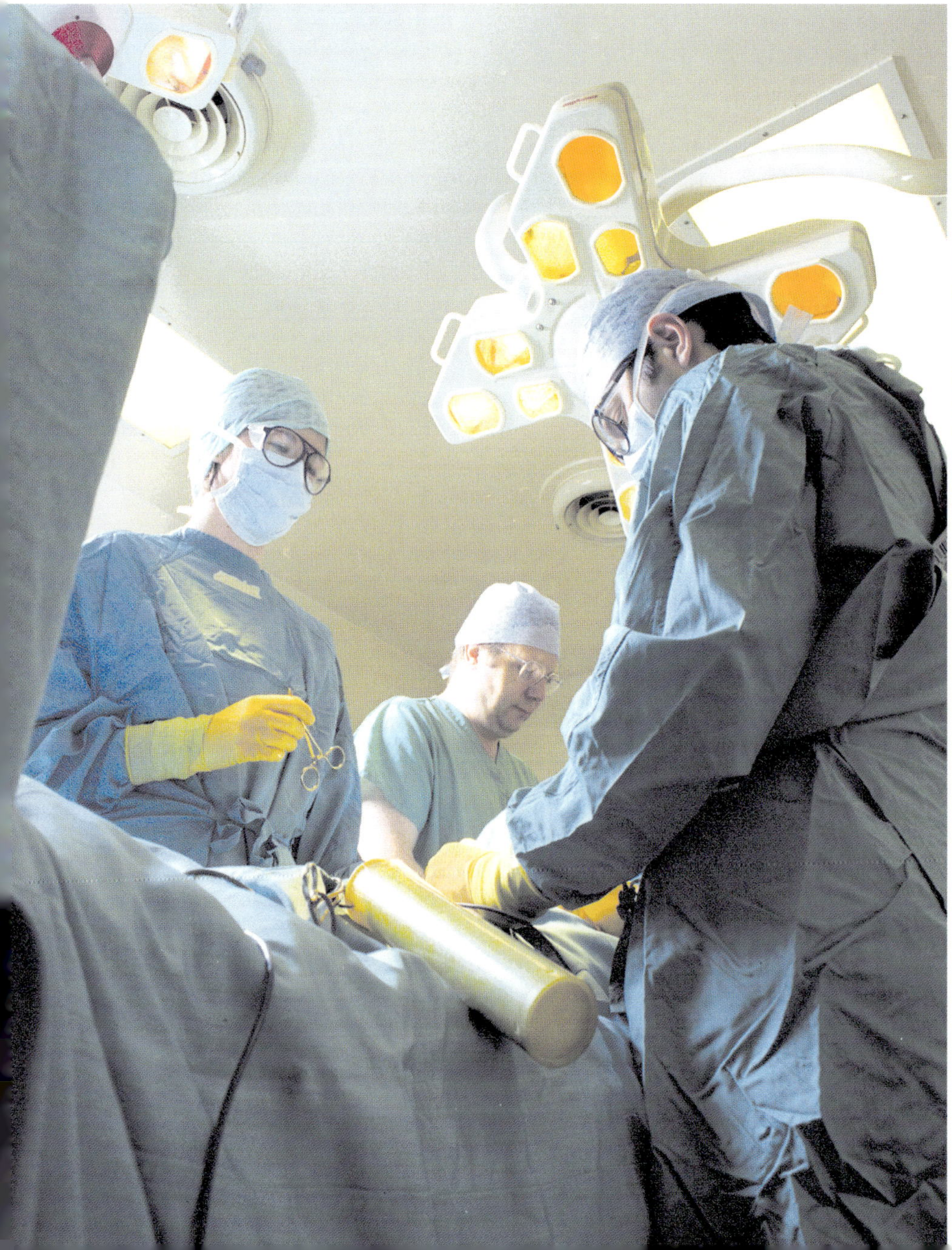
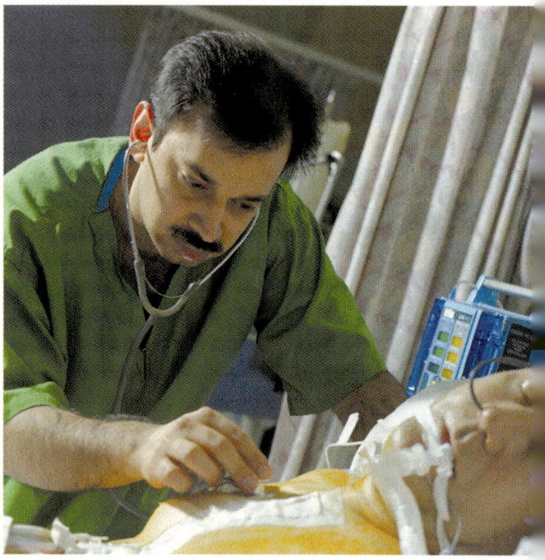
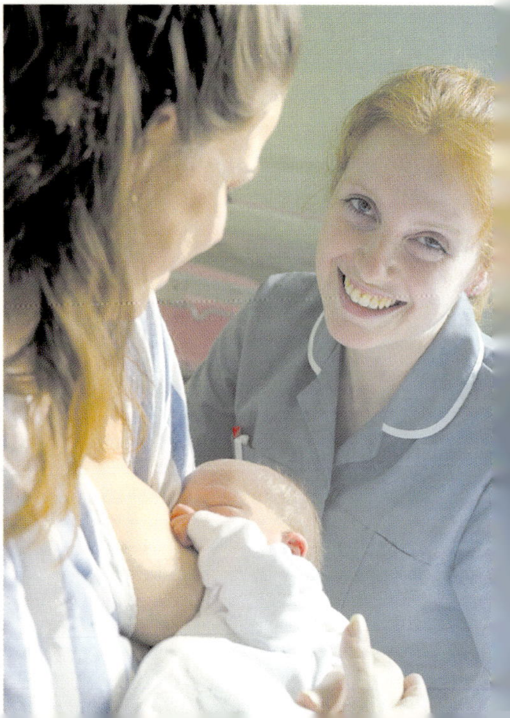

The People's Hospital

Meanwhile managers were delighted to announce in 1984 that a purpose-built operating theatre for burns patients - mothballed for four years because of cash restrictions - would finally open. Initially the theatre opened two days a week to relieve the severe strain on the main theatres. It was also confirmed that a 19-bed burns unit would be progressively opened.

The arrival of a cow in the outpatient department one Saturday morning brought a bit of comic relief during a time of squeeze and save. Ann Booth, personal Secretary to Professor Roger Cotton, recalled the incident. "I rushed in to tell Stephen Jones, who had a marvellous sense of the ridiculous, and we decided to go and explore. Firstly we tried a side entrance to outpatients but the door was closed. A frightened nurse responded to our knocks and said she wouldn't let us in as it was dangerous.

"Still not quite believing what was happening we took the alternative route to outpatients, approaching from the east. When we reached the intersection of the corridors with the inner courtyard in view, a young and frightened looking policeman blocked our way, his arms outstretched. He pointed to the inner garden in outpatients where a frightened looking cow stood unhappily in the far corner. The police refused to let us get any nearer and advised us not to move on the basis that if the cow saw us moving it might charge, smash through the windows and harm us and itself. The farmer eventually arrived to retrieve the animal. But it was so frightened and distressed that it had to be shot. A sorry end to a bizarre event."

Happier times came in 1986 when the Duchess of Gloucester unveiled a plaque to officially open the new Medical Research Centre. She was so absorbed meeting staff and patients along the main corridor that the royal programme overran by more than 20 minutes.

The Duchess spent half an hour visiting the laboratories, escorted by Dr John Fletcher, Consultant Physician and Chairman of the Medical Research Centre Management Committee. She also opened a new histopathology department and showed great interest in the cervical cytology service.

In 1988 a giant crane swung a portable breast screening unit into place. The purpose-built unit - the first of its type in the Trent region - had to be slotted into a confined space with only a few feet to spare. The accommodation included a reception area, changing rooms, dark room and X-ray room to replace the service started in 1979, as a charity established in memory of Mrs Helen Garrod. A second unit arrived six weeks later as part of the Government's new initiative to provide a breast cancer screening programme for women aged 50 to 64. Nottingham was one of the first places to run a screening centre and the City Hospital became one of the first four training centres in the country.

What was it like being a junior doctor in the 1980s? Dr Douglas Black, now a GP, was at the City Hospital in 1980 and from 1983 to 1986, says the long hours and being too tired to sleep, has been erased from his memory.

"What I do remember is the sheer buzz of life in the hospital, the vitality of the hospital corridor snaking down from Oxton and Gedling ('they're only temporary wards you know') past the Mess (Space Invader competitions, Rugby Internationals whilst on call on Saturday afternoons, where I was when I heard that John Lennon had been shot) up towards the theatres, X-ray, outpatients and onwards to pathology.

"During the day the corridor was alive, it was impossible to make even a short journey without some form of meeting and greeting, often minor yet occasionally very major pieces of business were conducted there in the midst of public bustle. It was a beautiful place to behold. And yet strangely even more beautiful at two in the morning, deserted except for the droning of the buffing machines, and the thought that it should be possible to roll a golf ball right down the middle of that highly polished surface. I bear witness that it is."

The opening of the 1990s saw the hospital enter one of the most important building periods in its history. It began with three of the four Bagthorpe workhouse wards being demolished at Sherwood Hospital. A purpose-built genito-urinary medicine unit opened, following the transfer of the specialist clinic from the Nottingham General Hospital.

Paediatric facilities were undergoing a transformation too. The refurbished children's outpatients' department opened in 1990 with generous backing from the City Hospital League of Friends. The

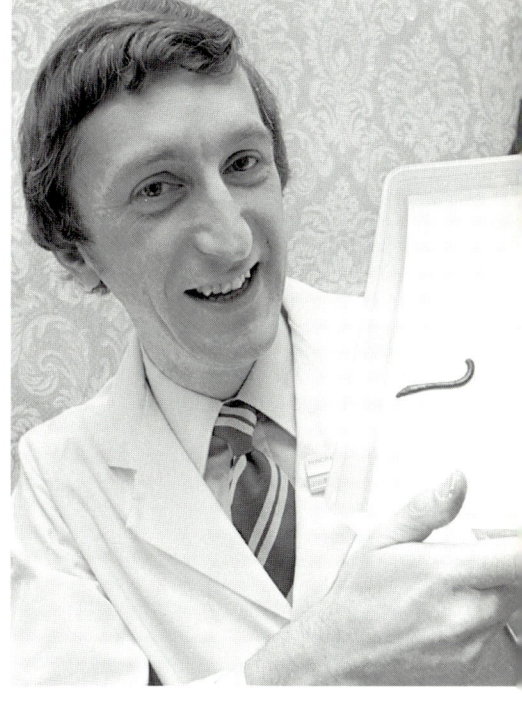

Principal Pharmacist John Gilby in 1982 when leeches were making a comeback at the hospital

Opposite page, top left and bottom left: Hospital theatre scenes
Top right: A patient undergoes an ultrasound scan
Right centre: A doctor and patient in intensive care
Bottom: Modern mums are encouraged to breast feed

following year cricketer Derek Randall opened the new trend-setting children's clinic, offering some of the finest facilities in the country.

Derek admitted that as a young boy he had been terrified of hospitals, but staff explained the secret of putting parents and patients at their ease from the moment they arrived. In fact the clinic soon proved so popular that youngsters protested when it was time to go home.

Six months later the clinic was visited by Health Secretary William Waldegrave and he was asked if services would suffer if the City Hospital became an NHS Trust. "I would argue," he countered, "that this kind of local management initiative will strengthen the services."

Unit General Manager Thelma Holland was burning the midnight oil, attending more than 50 meetings with staff to assess opinions and answer questions. Convinced that Trust status was the best way forward, she was determined to see £40m spent on developing the site over the next 10 years - and argued this was more likely if the hospital took control of its own budget.

By April 1, 1992 the concept had become a reality - Nottingham City Hospital was in the first wave of new NHS Trusts. A ballot of consultants and senior managers showed 71 per cent favoured the bold move. Miss Holland said: "If the ballot had resulted in a 'no' vote I would have

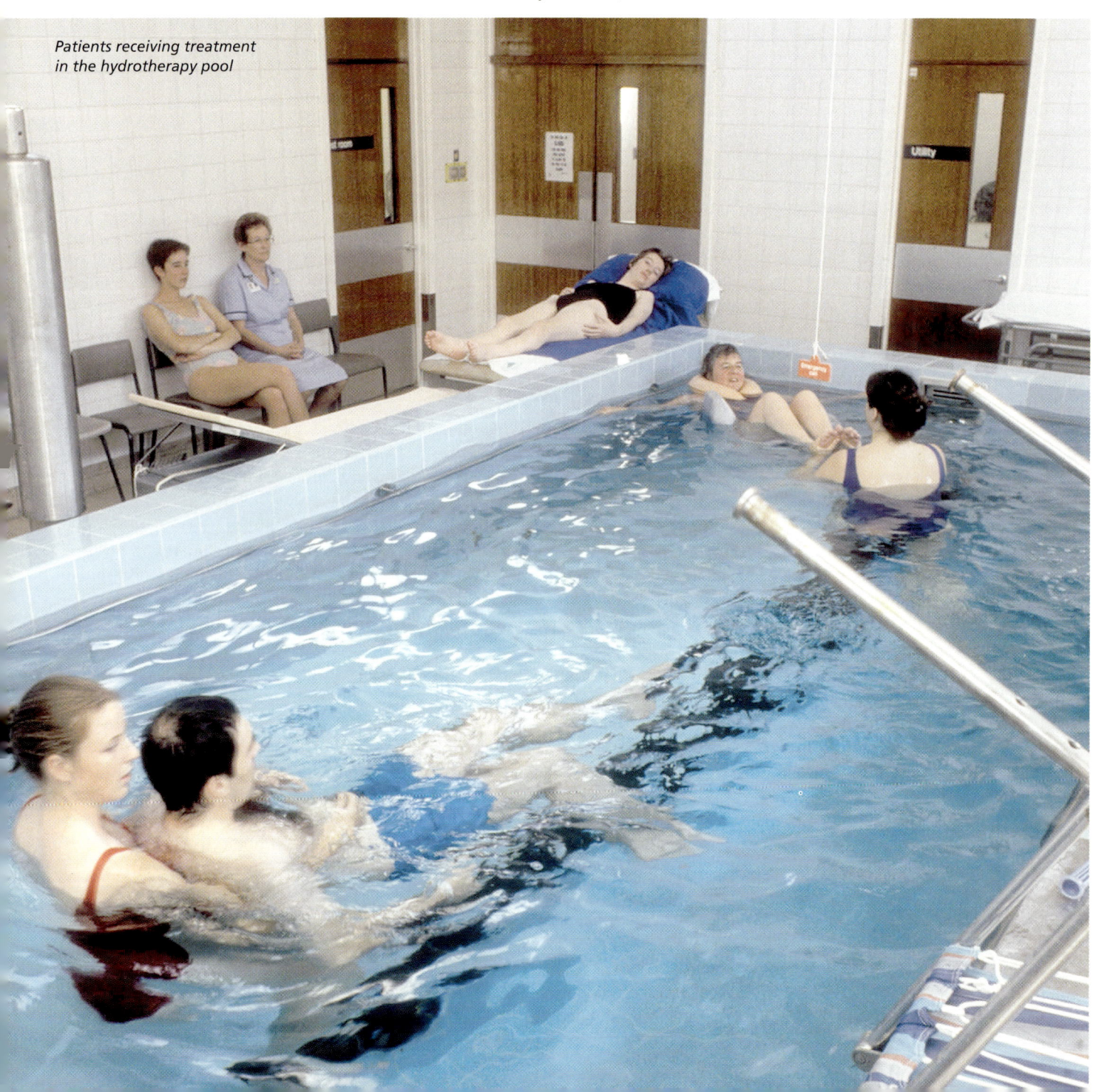

Patients receiving treatment in the hydrotherapy pool

The People's Hospital

withdrawn the application and we would not have proceeded."

She wanted to see the City Hospital make rapid progress. Having trained as a nurse at St Thomas' Hospital, London - the training school made famous by Florence Nightingale - Miss Holland went on frequent hospital 'walkabouts' to see what was happening on wards and in clinical areas.

Soon after taking up her new post in September 1990, she had to introduce tough economic measures - closing wards and beds, freezing vacancies and cutting the number of operating theatre sessions to prevent the hospital being more than £1.5m overspent by the end of the 1990/91 financial year.

She praised staff for helping the hospital break even. "Staff achieved that position - not without some hardship. They gave management tremendous support and pulled out all the stops."

By now the City Hospital was a £100m-a-year operation, with more than 1,200 beds - and more were on the way. Two former cancer sufferers, who owed their lives to the hospital's skilled medical teams, attended a turf-cutting ceremony to mark the start of work on the £32m renal/oncology building - one of the largest and most important projects ever developed in the Trent region. The unit, which opened in 1993, brought oncology and renal services under one roof and offered superb facilities for treating 2,000 new patients a year.

It also enabled the acute renal wards to be relocated alongside the dialysis unit in H Block. The state-of-the-art centre, serving more than one million people in Nottinghamshire and surrounding counties, put the city among the world leaders in cancer care and research. Clinical Director Dr Eric Bessell said: "Five thousand local people develop cancer each year. We're going to be able to provide them with first-class treatment in facilities that are as good as any in Europe."

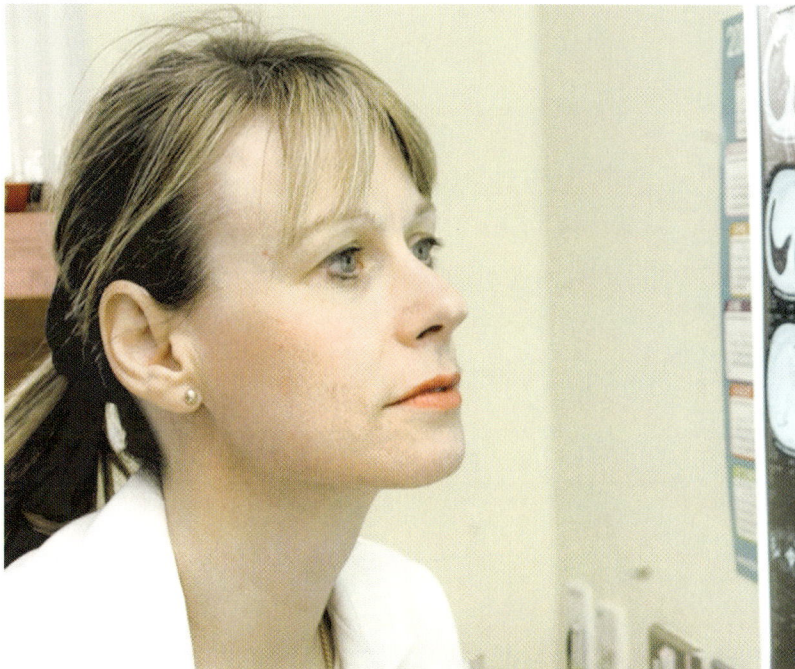

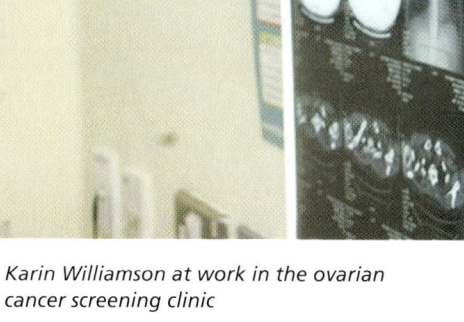

The radiotherapy suite contained the latest linear accelerators networked to verification systems to ensure optimum treatment for every patient. A selectron provided internal radiotherapy with closed-circuit TV so that patients could chat with staff and visitors. The chemotherapy treatment areas were also superbly equipped and included counselling and relaxation facilities. The unit, containing three 18-bed wards, also incorporated the Nottingham University Academic Department - one of only 10 in the country - funded by the Cancer Research Campaign and headed by Professor Jim Carmichael. The unit, also accommodating the Derby University School of Radiotherapy, was officially opened by the Duchess of Kent in February 1994.

A few months earlier an old, unoccupied building close to the No 3 entrance on Hucknall Road was successfully converted into the new medical genetics centre. Trent Regional Health Authority gave £1.17m, the City Hospital Trust pledged £10,000 of its charitable funds to the project and many donations came in from patients and their families. The scheme - aimed at creating a centre dedicated to

Karin Williamson at work in the ovarian cancer screening clinic

providing medical genetic services for more than two million people - was spearheaded by Professor Sandy Raeburn, Professor of Clinical Genetics and head of the Interdisciplinary Centre for Medical Genetics. The project extended the excellent work started by his predecessor Dr John Fitzsimmons, whose vision led to the early development in Nottingham of nurse specialists to visit families at home.

Work had already started on the University of Nottingham's £6m Clinical Sciences Building - its first purpose-built facility at the City Hospital. The development represented the university's biggest investment in medicine for 20 years. Built on the site of a former nursing home opposite the hospital's main entrance, it brought together the university's medical departments which were spread around the 90-acre hospital site.

University Director of Estate Management Chris Jagger said: "This was a vision: the co-operation and support of the City Hospital management team has made it a reality."

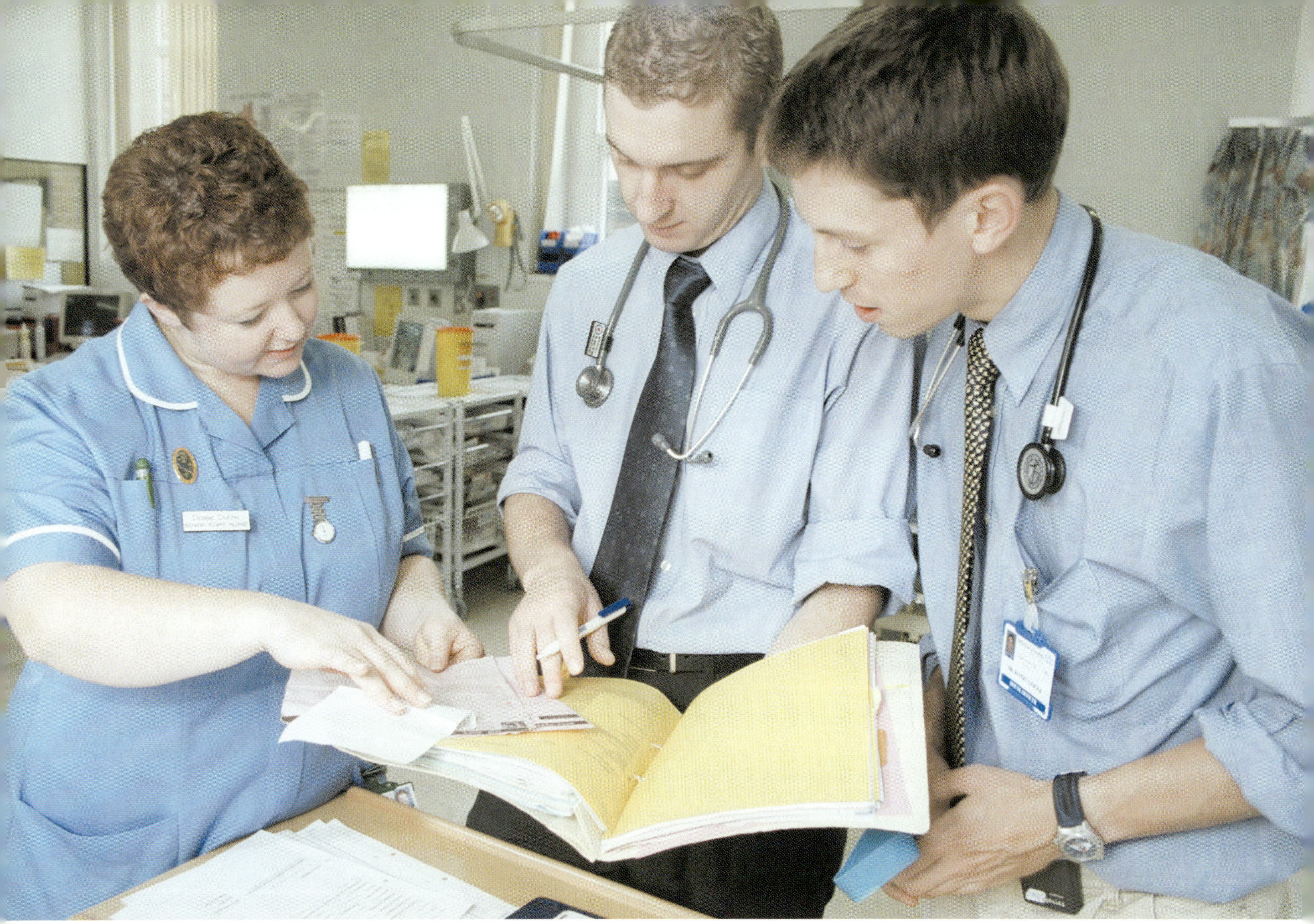

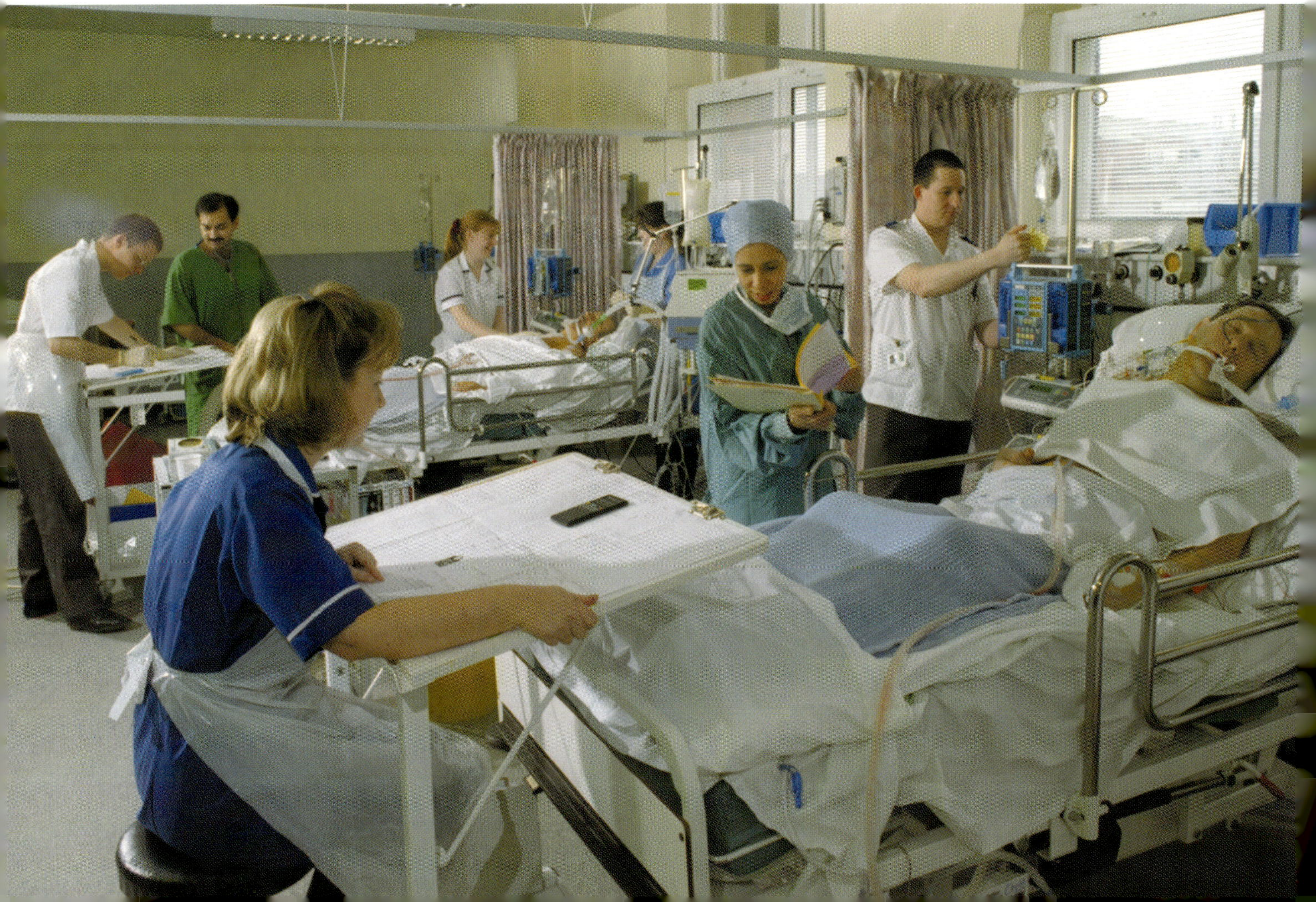

The People's Hospital

Among the facilities in the building is a 220-seat lecture theatre, seminar rooms, offices, research laboratories and practice rooms.

Meanwhile the City Hospital's neonatal unit was making headline news in caring for the world's smallest baby, who weighed just 11 ounces and was only six inches long after being born 11 weeks prematurely.

Consultant Paediatrician Dr David Curnock explained: "Technology is improving the survival rates of babies born 16 or even 17 weeks prematurely.

"But standard technology is not going to push the boundaries any further back than that. You can have all the machinery and expertise in the world. But you must never ignore the feelings of the mother and father. We try to care for the whole family. There are two parts to intensive care. One is high technology and the skills of nurses and doctors; the other is keeping together mother, father and baby right from the start. With the technology, but without the human side, you will end up with frightened, estranged parents and a baby who behaves differently when he or she goes home."

Meanwhile the hospital's new £10m maternity unit was winning plaudits from patients. The three-storey unit - replacing an asbestos-clad maternity unit built in the 1970s - contained two obstetric theatres, a 28-cot neonatal unit and 17 modern delivery rooms.

Three maternity wards provided 81 beds and mothers could look forward to post-delivery care in the purpose-built Patient Hotel - the first in the UK.

Based on a Scandinavian idea, the sophisticated hotel offered five-star treatment to new mums an other patients, relatives and visitors who would benefit from the more relaxed surroundings. Each of the 52 beautifully decorated hotel rooms was equipped with TV, tea and coffee-making facilities, radio, telephone and en-suite bathroom and the hotel has its own restaurant with sumptuous meals and eye-catching views over Nottingham.

The hotel released precious beds on hospital wards by allowing not-so-sick patients to get well in its cosy, self-care surroundings.

The Patient Hotel and new maternity unit was officially opened in 1996 by Health Secretary Stephen Dorrell.

As the hospital tried to come to terms with escalating traffic, parking charges were introduced in 1995. Revenue from the scheme would help pay for a package of measures aimed at cutting car crime, tightening security and reducing congestion.

It's ironic that while serving on the No 2 Management Committee in the 1960s, Consultant Thoracic Surgeon Mr Robert Barclay expressed concern about the growing number of cars using the City Hospital site. But when the issue reached the regional board in Sheffield he was brushed aside and told that parking would never be a problem on a site as large as the City Hospital!

In 1996 the last vestige of the City Hospital's workhouse origins disappeared when the final Sherwood ward was demolished to make way for a new endoscopy unit. The League of Hospital Friends of Sherwood and St Francis decided to wind up after raising large sums of money for the comfort of elderly patients for the previous 30 years. The hospital opted to change the name from Sherwood Hospital to South Corridor to end reminders of the old Bagthorpe workhouse.

Between 1992 and 1997 the City Hospital site changed dramatically with £46m spent on new buildings. The biggest slice went on the creation of the £30m renal/oncology department, the new maternity unit and Patient Hotel (£13m). Other important new developments included a £2m day surgery unit, the women's endoscopy unit and a £1m link corridor scheme from the hospital to the new maternity unit. In 1995, £1m was spent redeveloping facilities to allow patients who would previously have had to travel to Sheffield or Leicester for heart surgery to have their operations in Nottingham. Around £14m was also spent upgrading outpatients, orthopaedic wards and cardiac intensive care.

The site was landscaped and hospital managers were proud of its green and friendly feel. New signposting was put in place and a park-and-ride scheme was established to help people get from one side of the site to the other. Buses began running through the hospital grounds for the first time - stopping at key

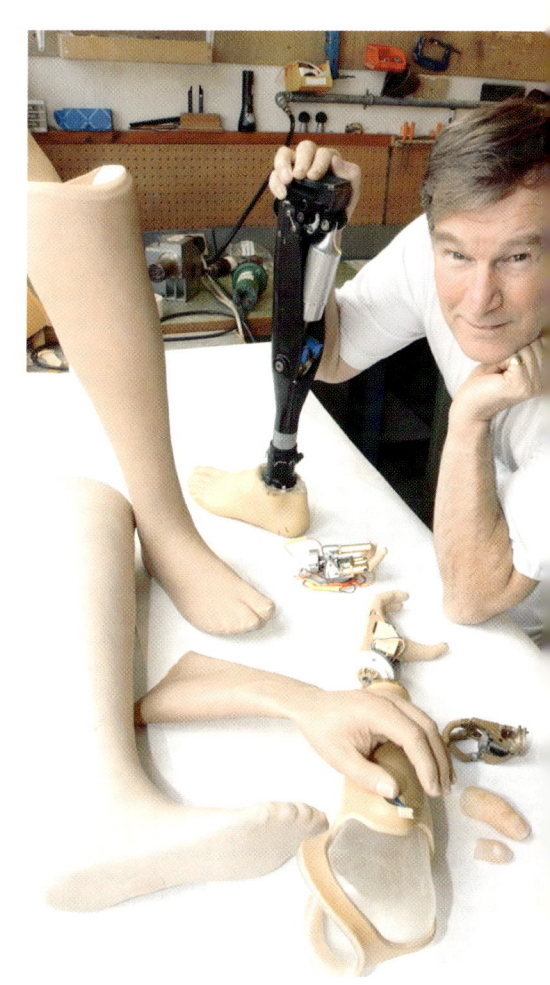

Above: Prosthetics Manager John Ronald, pictured in 2001 with a selection of false limbs and mechanical aid devices manufactured from scratch from carbon fibre, titanium, silicon, polyester resin, aluminium and using advanced electronics

Opposite page, top: Two doctors and a nurse discuss a patient's notes in the assessment unit in 2001
Bottom: Staff at work in the cardiac intensive care unit in 1999

The People's Hospital

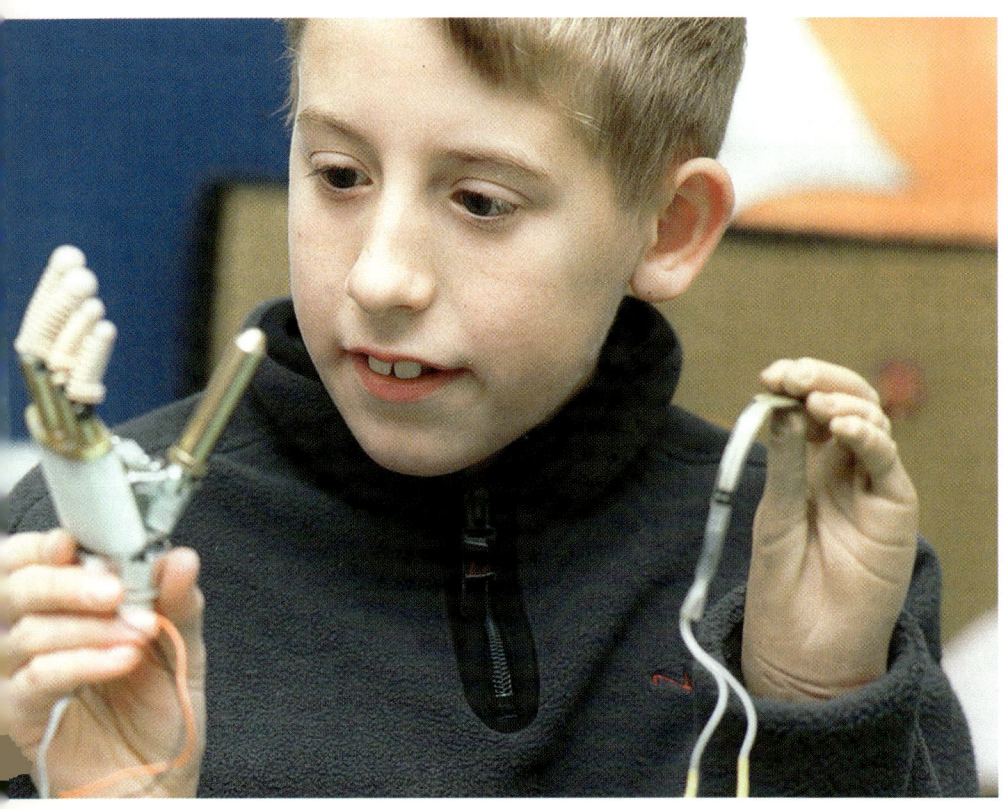

points to encourage patients and visitors to leave their cars at home.

At long last the hospital was putting on a modern face to match its reputation. A £60m package, unveiled in 1995, contained major developments - a £5m state-of-the-art breast institute to open in 2003 and new surgical wards to replace dilapidated mobile units and rundown 1920s buildings. A new £7m road layout aimed to make it easier to get in and out of the 90-acre site. The project also included plans for a new one-way system, roundabouts and improved parking and new accommodation for medical staff. Director of Service Development

Left: Jeremy Driver, 11 from Nottingham, one of six children to take part in the country's first clinical trial of the Prodigits 'bionic hand' project in 2000

Below: Children at play on a paediatric ward

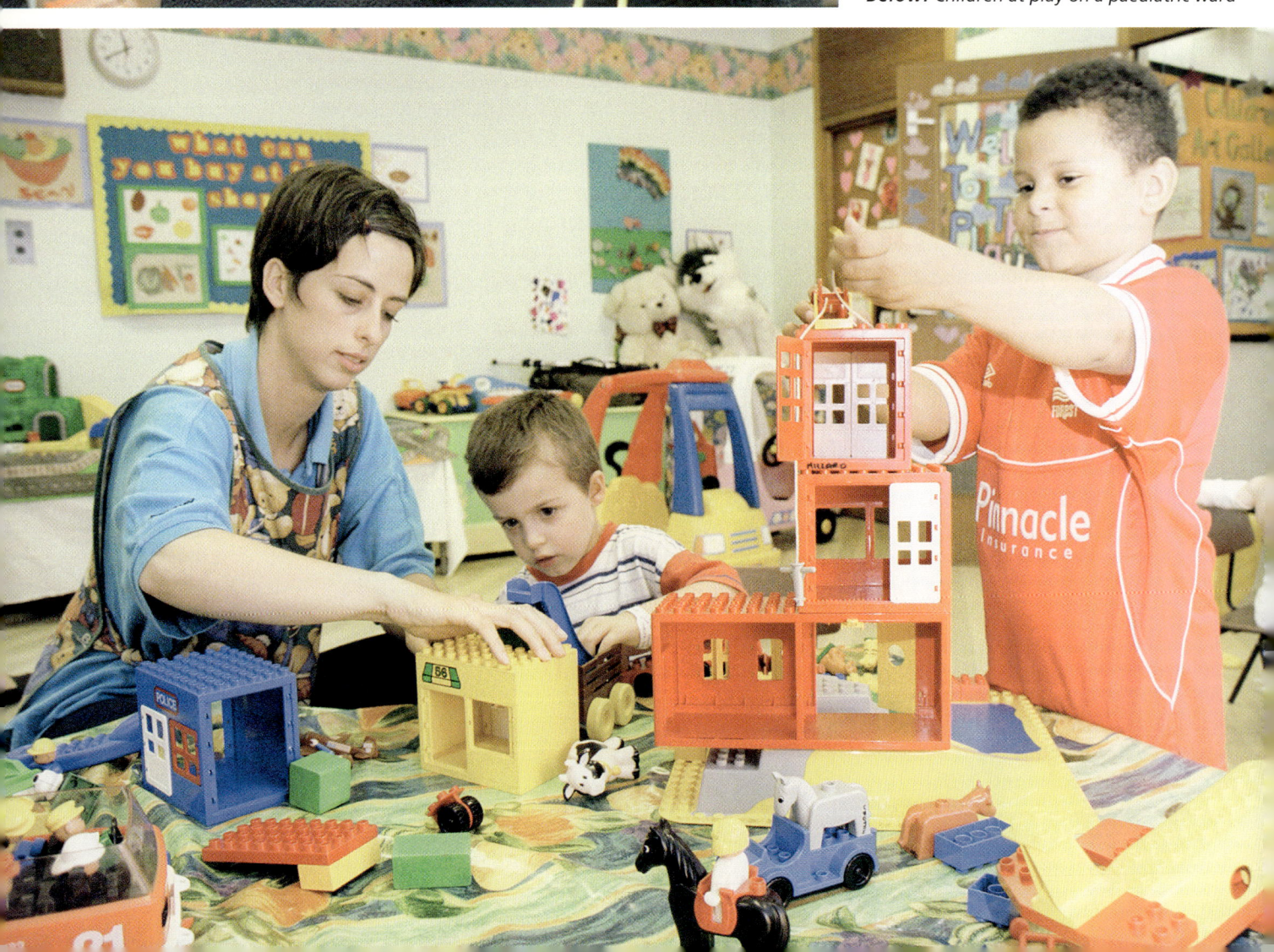

The People's Hospital

John Gilby said: "A great deal has been done at the City Hospital but we are aware that a considerable amount of investment is still needed."

In these exciting times there were changes at the top. Norman Deakin, who had made a significant contribution to hospital development, stepped down as Chairman. He was succeeded in 1998 by Christine Bowering, former head teacher of Nottingham High School for Girls, who had served five years as a non-executive director at the Queen's Medical Centre. She believed her professional background would "have an important role in bringing the hospital and the local community closer together."

As the hospital's centenary drew nearer, support grew for the establishment of a formal archive. And one of the many artefacts worthy of inclusion in the collection could be an original pair of forceps designed and used 70 years ago by the City Hospital's first thoracic specialist Laurence O'Shaughnessy. The forceps - believed to be the only pair of their kind in the world - were found in a medical storeroom in 1998 by David Richens, head of the cardiac surgery unit. "I couldn't believe it," he said. "This means that heart surgery was being carried out in Nottingham as early as the 1930s - much earlier than we thought. O'Shaughnessy was an icon in the world of early heart surgery. He designed the special curved forceps, known as O'Shaughnessy forceps, which are still used in every operating theatre, and we now have a pair of the original ones he used." Mr Richens also discovered in the hospital medical library one of the first text books on heart surgery, written and signed by O'Shaughnessy, dated 1934. Both items went on view in the City Hospital's new cardiac training centre, where they contrasted with the latest computerised equipment used in heart surgery today.

Innovations and developments continued to come thick and fast. In 2001 the hospital opened a pioneering clinic to help patients get over the psychological effects of their life-saving treatment. About 500 patients are treated annually in the hospital's intensive care and high dependency units - and almost half suffer physical and psychological problems such as nightmares, insomnia, panic attacks, anxiety, memory loss and relationship difficulties. Cheryl Crocker, Nurse Consultant in critical care, said: "These problems are not picked up in the community, as patients are reluctant to go to their GP because they think they are going mad. But their experiences are perfectly normal." About 200 patients were expected to benefit from the fortnightly clinics when patients can see a nurse and doctor, an occupational therapist, a physiotherapist and a hospital chaplain, who is a trained counsellor.

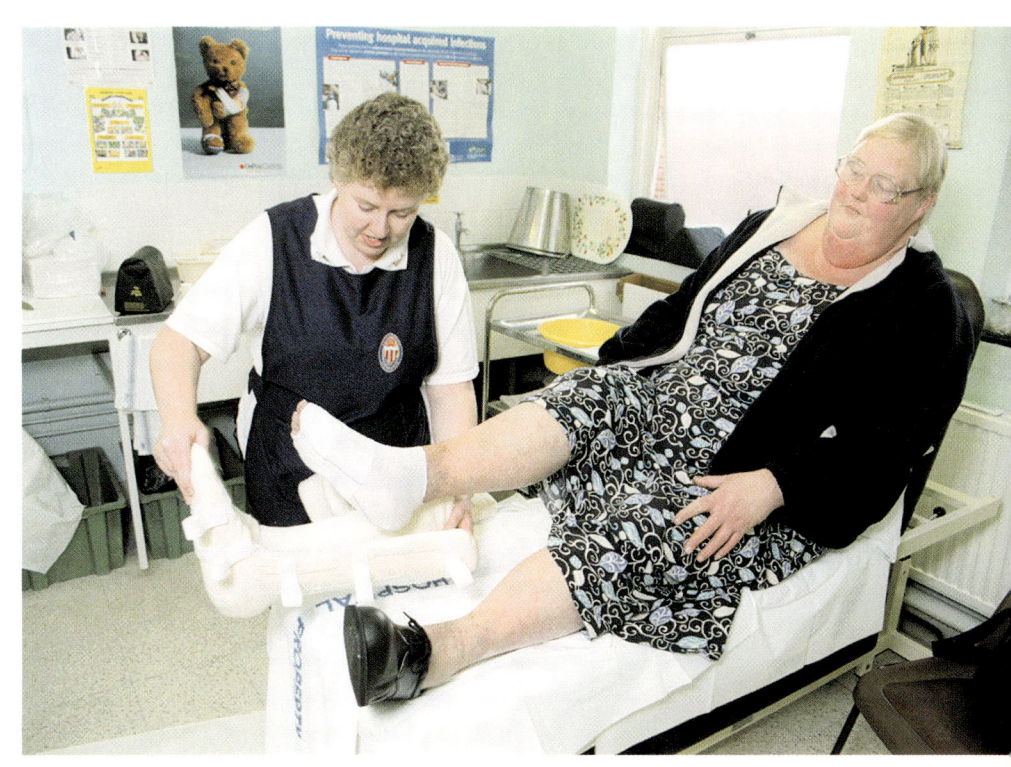

Young people set up the country's first youth club for hospital patients, helping themselves and learning valuable new skills along the way.

Above: *Patient being fitted with a leg cast in the plaster clinic*
Right: *At work in the pharmacy*

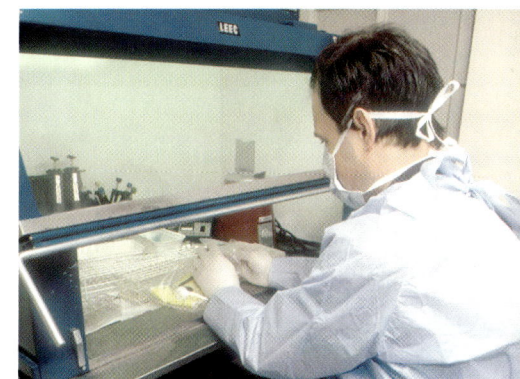

The initiative helped earn Donna Hilton the 'Outstanding Achievements with Youth Work' honour at the Action for Sick Children Awards. Donna is one of only a handful of dedicated hospital youth workers in this country.

In March 2000 Chief Executive Thelma Holland laid the foundation stone for a new £3m endoscopy centre. When it opened in 2001, it replaced the cramped and outdated facilities at the City Hospital for patients who suffer from bowel and stomach problems. And it enabled surgical, medical, diagnostic and outpatient facilities to be brought under one roof.

It was one of Miss Holland's last official ceremonies before leaving to

The People's Hospital

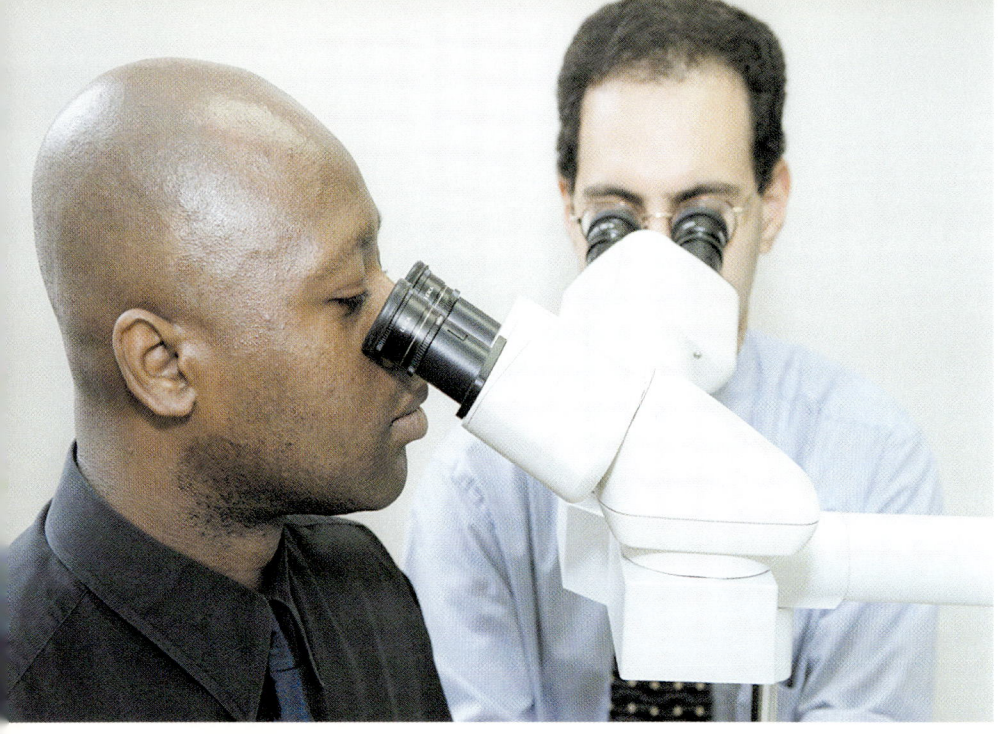

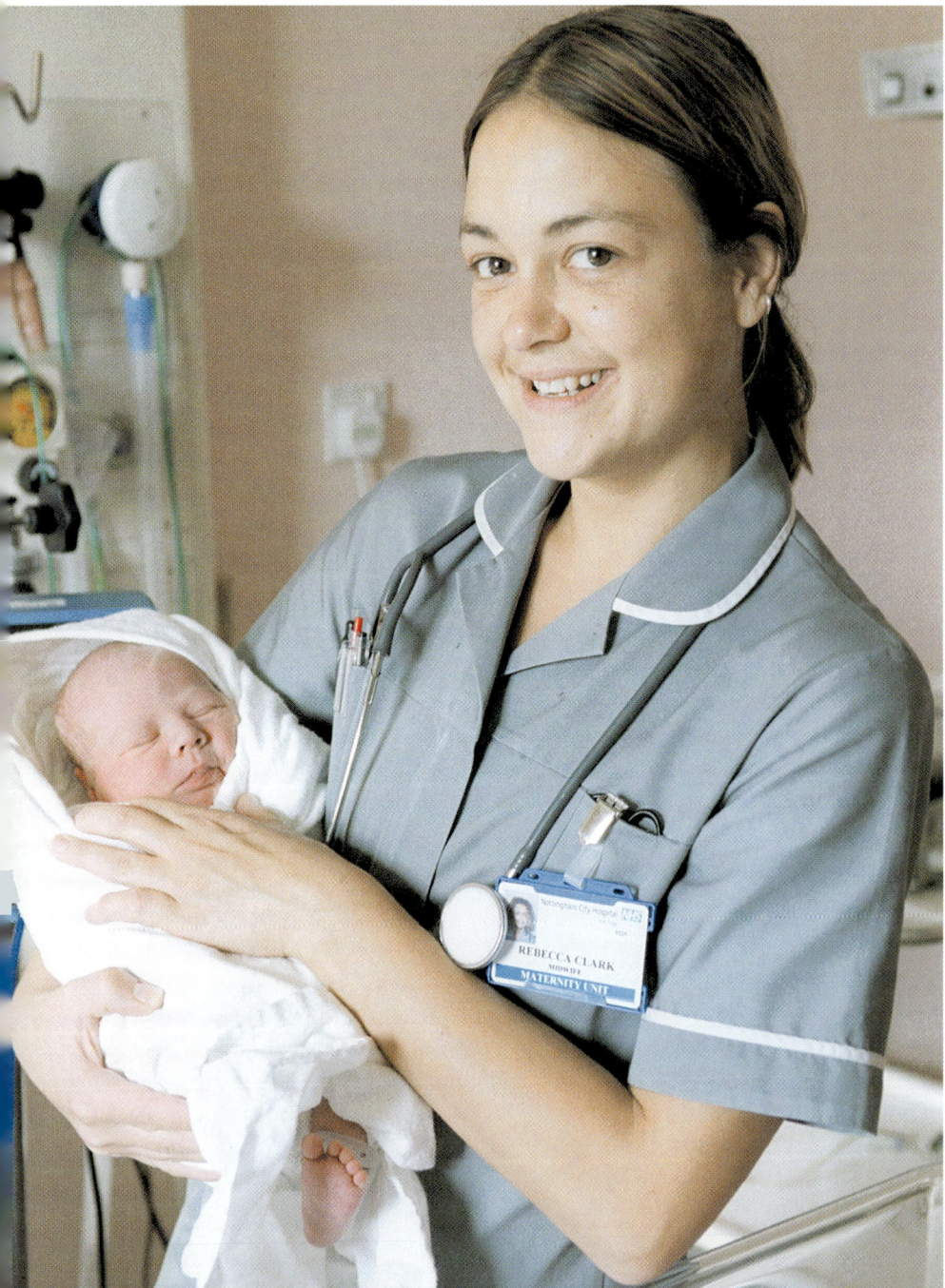

become Chief Executive of Cornwall and the Isles of Scilly Health Authority.

She said she had enjoyed 10 wonderful years at Nottingham City Hospital.

Gerry McSorley took over as the new boss. He had previously been Acting Chief Executive at the University Hospitals of Leicester Trust after being in charge of Derby City and Leicester General Hospital.

Talking about his new role he said: "There is enormous scope for the development of services in Nottingham as a whole, particularly in respect of the closer collaborative working style being cultivated between the City Hospital and Queen's Medical Centre, as well as the links with primary care and social services.

"The hospital is known by local people for its friendly atmosphere, yet it also commands respect as a large, dynamic, excellent teaching hospital, with a reputation for high-quality services and leading edge research."

Before handing over the reins Miss Holland had led the first steps towards closer links with Queen's Medical Centre.

The two trusts were planning to combine many of their acute services and her last job before leaving was to draft a report on proposed changes.

She said: "The new collaborative process between Nottingham City Hospital and the Queen's Medical Centre will lay the foundations for the city's hospital healthcare over coming years.

"Our two hospitals have developed a strong working partnership and we believe that this type of co-operation between us will ultimately lead to better care for our patients for many years to come."

New records were celebrated. In

Above: Two staff screening slides in the histopathology department
Left: Midwife Rebecca Clark cuddles one of the maternity unit's newest arrivals

The People's Hospital

2001 British medical history was made when a new technique for repairing heart valves using keyhole surgery was performed by Cardio Thoracic Surgeon David Richens at the City Hospital. In August 2002 Norman Parker became the hospital's 1,000th kidney transplant patient.

The hospital is a centre of excellence for children born with a cleft lip or palate. In October 2001, a six-month-old Romanian baby was flown to Nottingham for her initial operation to correct her cleft lip and palate. Burton Joyce couple Peter and Phyllis Sturgeon raised the money to bring tiny Cristina Cocor to this country for special treatment and hospital staff agreed to carry out the life-changing operation. The surgery was a great success, and just a few weeks later she returned home with her overjoyed parents to begin her new life.

The dedication and expertise in the operating theatre is mirrored in departments across the whole hospital. Every member of the team at Nottingham City Hospital makes a special contribution to the quality of care, and this evokes particular pride when they are recognised by people outside the trust. For example Vanessa Martin, cleft lip and palate Nurse Specialist, was named Nurse of the Year and waitress Maggie Landy was declared an 'Unsung Hero' for the first class service she has provided to staff, patients and visitors in the hospital restaurant and snack bars for the last 20 years. The hospital attracted positive, world-wide publicity after testing a pioneering 'bionic hand' on five young children who had no fingers of their own. It enabled them to do new tasks and an ongoing trial with an adult is producing very encouraging results.

More good news came in July 2002 when the Government confirmed a new £1m linear accelerator - used in the treatment of tumours - was coming to the City Hospital. It will replace an existing 10-year-old machine and is expected to be in service in 2004. The City Hospital has three linear accelerators which target high-energy radiation beams to destroy tumours. The hospital sees around 2,600 patients a year who receive treatment ranging from a single dose to up to seven weeks of daily treatment.

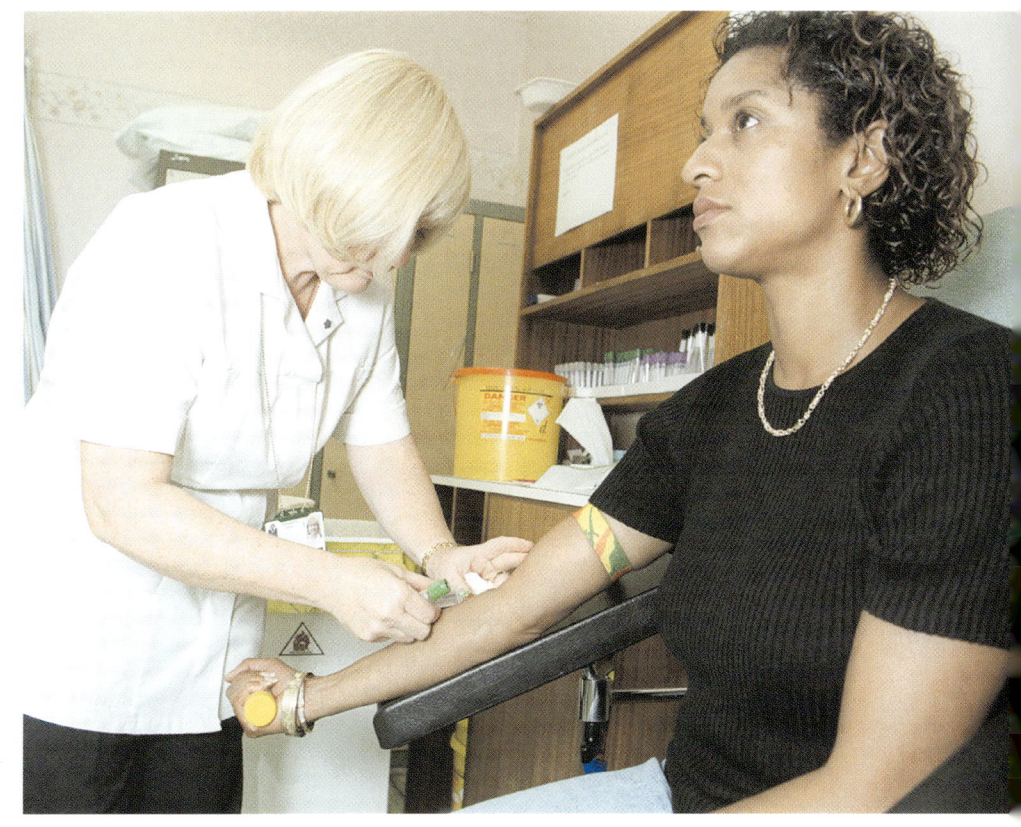

Kim Fell, Manager of the Nottingham Cancer Centre, said: "We are seeing a lot of investment in cancer services in Nottingham and that has to be good news for our patients. Demand for radiotherapy is increasing and patients need to start their treatment as quickly as they can in order to achieve the best results."

And in spring 2003, Nottingham City Hospital outlined an exciting package of revelopment to take place on the site, modernising services and replacing many of the outdated buildings to help staff provide the quality of care which is expected in the 21st century.

Proposals include reconfiguring services, providing care in different ways and improving the physical environment, while at the same time protecting the hospital's green areas

A patient gives a blood sample in the haematology department

and preserving the architectural and historical integrity of the site - and most importantly - the spirit of the people who work there.

If the scheme is approved it will be one of the largest capital projects in the region, with present estimates at around £500m. It will involve the complete redevelopment of large parts of the hospital, particularly focused on the North Corridor area, and will deliver much-needed additional capacity for inpatient beds and theatre facilities.

A dedicated emergency admissions unit is proposed to help manage the increasing number of patients who come to the hospital as emergencies and clinical and support services will be grouped together to make it easier for patients and staff to move between them.

It is appropriate that the hospital should choose to launch its proposals for the next 100 years of acute health care in Nottingham during the centenary, and these plans indicate that exciting times lie ahead.

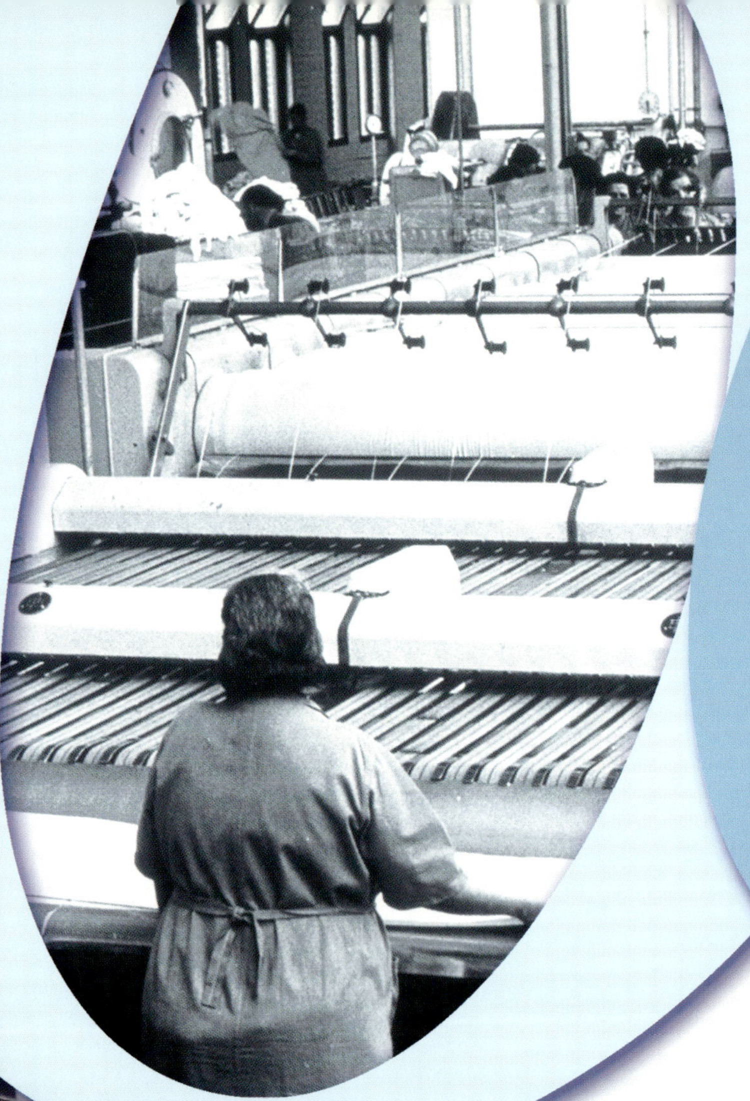
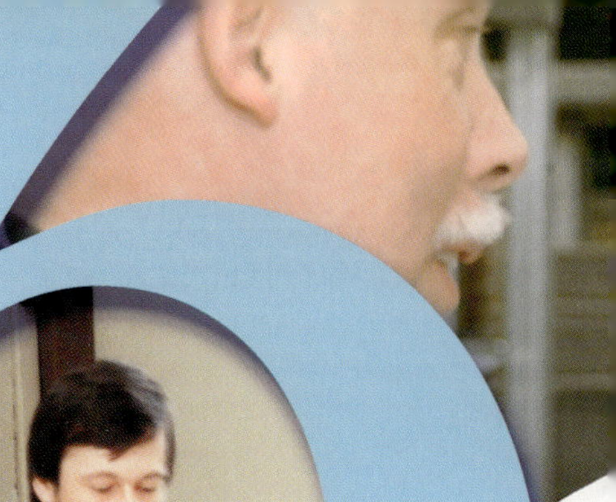
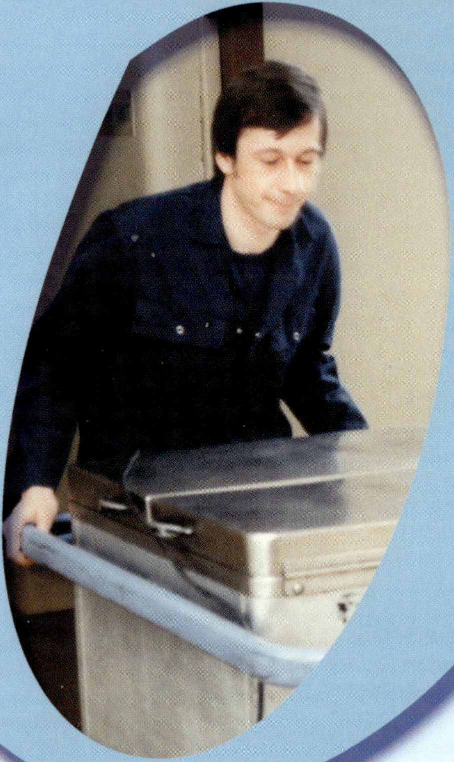
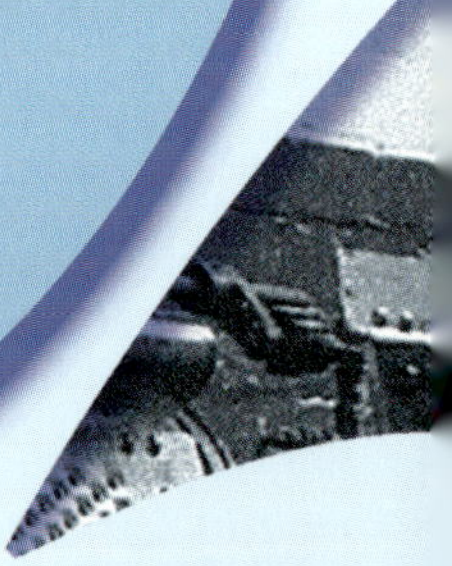
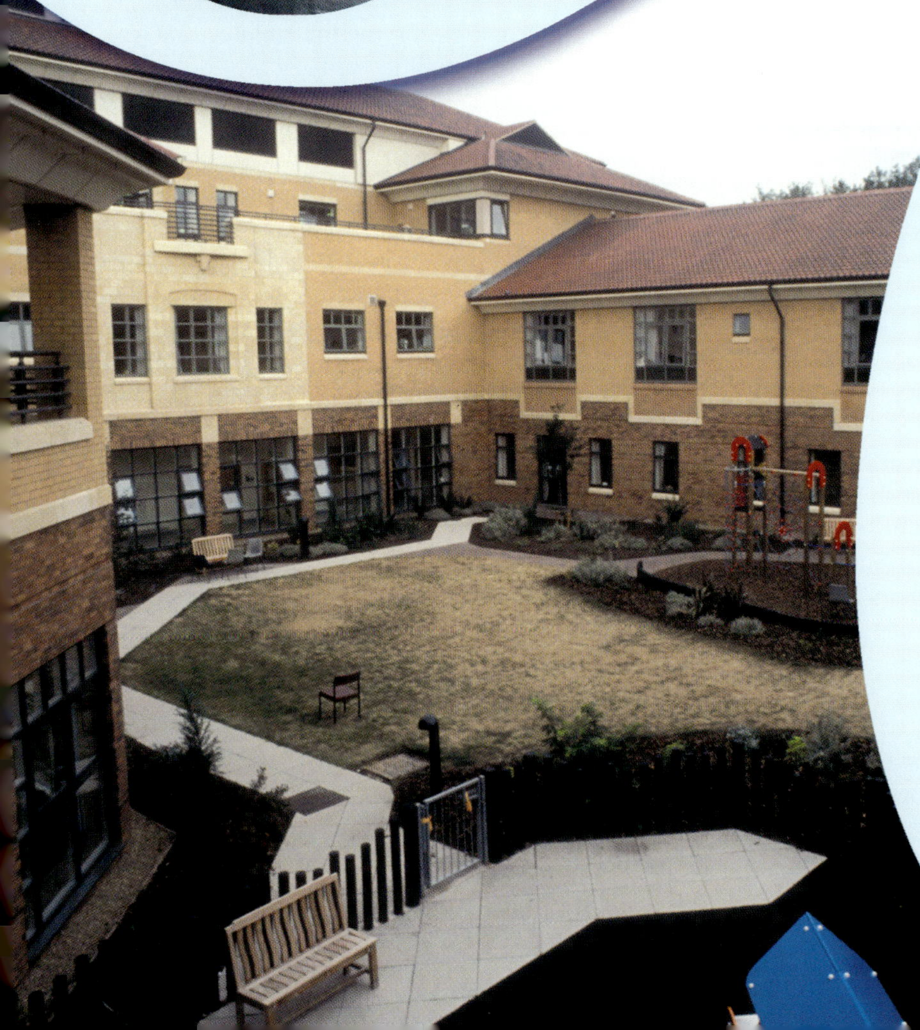
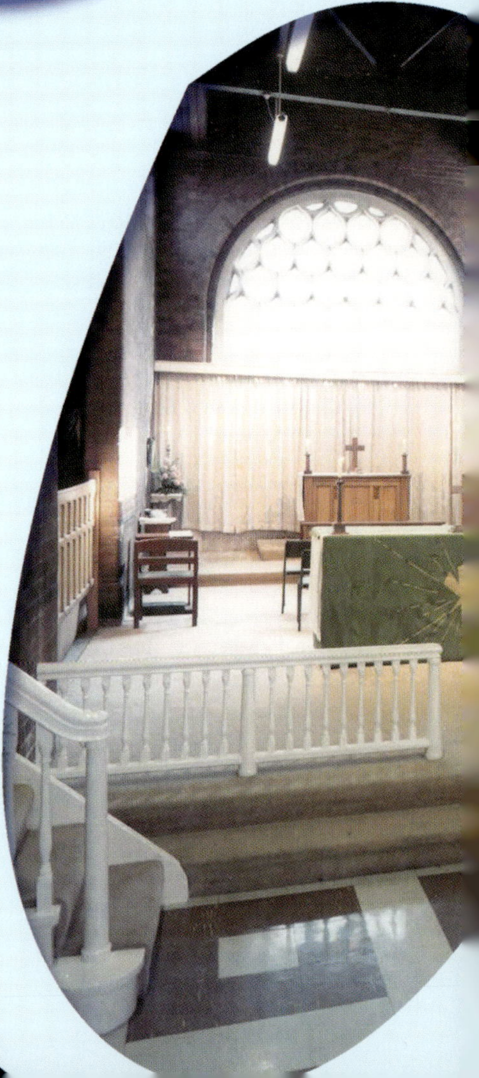

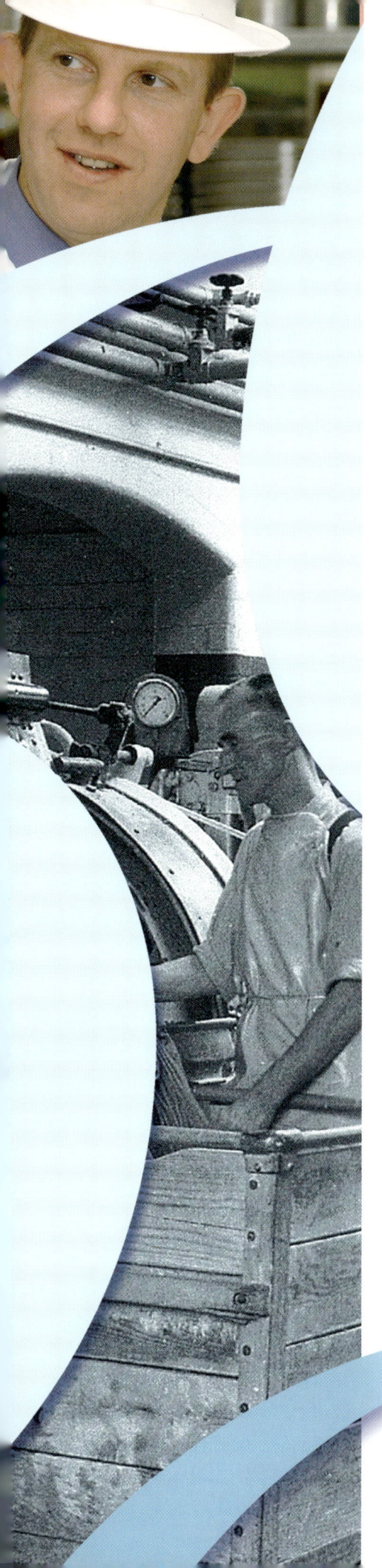

Support Services: A winning team

Working together to keep the wheels turning

A HUGE team effort by more than 5,700 people is involved in delivering high standard services at Nottingham City Hospital. While medical staff are very important and nurses form 50 per cent of the workforce, they cannot work in isolation. They cannot care for patients unless meals are being cooked, walls and floors cleaned, sheets laundered, investigations carried out and 1,001 other jobs are performed efficiently. This section turns the spotlight on some of the behind-the-scenes support services.

Sterile services

THE department supplies surgical equipment to all the City Hospital's operating theatres, as well as providing services for other local health organisations. Last year the department decontaminated 2.5m surgical instruments and distributed more than five million sterile items.

The department opened in 1954 when the twin theatre suites were brought into use. The two departments were directly linked for the supply and return of sterile packs of equipment, instruments and dressings by separate 'clean' and 'dirty' corridors.

In 1997 the team's high standards earned a European award - the first to be given to a major British hospital. It received the Lloyds Register of Quality Assurance award - recognising the quality of the management system, its procedures and written records.

The award was presented to the department's longest-serving staff members, Margaret Sorsby and Monica Swain, who between them have worked in sterile supplies for more than half a century.

Laundry

THE Sherwood laundry, an important feature of the hospital complex from its earliest days, developed over the years. The current laundry service was established in the 1970s when it was handling 250,000 items a week for health organisations locally and across the region. In the mid-1990s capital charges were introduced which compromised the laundry's ability to provide a competively priced service and many contracts were placed with other laundries, impacting on the cost effectiveness of the service.

Numerous other hospitals across the country have already closed their laundries and agreed contracts with external companies to provide their linen services. Nottingham City Hospital is probably one of the few trusts which continues to retain the facilities and skills in-house.

The laundry currently employs 46 staff who provide a washing and ironing service for Nottingham City Hospital (64,000 pieces of laundry each week) and a service for Nottinghamshire Healthcare Trust (10,000 pieces a week).

In July 2001, laundry staff received a big boost when the in-house team won the hospital's three-year washing and ironing contract against tough competition from private firms. The laundry, previously occupying a prime location in the middle of the campus, moved to a smaller building on the site at the end of 2002.

Administration and management

FROM 1948 until 1974, the City Hospital was managed by the Nottingham No 2 Hospital Management Committee, which was responsible for 10 hospitals. Committee members were appointed by the Regional Hospital Board based in Sheffield. All capital expenditure was controlled by the region, which itself was accountable directly to the Department of Health.

A supervisor and a member of staff at work in sterile services

A big reshuffle followed health service reorganisation in 1974 when the City Hospital became part of the North Nottingham Teaching District under the Nottinghamshire Area Health Authority. Roy Batterbury was appointed District Administrator and, according to Dr James Macfie, author of a City Hospital history, he brought a new enthusiasm to administration on the campus.

But there was much to do.

Reviewing the 13 years he spent on site from 1969 to 1982, Roy recalled: "Massive management changes were occurring at the same time as we were having to develop the City Hospital rapidly for its new teaching role. The style of management changed to what was known as consensus management in which any individual member of a district management team could object to decisions taken by the team by referring it to the area authority. A district management team comprised the district nurse, the chairman of the medical staff, the district medical officer, a university representative, the district treasurer and the district administrator.

"Until 1969 only two capital developments of any note had been completed since 1948 - the extension to the outpatients department and a new twin operating theatre block.

"But planning had begun in the late 1960s for a new 160-bed maternity unit and a new physiotherapy department which were built in the early 1970s.

"All the wards required serious upgrading. Acute beds were based in the three original buildings of the workhouse infirmary and the obstetric department was mostly housed in First World War huts.

"Sherwood housed the beds for older people and in the early 1970s Heathfield Hospital (the original isolation hospital) was still being partly used for a few TB patients and some dermatology beds.

"Between 1971 and 1973 discussions took place at regional and national level over the development of a major ward block to replace the

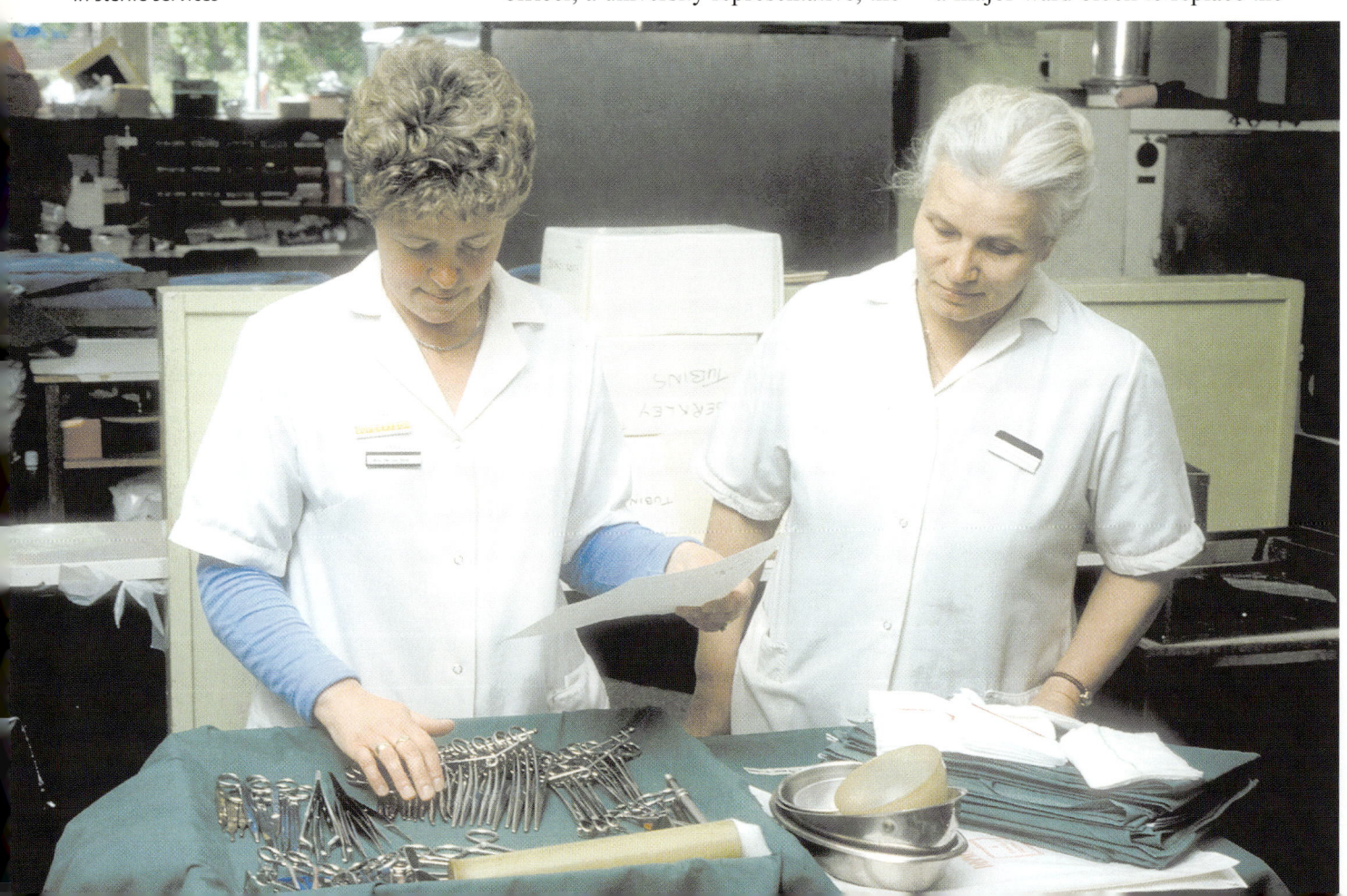

The People's Hospital

very inadequate accommodation for plastic surgery and burns services, the renal services and paediatric services, including paediatric surgery. The new facilities were opened in 1979.

"The first phase of a new radiology department was planned and built during this period and planning commenced on the replacement of the facilities for histopathology and cytology services, including a new mortuary. These facilities were opened in the early 1980s.

"Medicine does not stand still and so often current workloads outstrip facilities, especially those which have been converted from old buildings some years ago. Modern developments can provide for expansion as long as the site chosen for such developments permits this.

"The old workhouse bed blocks in Sherwood Hospital, now integrated as City Hospital (South Corridor), were being replaced and the new oncology department in the 1990s enabled the remaining two blocks to be demolished. These old wards had been a painful reminder to many older people of an obsolete regime.

"Other clinical-related developments also took place including expanded accommodation for other pathology services such as haematology, biochemistry and immunology. Facilities for a department of medical genetics were also developed.

"Staff deserve the highest praise for their efforts and co-operation in coping with the difficulties arising from the new building and conversions while providing a first class service to the patients."

Finance

THE hospital's finances were originally conducted by the Board of Guardians, then by the City Treasurer's Department. From 1948 to 1974 No 2 Hospital Management Committee had its own finance department in Sherwood Hospital. These responsibilities were then taken over by Nottinghamshire Area Health Authority, although services for the City group of hospitals continued to be based in offices at Sherwood HQ.

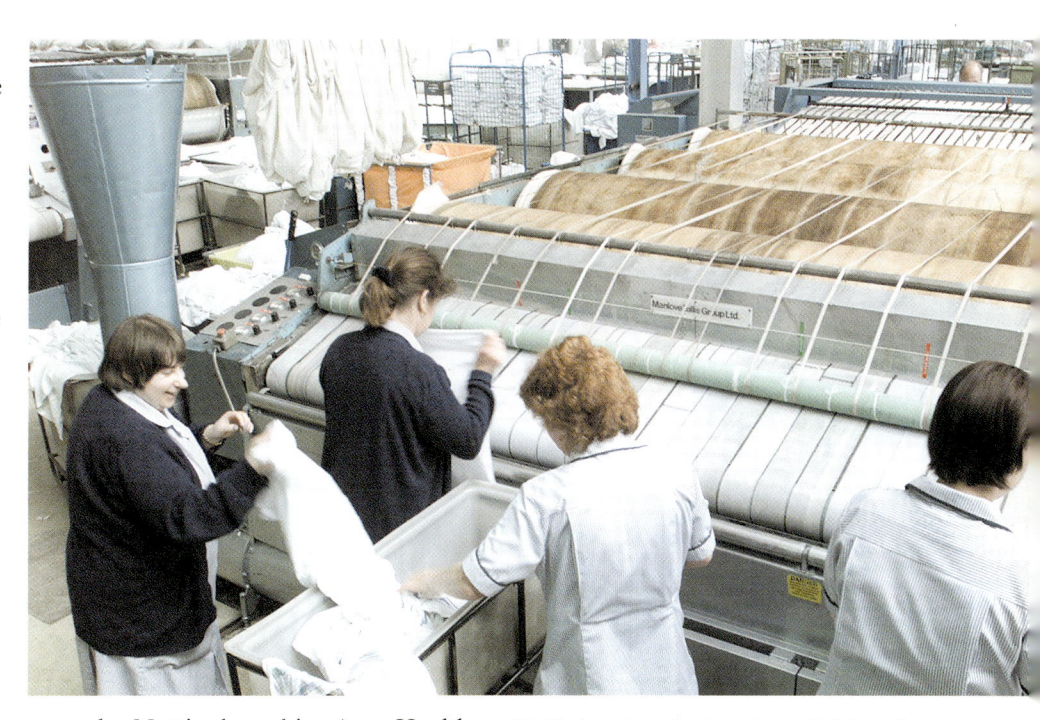

This period saw completion of the transition from manual methods of accounting to the use of local computer terminal facilities linked to the regional main frame computer. In 1982 the new District Health Authority took over and this continued until 1992 when the hospital achieved Trust status and financial services were transferred to a team of staff based on the hospital site. Since then the finance department - currently based in accommodation at St Francis - has continued to provide a high quality service to the Trust.

It is now a modern, forward-looking department which has a programme of professional and NVQ training for staff. It also acts as host trust to the Nottinghamshire Consortium for the National Financial Management Training Scheme. Each year the Trust produces an annual report which outlines the achievements of the past year and presents the accounts which has always been produced within the deadline and received an unqualified opinion.

Staff at work in the laundry, which handles over 70,000 items a week

Information, communication technology services

THE hospital's ICT department recently celebrated its birthday as the service notched up its first decade.

The department's first project was originally called the Hospital Information Support System (HISS). Nottingham City Hospital was one of only three hospitals chosen nationally to host the HISS project. HISS meant that for the first time patient information was stored on a central computer database rather than being spread over many different computer systems across the site.

When the first part of the system went live in July 1992, the network was the largest of its type in the NHS, supporting several hundred terminals and printers. Next came the 5 Unix based Pyramid computer systems, which hosted the Uniplex office automation package.

Uniplex went live shortly afterwards, and provided a common word processing package and email facility to users across the site. The HISS patient database came on-stream in March 1993 and still forms the backbone of today's main patient database.

Since 1992 the network and main computer systems have all been replaced, and of the original staff that were based at Heathfield House 10 years ago, only six remain. Today a gigabyte per second network replaces the original network, PCs and Winterms are replacing the older terminals, and the original Pyramid computer systems have been replaced by Siemens Unix systems to host the main patient database. There are also a growing number of NT servers, which also support email, patient based systems and internet/intranet access.

In the future ICT at the hospital is set to change again, as the service merges with that at the Queen's Medical Centre. This will provide a unified strategy for both hospitals, which will deliver value and consistency in patient care information systems for the future.

Matron's maid

IN the early days of the NHS, hospital matrons were expected to live on site. Their accommodation ranged from purpose-built properties to a suite of rooms, say in Sherwood Nurses' Home.

They also had accommodation within the hospital, including an office and a sitting room, where VIP visitors would be seen. Early plans for the hospital HQ show matron's sitting room and bathroom.

Matrons also had the support of two maids. When a maid had a day off, her opposite number worked a long day to ensure that coal fires were laid, early morning tea, breakfast, lunch, afternoon tea and dinner were served. Maids also did matron's laundry and ran errands.

If matron had a dog, it was walked by the maid and the dog's special dietary requirements were met by the Sherwood kitchen.

Matron's maids also lived on site. Although they did not have the same standard of accommodation usually afforded to the matron, resident maids did have their own dining room where their meals were served. There were separate dining rooms for doctors, sisters and nurses - and often silverware was provided for the sisters and doctors!

Cleaning services

THE second largest staff group to nurses in the hospital are the staff who provide the cleaning services. Each week the equivalent of 142,000 square metres are cleaned. Over the years there have been many changes. Today's cleaning technology includes ride-on machines that can scrub and burnish floors. Years ago, much of this would have been carried out on hands and knees with a scrubbing brush and bucket.

Over the years, professional qualifications have become available for staff. It is also worth noting that cleaning staff at ward level and the ward waiters/waitresses who serve patient meals, are valued by the patients for the contribution they make towards improving the patients' environment and experience.

The important role cleaning staff play at ward level is recognised in the recently published NHS Cleaning Standards.

Hotel Services receive many letters of appreciation from patients, naming individuals who have gone the extra mile and always enjoy passing the time of day with the support staff while carrying out their work.

Left: Patient escorts outside the North Corridor main entrance

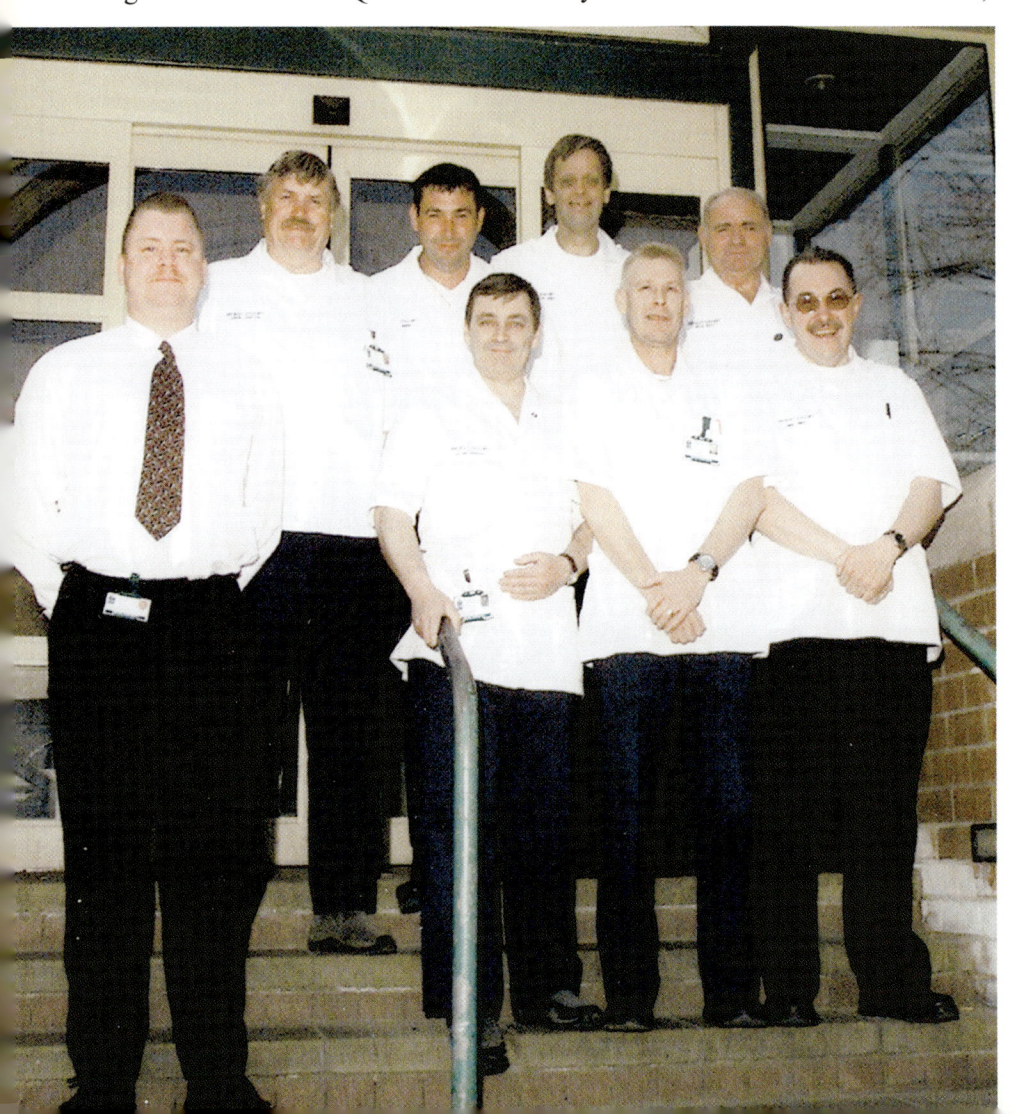

The People's Hospital

The porters/patient escorts

THE job of the hospital porter has come a long way since the days when the job meant being the guardians of the gate to the workhouse and infirmary. Today the change of title to patient escort reflects that the job is now more patient-orientated.

Once the patient has been seen by the doctors and nurses and it's time for them to be either taken to the X-ray department for further investigations or to be admitted onto a ward, the hospital porters are called in. It's their duty to see the patient safely escorted, either in a wheelchair, on a trolley or a bed, to wherever the patient is next required.

It used to be said the hospital porter was a jack of all trades. Before the logistics department was established to deal with all non-patient movement, the porter was required to do all the manual jobs.

This could involve clearing out doctors' and nurses' residences before they were re-decorated, taking meal trolleys to wards from the hospital kitchens, removing confidential waste from offices, removing patients' case notes from secretaries' offices as well as escorting patients to and from wards and departments.

Porters see life at the sharp end, resulting in a wealth of funny stories, experiences and anecdotes.

They retrieve expectant fathers who have fainted in the maternity unit delivery rooms. And one day they rescued a consultant who had fallen into the swill bin on the hospital's North Corridor.

And they still talk about the Saturday in November 1998 when 23 members of the portering staff won £1.9m on the National Lottery, which shared between them all amounted to £78,500 each.

Local and national media went into a frenzy with stories about porters being woken to be given the good news. In fact the adrenalin rush after 8pm that evening was so great that many couldn't sleep.

However it did make the return to work on the Monday morning a very happy experience. Other members of the hospital staff were very complimentary about their good fortune, and strangely enough not one member of the portering staff was off sick that day.

The actor Kevin Lloyd, playing DC Tosh Lines in *The Bill*, once said: "If you want to know the way around a hospital, don't ask the nurses, ask the porters."

This is true and one thing is certain. Whatever changes are made to the hospital the porters will always be needed.

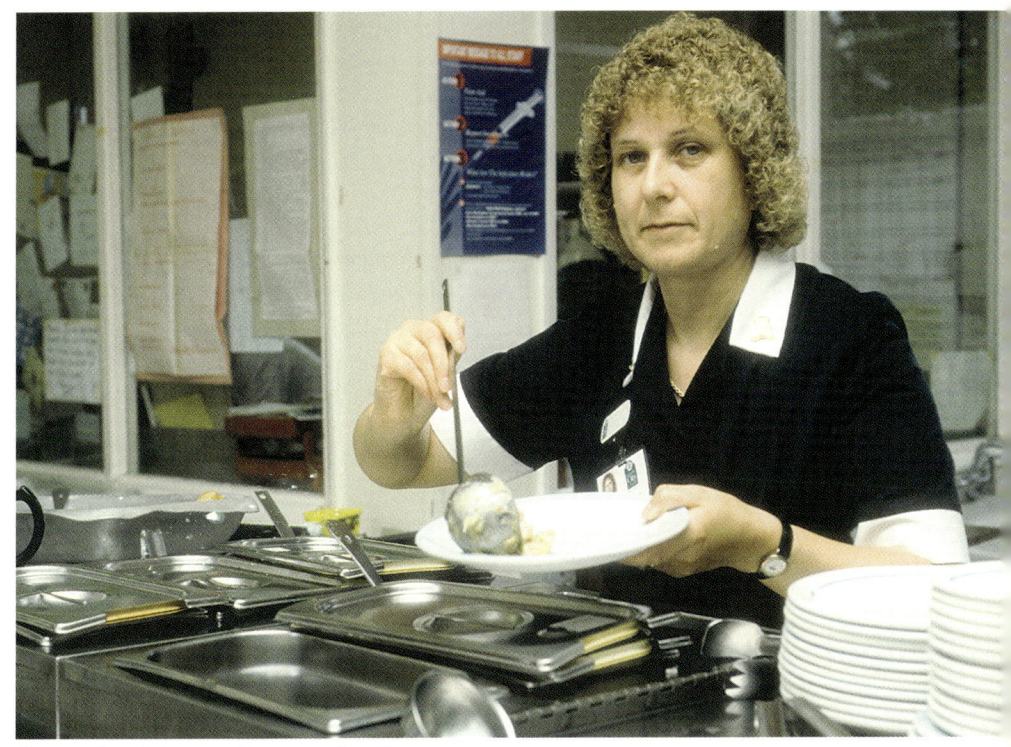

Above: *Lunch is served by a ward waitress*
Right: *Catering Manager John Hughes (right) discusses the menu of the day with Chef*

Catering services

HOSPITAL food is an important part of a patient's care. When the workhouse and infirmary opened 100 years ago, breakfast was a bowl of gruel and dinner was bread and cheese or suet pudding. Now the Nottingham City Hospital catering staff aim to tickle the patient's tastebuds. Today's typical main meal could include braised lamb in cider with parsley dumplings, seafood pasta and butterscotch tart.

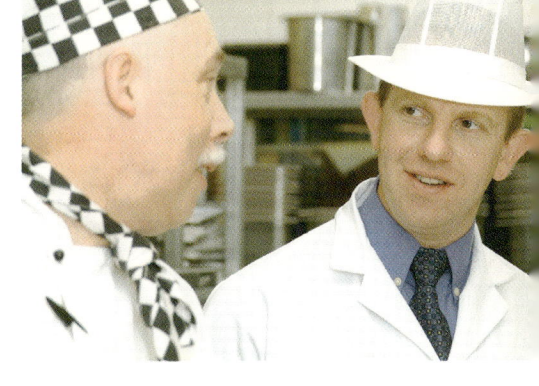

The national NHS menu provides a welcome and tantalising variety of dishes, which have proved popular with both patients and staff. The catering department works closely with doctors, nurses and therapists to get the right balance when preparing menus. Dishes are created with vegetarian and cultural needs in mind and the emphasis is on nutritional value for patients who are feeling unwell.

Catering Manager John Hughes says: "Food is a really important part of the care we give to patients during their stay and there is evidence to show that it plays an integral role in their rate of recovery. We have carried out a lot of work to improve the choice, variety and availability of meals for patients."

A new staff dining room, known as the City Side Restaurant, was opened in 1992. About £120,000 was spent turning the 1970s-style canteen into one of the country's best hospital restaurants, incorporating a carvery and self-service counter for staff, patents and visitors. The former staff canteen is now in use as a cardiac surgery training unit.

Until about 10 years ago, the catering department provided an on-site butchery service to ensure the provision of meat to the hospital's food production kitchen. Two qualified butchers were needed to provide this service. In earlier years the hospital had its own farm, where vegetables were grown and pigs were kept. Indeed the Whitley Council section for Ancillary Staff Allowances, has an allowance for the slaughter of animals.

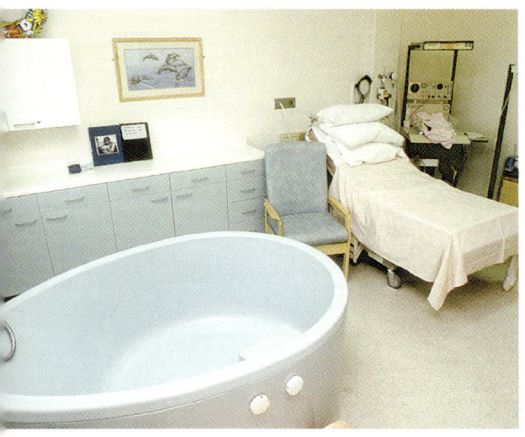

Patient Hotel

THE Patient Hotel was opened in November 1994. Based on a Swedish concept, it was the first purpose-built patient hotel in the UK.

The hotel accommodates patients who do not require the full facilities of a ward but need less intrusive care in safe, secure, restful surroundings. Some of the 52 rooms are twin or family rooms.

The maternity department reserves rooms for mothers who have had a straightforward pregnancy and delivery. Midwives are based in the hotel to look after these mothers and babies during their stay.

Left and below: Two rooms in the Patient Hotel

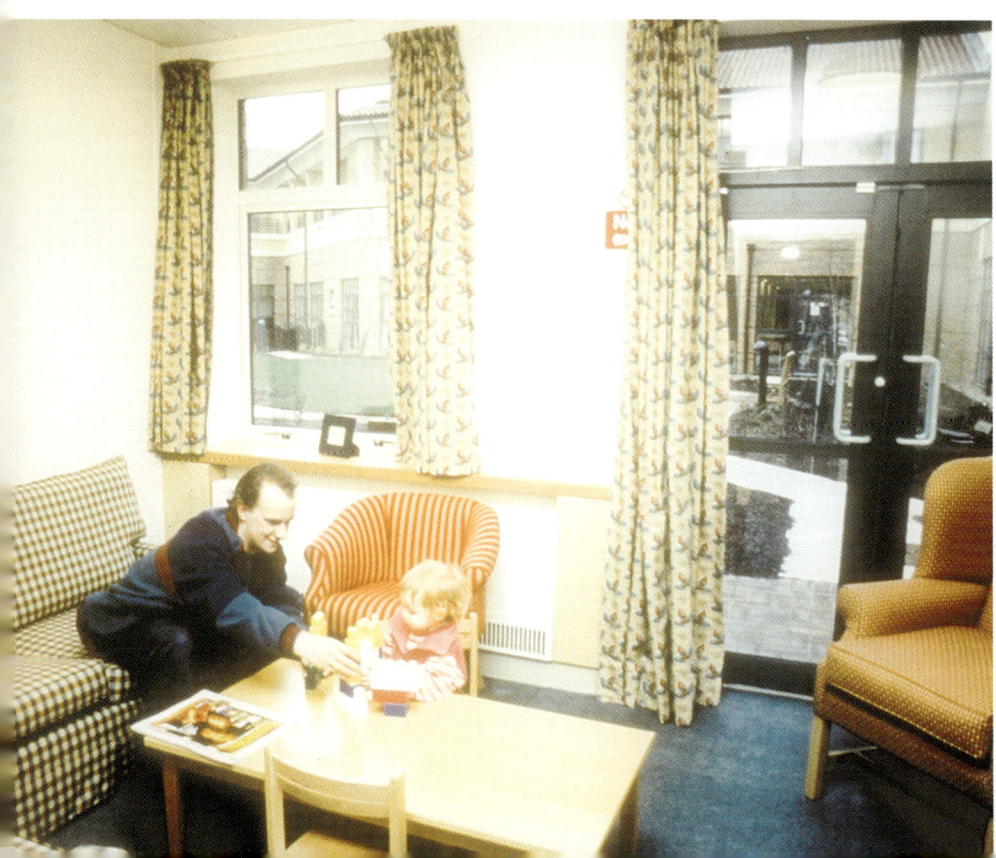

Patients are also referred from several other wards and departments within the hospital - in fact any patient may be referred from any department as long as they are able to take care of themselves within the hotel environment. A registered general nurse (RGN) co-ordinator is based in the reception area 24 hours a day to assess patients' suitability for admission and to monitor their health during their stay. The hotel also accommodates relatives of patients who may be in the hospital or people attending courses.

The hotel is a self-contained department with its own licensed restaurant, kitchen and catering team, comprising chefs, catering assistants and kitchen assistants. There is also a team of housekeepers, and a reception team comprising the RGN co-ordinators, administration and clerical staff and hotel assistants.

Property services

PROPERTY services have come a long way since estates department staff issued half candles to wards during power cuts.

That was the contingency policy during and after the Second World War when the hospital used to generate its own electricity.

Technical supervisor John Chambers, who retired in 2002 after nearly 30 years service, was told the story by a colleague when he joined the department.

John said: "If the supply failed, the wards were issued with half a candle each. Once power was restored they were collected up again."

Much of the hospital remained on DC electricity supply until 1952. It meant, for example, that if portable X-rays had to be carried out in some wards, a bulky rotary convertor had to travel with the X-ray machine. Special lines also had to be rigged up to operate the mechanical respirators.

John recalls that until the 1970s, sub-station five was based in what is now the fitters' workshop. In the event

The People's Hospital

of a power cut, estates staff had to run back to that area to manually make the changeover.

In the early days the hospital grew most of its own vegetables, kept pigs and employed its own butcher. John also remembers the times when five barbers were kept busy on site giving haircuts to longer stay patients on the campus.

One of the major on-site engineering improvements was commissioning a new dual fuel boilerhouse around 1973.

Local housewives often grumbled that the hospital's 170ft boiler house chimney was the reason for smuts on their washing - until three demolition workers spent more than a month in 1981 taking down the 250-ton landmark brick by brick.

Now property services employs 90 staff and is responsible for the maintenance of vital, high-tech services in a vast array of buildings across an ever developing site. Innovations and improvements are continually in progress.

Ambulance service

EVERY day hundreds of people travel to and from Nottingham City Hospital by ambulance to attend day centres, outpatient clinics or benefit from the extended hours dialysis service.

The ambulance liaison point in the outpatient department was introduced about 20 years ago in response to the growing number of patients needing ambulance transport. Five liaison staff take bookings from outpatient clinics and organise this vital support service.

Chaplaincy

WHEN the hospital church opened in 1902, all mobile residents and patients were obliged to attend services on Sundays and Saints Days. Baptisms were a regular event - there were 86 alone in 1904. Up to 1939 the Church of England, Free Church and Roman Catholic chaplains were all part-time. In 1939 a Free Church chaplain was appointed to serve the institute and infirmary. This appointment became full-time after 1971 and the Church of England chaplaincy became full-time in 1944.

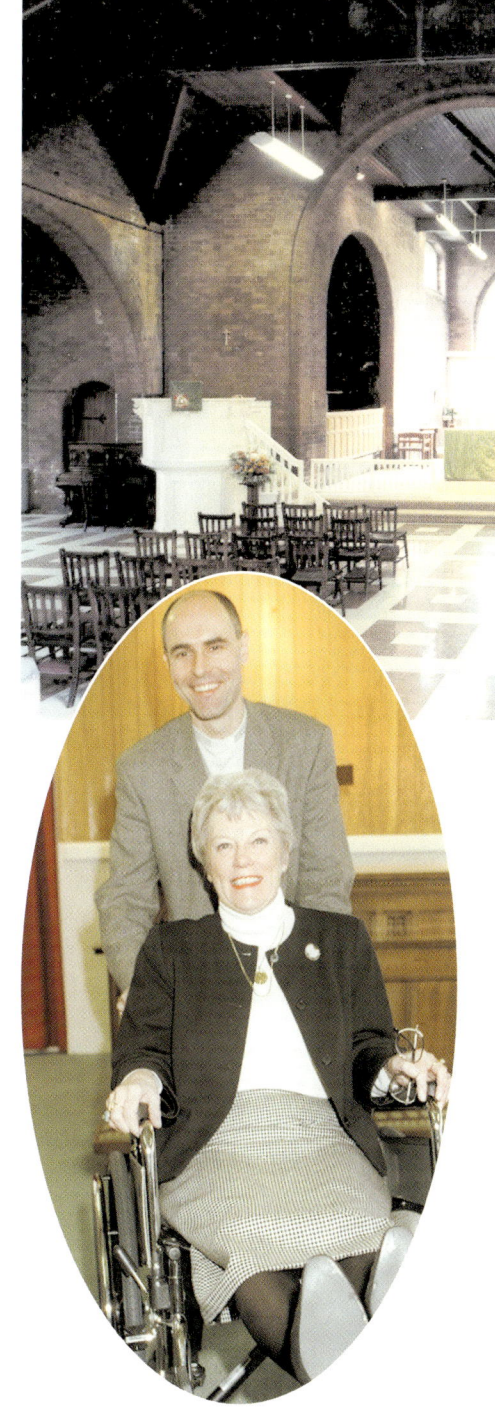

Carol singing was much appreciated as nurses, doctors and chaplains visited the wards with lighted lanterns on Christmas Eve. Attendances at services fell over the years, particularly after compulsory attendance was stopped, and in 1975 the church was renovated, reduced in size and had central heating and better lighting installed. It was officially named the Hospital Church of St Luke in 1978. The Archdeacon of Nottingham the Venerable Roy Williamson, who later became a Bishop, re-dedicated the church and gifts, including a restored painting given in 1904 by Mrs Mary Thorpe when she retired from the Nottingham Board of Guardians. The hospital church has been closed since June 1988.

Today a team of chaplains (four of them are full-time) and volunteers enable individuals and groups to respond to spiritual and emotional needs generated by experiences of life and death, illness and injury. They offer counselling, pastoral support and religious services, as well as inputs to training and to ethical issues.

Above: A view of the hospital church
Left: Senior Chaplain the Rev Martin Kerry is pictured with Joan Westwood, a member of the Nottingham and District Blood Donors Association, who presented two wheelchairs to the hospital in 1997

7

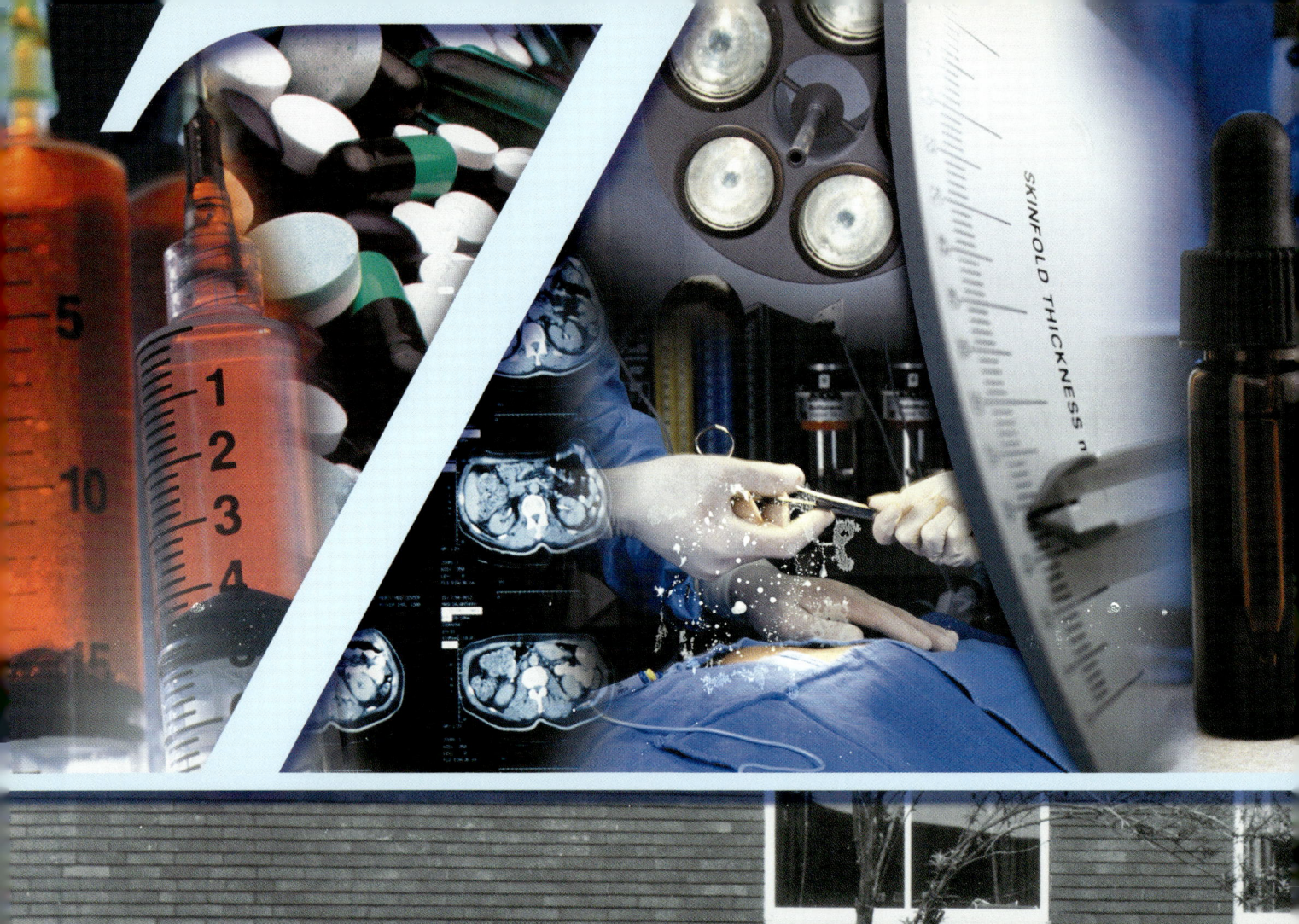

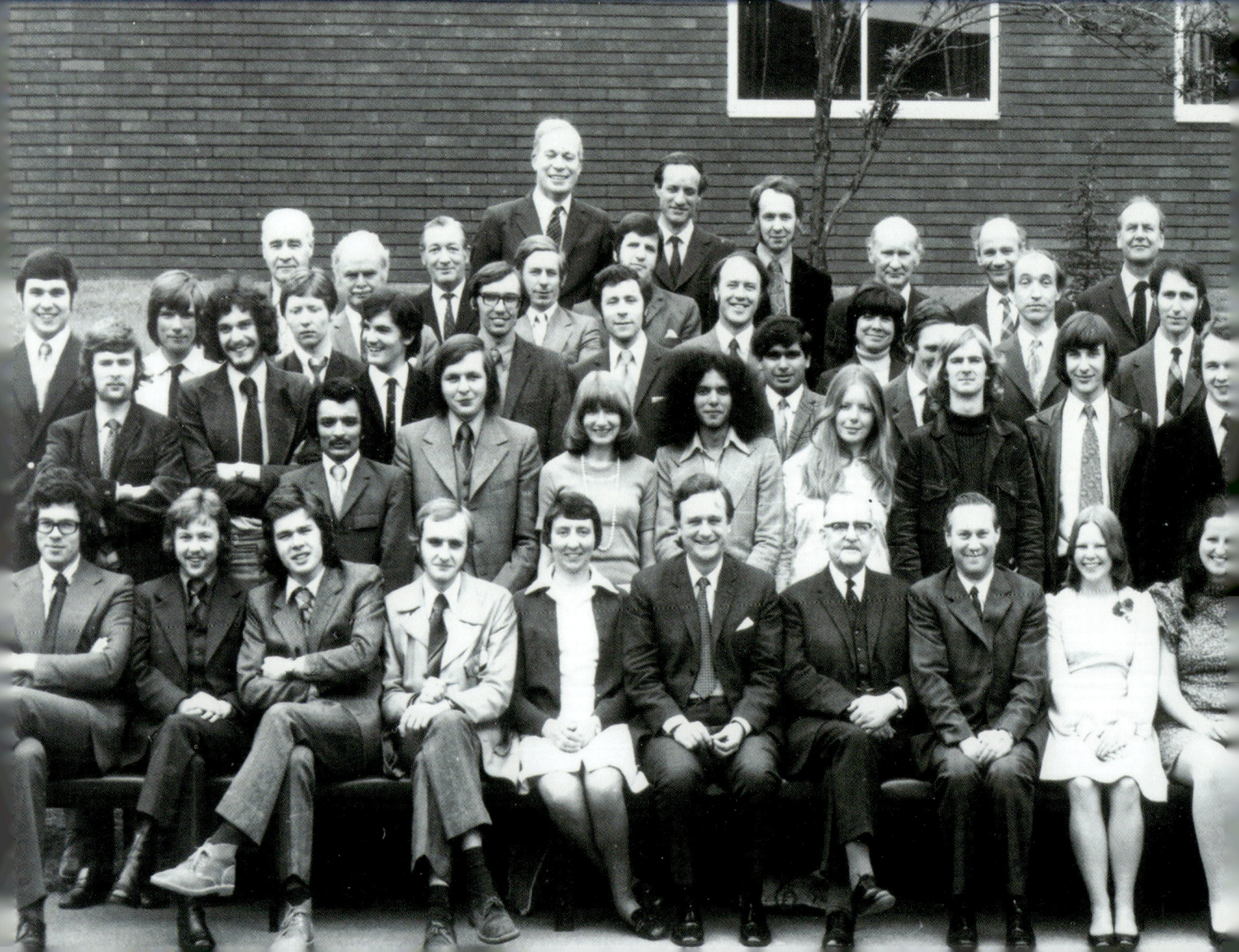

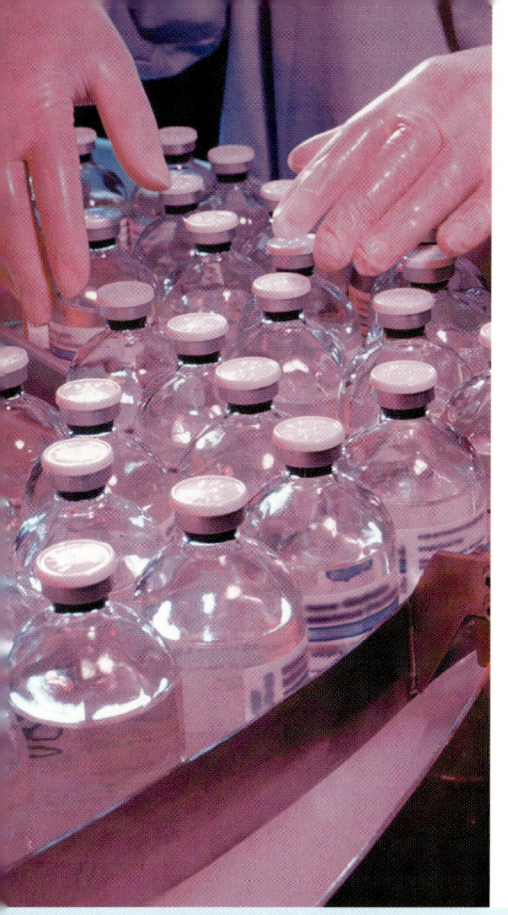

Medical training: major benefits for everyone

Integrated approach to education brings real gains to patients, students and services

By Robert Graham, Roy Batterbury and Professor Anne Tattersfield

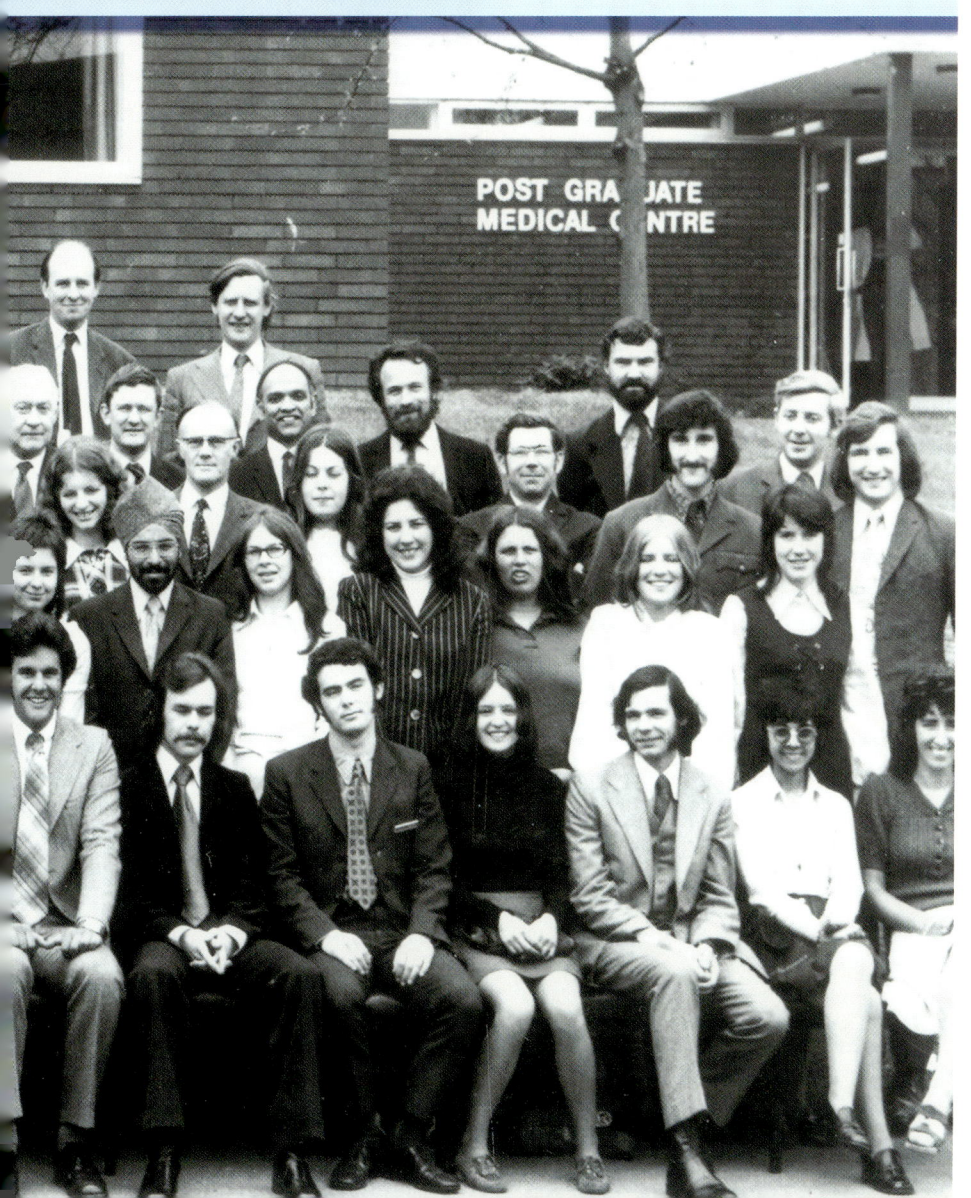

THE Government announcement in the mid 1960s that an integrated hospital and medical school would be established in Nottingham brought a flurry of activity. The first students entered the Medical School in 1970 and were housed in temporary accommodation on the University of Nottingham campus. They were due to start their clinical training and ward practice three years later in 1973.

But the delay in the building and completion of the University Hospital meant the City Hospital would play a much larger part in the training of clinical students than originally envisaged.

Facilities at both the General and City hospitals urgently needed to be developed and planning and liaison between the various parties was intense. Foundation Chairs for the new Medical School were filled and additional consultants appointed. Malcolm Symonds, Foundation Professor of Obstetrics and Gynaecology and David Hull, Foundation Professor of Child Health, moved into the new professorial suite

Left: *The first group of 44 clinical students with some of their teachers outside the Post Graduate Medical Centre in April 1973*

in the City Hospital maternity unit in 1972.

The first group of 44 clinical students arrived on the City Hospital campus in April 1973. They assembled in the lecture theatre in the Post Graduate Centre with their teachers - and the first clinical course was under way. All consultant staff in Nottingham were appointed part-time clinical tutors and the University doctors became honorary NHS clinicians. This integration of academic and clinical medicine had great benefits for patients, students and the development of services.

For the first 10 years the bulk of clinical teaching was shared between the City and General Hospital. As clinical departments moved into the University Hospital in the early 1980s so the City's share of the total teaching load dropped. This created a feeling of some resentment, particularly when child health, obstetrics and gynaecology, microbiology and therapeutics moved to their custom-designed accommodation at the University Hospital as foreseen in the Pickering Report of 1965. Fortunately this feeling was fairly short-lived. Professor Tom Arie, Foundation Professor of Health Care of the Elderly, established his department in the City Hospital for several years. Roger Blamey had already moved to the City Hospital and Professor Anne Tattersfield joined the staff as Foundation Professor of Respiratory Medicine in 1984.

Robert Graham, former Registrar of the Medical School, recalls: "The role of the City Hospital in acting as 'midwife' to several clinical departments in the earliest years of the Medical School was critical to the success of the School. The City has continued to provide superb clinical teaching support and all the developments in the academic staff and facilities at the hospital since I retired 10 years ago bear witness to the fact. It is very much a large teaching hospital in its own right."

Today there are between 65 and 91 students on the City Hospital campus at any one time and the Medical School intake is now 250 a year.

Professor Tattersfield says: "Many specialist areas and services are based at the City Hospital so that students can obtain experience here, for example, dialysis and renal medicine, cystic fibrosis, thoracic and cardiac surgery, dedicated hospice care within a hospital, haematology (particularly leukaemia and lymphoma), rheumatology, medical oncology and radiotherapy.

"Facilities for teaching improved in 1998 with the opening of the new Clinical Sciences Building. Teaching has changed over the years. There are more students but smaller groups. There is more focus on attitudes, communication, problem solving, personal and professional development, reflective learning, more interactive teaching, more continuous assessment and increased objectivity in examinations."

A pleasing aspect is the close collaboration that now exists between the City Hospital and the Queen's Medical Centre. This partnership, building on each other's strengths and fostering a co-ordinated approach towards the development of skills and services, will ensure patients can look forward to better local NHS care and treatment in the future.

Post Graduate Education Centre

By Professor Roger Cotton, Professor John Fletcher and Dr David Banks

LONG before the advent of the Medical School, post graduate teaching was well established in Nottingham. Credit for that must go to Consultant Physician Dr James Macfie and Orthopaedic Surgeon Mr Peter Jackson. 'Grand rounds' instituted by Dr Macfie in the late 1960s and held anywhere in the hospital that could accommodate the

Left: *Medical students taking part in a sponsored bed push*

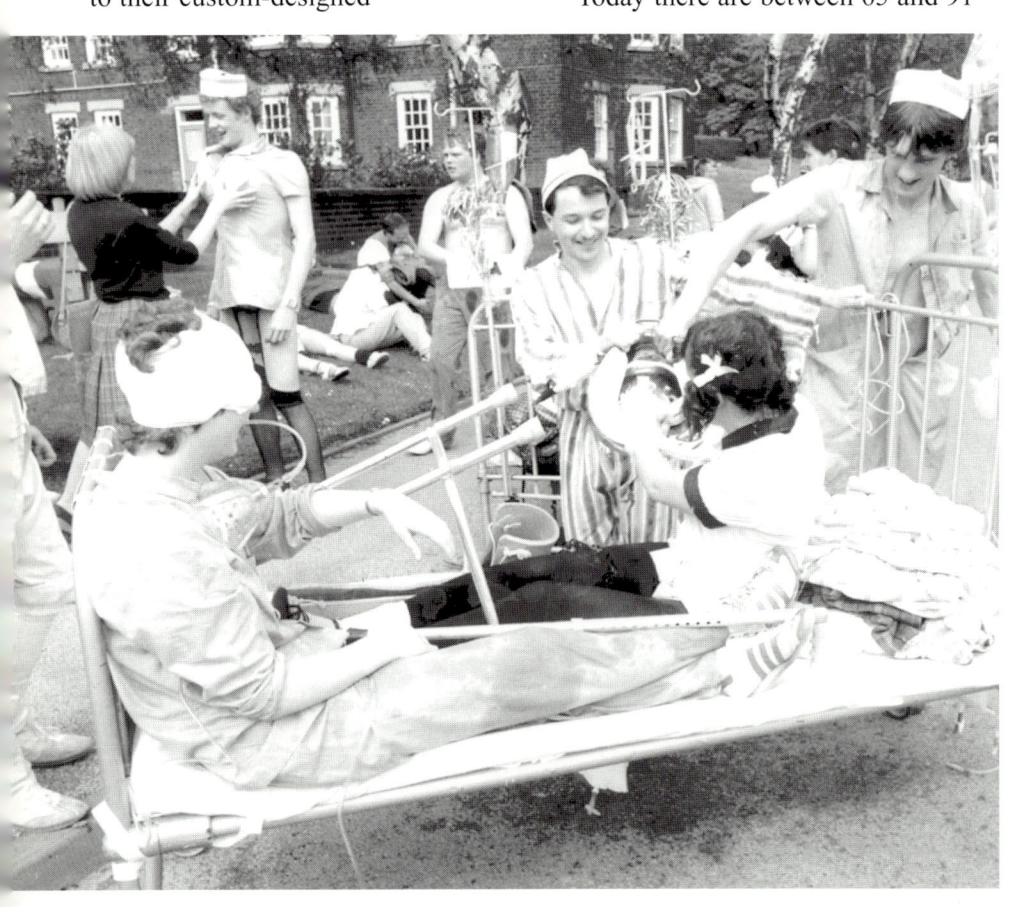

The People's Hospital

assembly, allowed cases to be discussed.

Professor John Fletcher recalled: "James Macfie had taken upon himself responsibility for what is now called 'continuing medical education.' He organised a Wednesday morning grand round for hospital staff with an occasional invited speaker. He also organised a Sunday morning session for general practitioners which counted towards their seniority payments.

"The GPs were required to sign an attendance book that James refused to put out until the end of the meeting. If it contained names of doctors whom he knew had not been at the meeting he would write to them asking for their opinion about what they had (not) learned. James' contribution to medical education was later recognised by the university when he was awarded an honorary doctorate degree."

Professor Roger Cotton recalled that pathology sessions, which included 'puzzle of the week', were added later and they were an early form of clinical audit because the pathologists could show any abnormalities present.

The new Medical School attracted a large number of young, bright doctors, who needed to pass post graduate diploma examinations to progress their careers. Many members of the senior staff helped them by organising clinical teaching sessions. For many years no junior doctor left the City Hospital without a higher diploma - a remarkable achievement as the overall pass rate was of the order of 30%.

The Post Graduate Education Centre was opened in 1972 with joint funding from the Nottingham Medico-Chirurgical Society, local doctors and the Regional Health Authority. This allowed the 'grand round' to have a permanent home. Purpose-built as a Nottingham district-wide facility for the teaching of dental and medical staff, including general practitioners and hospital doctors, it later came under the direct supervision of the City Hospital.

Key figures in getting the project off the ground were Dr (later Professor) Roger Cotton, Dr Ian McCallum (Dermatologist and subsequently a Chairman of North Nottingham District Medical Committee) and Mr Harold Malkin (retired Consultant Obstetrician), who chaired the relevant committees.

Some favoured the centre being built near the General Hospital but the committee convinced regional officers that the City Hospital was a much better site. Subsequent events proved this was a good decision and an appropriate one following the post graduate educational initiative taken by City Hospital consultant staff. It had an enormous impact on changing of attitudes about the City Hospital. The Medico-Chirurgical Society voted to move its operations from St James' Street into the new centre, where it could maintain its independence and a room was allocated for its sole use.

The centre was opened by the then Vice Chancellor of the University of Nottingham, Professor John Butterfield.

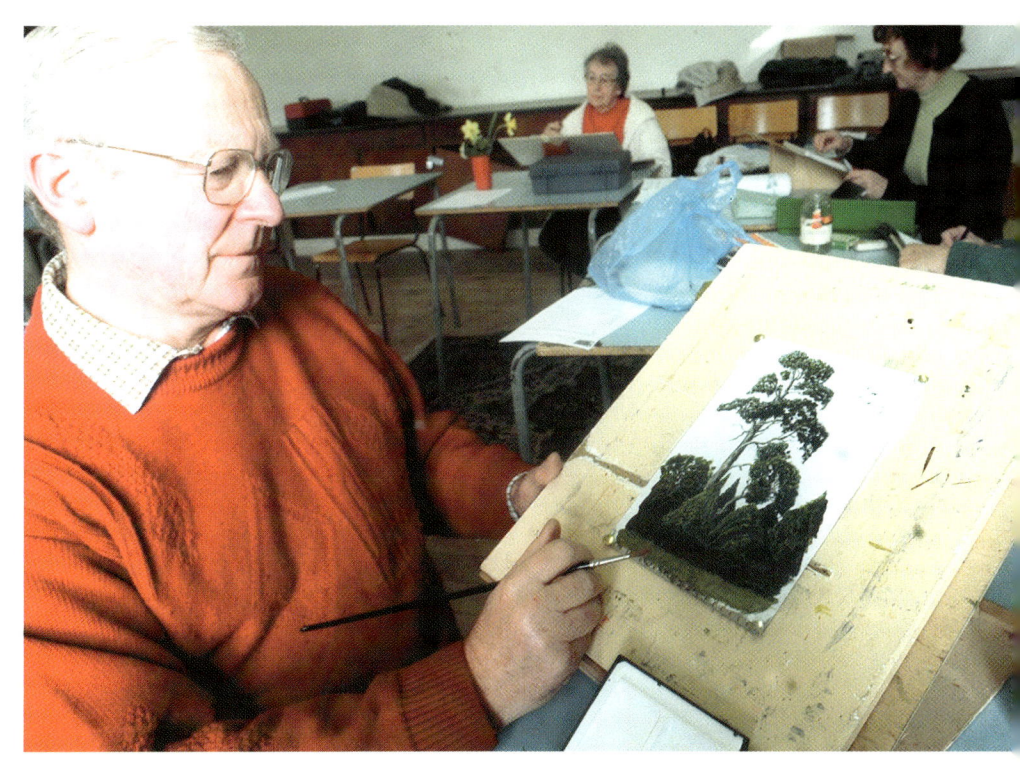

Dr Peter Toghill, a keen amateur artist, puts the finishing touches to an acrylic painting

In 1982 Dr David Banks started an innovative annual, week-long refresher course for GPs. Initially intended for the alumni of the Medical School, it gradually grew to accept all-comers. It became very popular, attracting doctors from all over the country. Some booked from year to year and attended several years running.

At about the same time the centre became the base for the GP vocational training scheme. As post graduate education became more organised and structured, Dr David Bossingham was appointed Clinical Tutor. When he emigrated to Australia, Dr William Jeffcoate, and more recently Dr Christine Bowman, took over. During Dr Jeffcoate's period of office he set up a second week-long course for GPs, which was held in the autumn to complement the spring course, and proved extremely popular.

In the late 1990s, following the lead given by general practice, hospital consultants and others were encouraged to undergo continuing medical education in a more formal manner. Dr David Banks set up a week-long consultants' course, which attracted specialists from all over the country. Profits from these courses, plus revenue from charging non-City Hospital users of the centre, went towards necessary extensions to the centre. This ensured it remained a premier post graduate centre with up to date equipment and multiple rooms, enabling it be used by many different groups of people. Much of this has been possible because of the excellent management by Mrs Sue Hodson.

Developments at the Post Graduate Education Centre (1986 to 1998)

By Susan Hodson

IN 1986 the Administrator Mrs Cayley retired and I took on the post, staying until I retired in 1998. As the centre and its staffing grew, my role changed to that of manager. The clinical tutors (initially Dr David Bossingham, then Dr William Jeffcoate and later Dr Christine Bowman) took an increasingly active part in post graduate education at the hospital and driving forward developments at the centre.

The introduction of a Post Graduate Education Allowance by the Government in 1990 brought considerable changes.

General practitioners (later hospital doctors) were formally required to participate in on-going teaching and it rapidly became apparent that an expansion in teaching facilities was required. Over the next decade several extensions were built. During the early 1990s the centre's role extended to providing a venue for undergraduate and post graduate teaching for other hospital staff - nurses, therapists, laboratory and non-clinical staff. At that time the name was changed to the Post Graduate Multidisciplinary Centre, later contracted to the present Post Graduate Education Centre. A change in emphasis from formal lectures to learning in syndicate groups meant there was an increasing need for more 'break out' rooms in which small groups could meet and learn.

Several important extensions were built between 1993 and 1996. A corridor was incorporated into the lounge and later it was extended to the rear to provide a new dining area.

A new entrance was built on the site of a former rose bed and the office size was doubled. Later an even larger entrance hall and reception area was built, together with a permanent office for the clinical and college tutors. A large extension was built to the medical library, providing a sizeable reading/quiet study area and enclosed audio-visual room. A wheelchair lift was installed to enable access to those who found stairs a barrier.

The midwifery education department moved into its purpose-built extension at the centre in 1994. This extra space and strong foundations downstairs now allowed the upstairs teaching room to be almost doubled in size, providing a much-needed intermediate sized

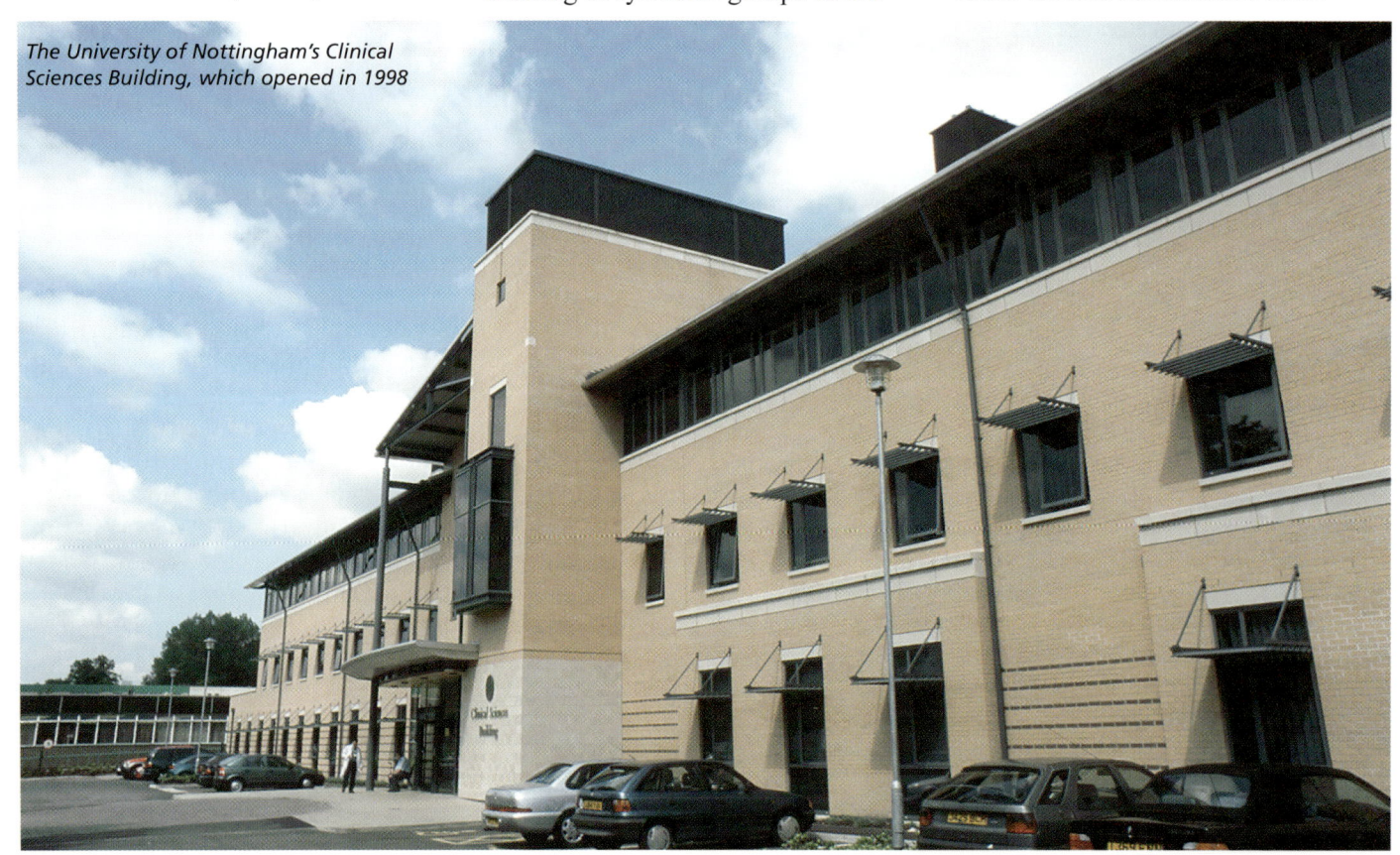

The University of Nottingham's Clinical Sciences Building, which opened in 1998

lecture room. It seemed in 1998 as though the site was 'saturated' with no more room for expansion, but the content of courses and quality of the teaching means the Nottingham City Hospital Post Graduate Education Centre continues to be a centre of excellence and a 'model of its kind.'

Nottingham Medico-Chirurgical Society

By Dr Peter Toghill

SINCE 1972 the Nottingham Medico-Chirurgical Society has been based at the City Hospital Post Graduate Education Centre, where it holds most of its meetings and has a handsome Council Room. The society has met regularly since 1828, making it one of the oldest medical societies in the country. Its membership of more than 700 embraces doctors from general practice, hospital specialties, academia, research and occupational medicine. The society is the chief meeting place for Nottingham's medical profession and offers a blend of education, vocational training, good fellowship and social activities.

From 1910 it met in a Georgian house at 64 St James's Street, Nottingham.

Because of overcrowding at meetings, difficulty in parking and the deteriorating fabric of the building, a decision was made at the annual general meeting in 1967 to negotiate new accommodation at the proposed Post Graduate Centre at the City Hospital.

In the last 20 or 30 years the society has grown in strength, size and influence. It provides common ground for general practitioners, academics and hospital consultants. A pleasant tradition has developed in that the presidency alternates between general practitioner and hospital consultant.

Fresh ground was broken when in the 1989/90 session Professor Tony Mitchell, Foundation Professor of Medicine accepted the invitation to

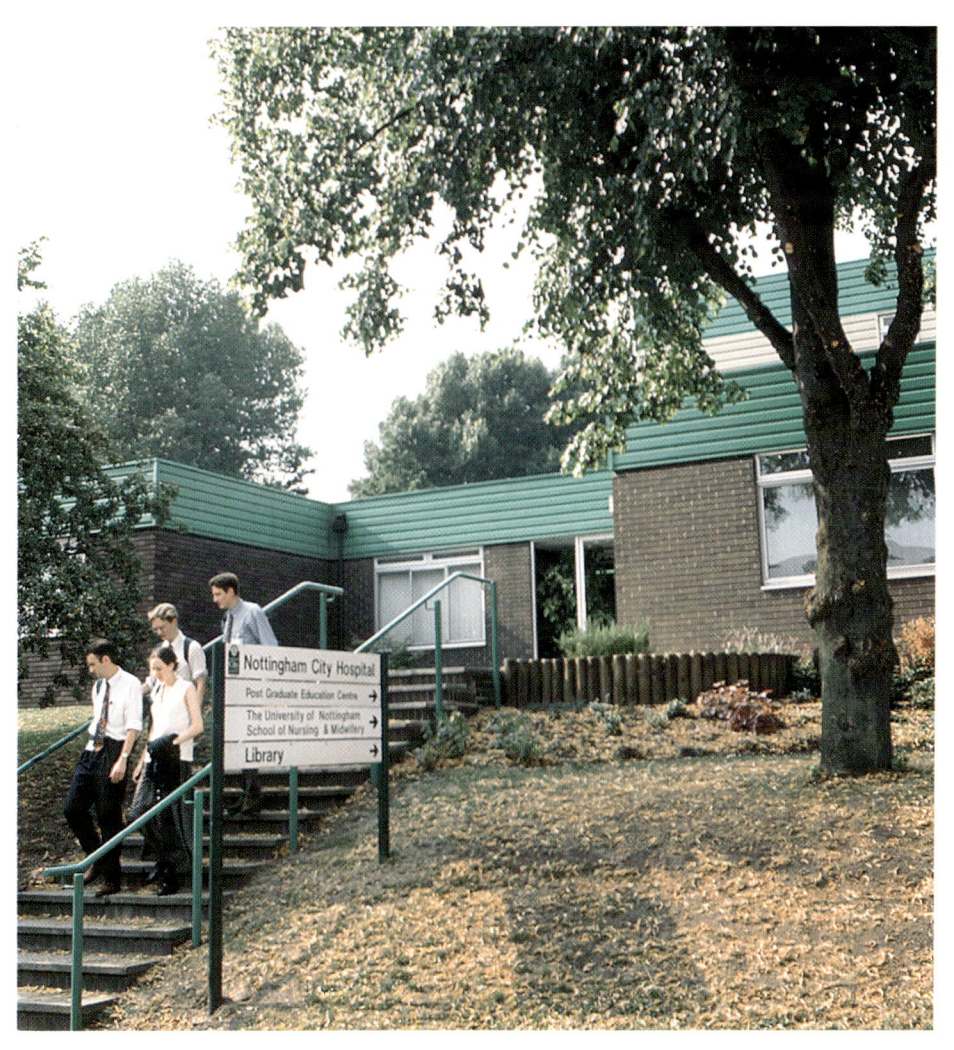

Post Graduate Education Centre

Right: Laura Peters, 11, of St. Wilfrids School, Calverton listening for breathing during a demonstration on National Anaesthesia Day in the Post Graduate Education Centre in 2002

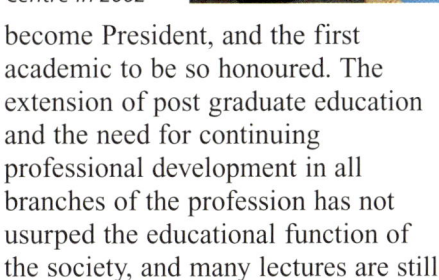

become President, and the first academic to be so honoured. The extension of post graduate education and the need for continuing professional development in all branches of the profession has not usurped the educational function of the society, and many lectures are still given which bring members up to date with branches of the profession other than their own. However, in the wider sense, the society hears from clerics, broadcasters, writers and explorers. And how wonderfully entertaining they have been.

The society lives on.

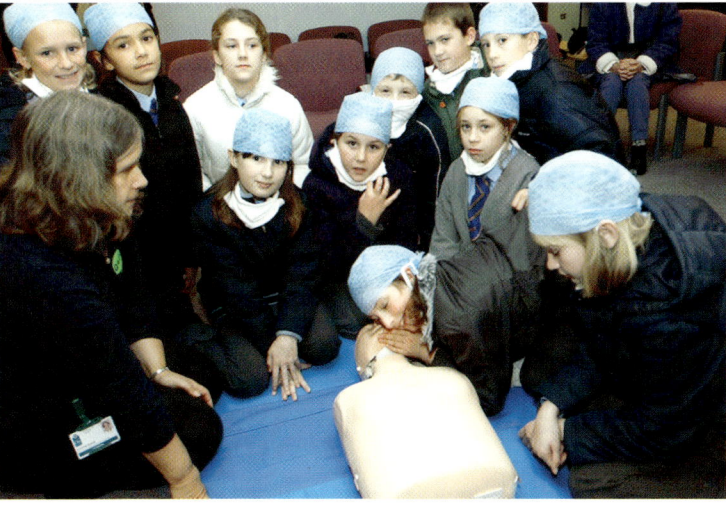

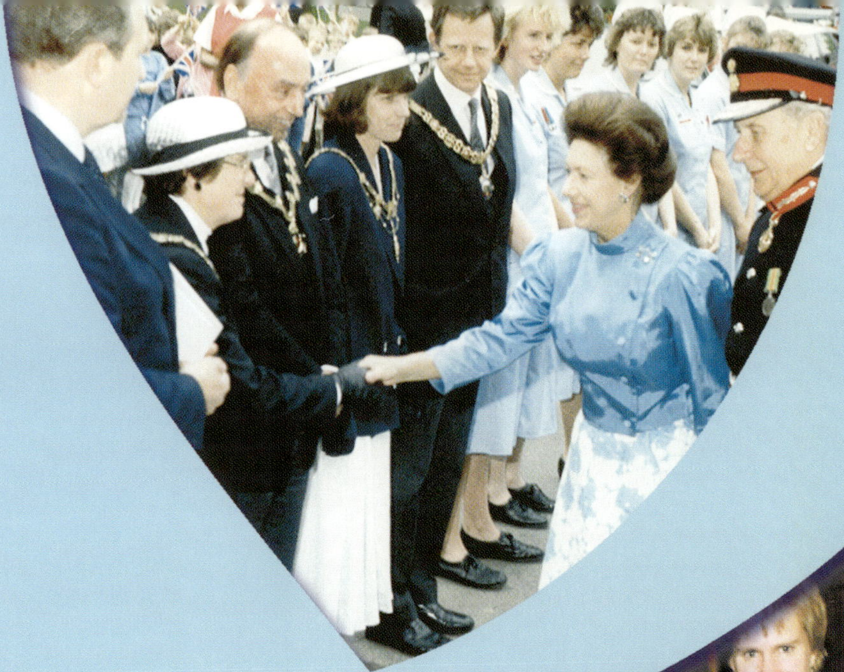

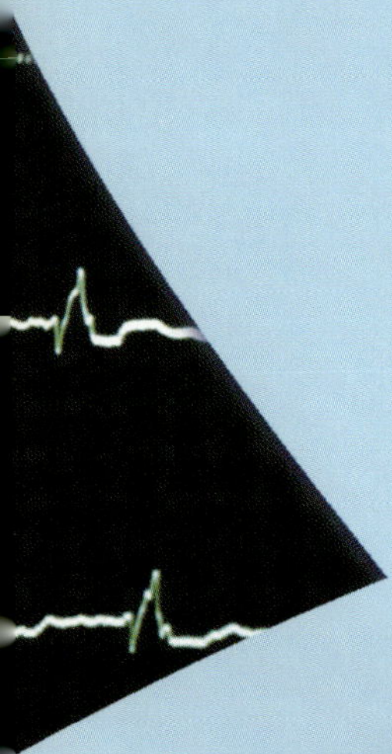

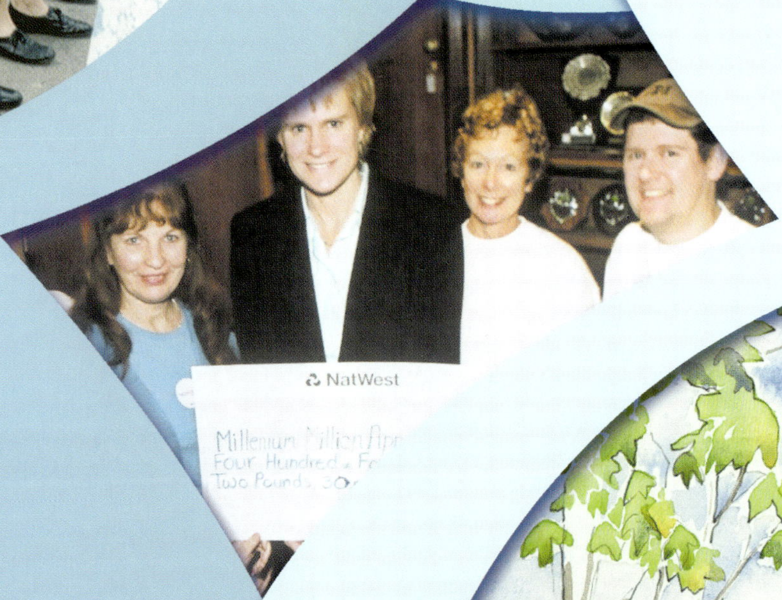
NatWest

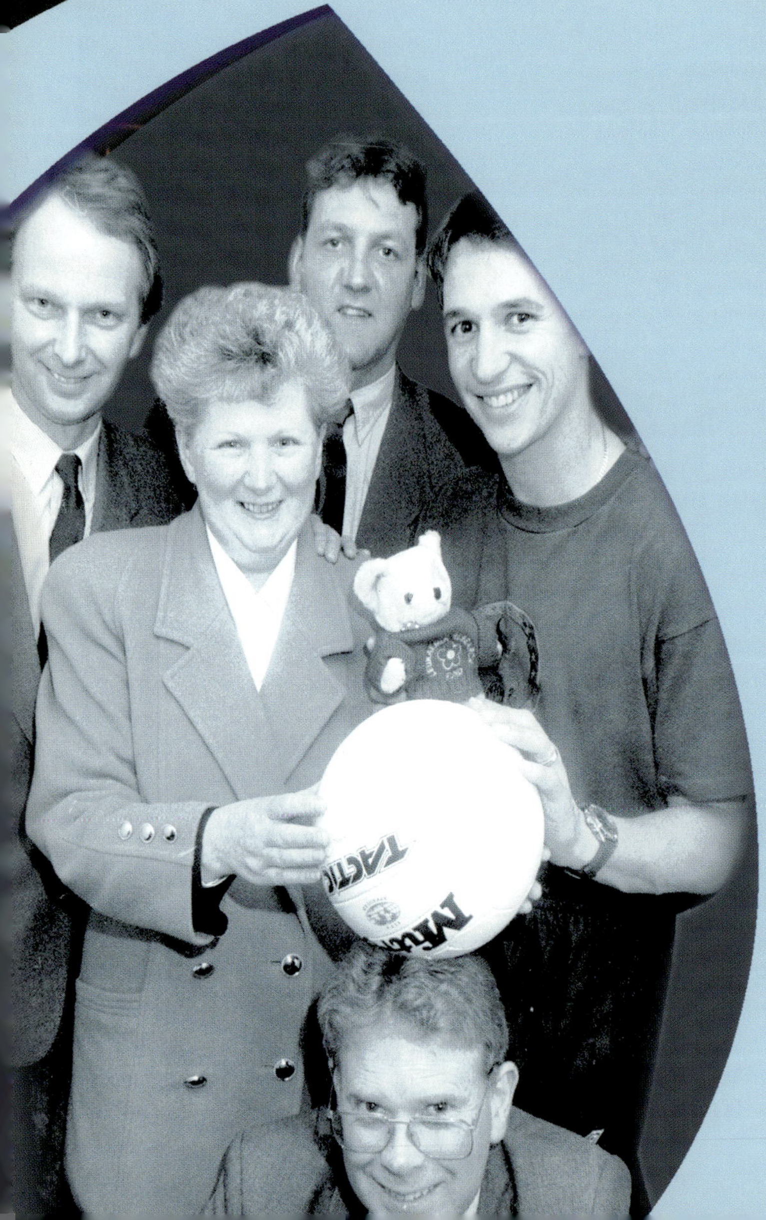

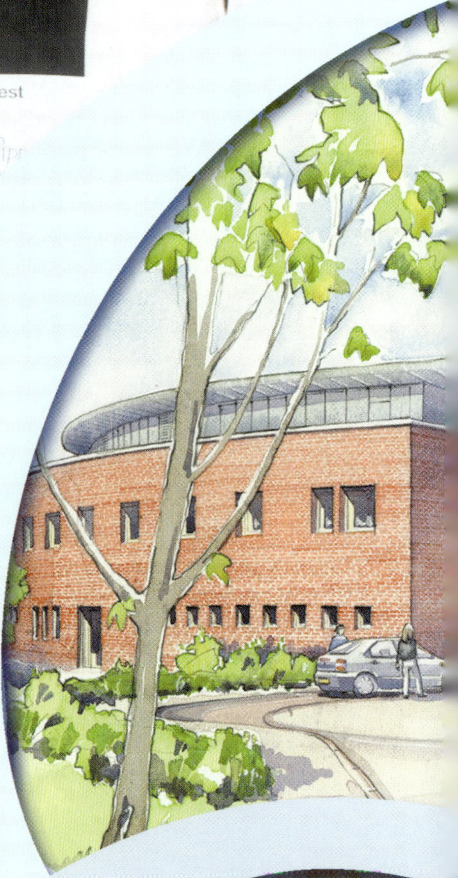

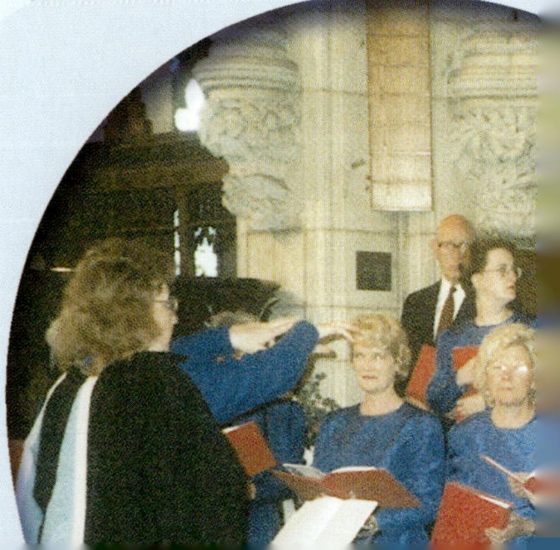

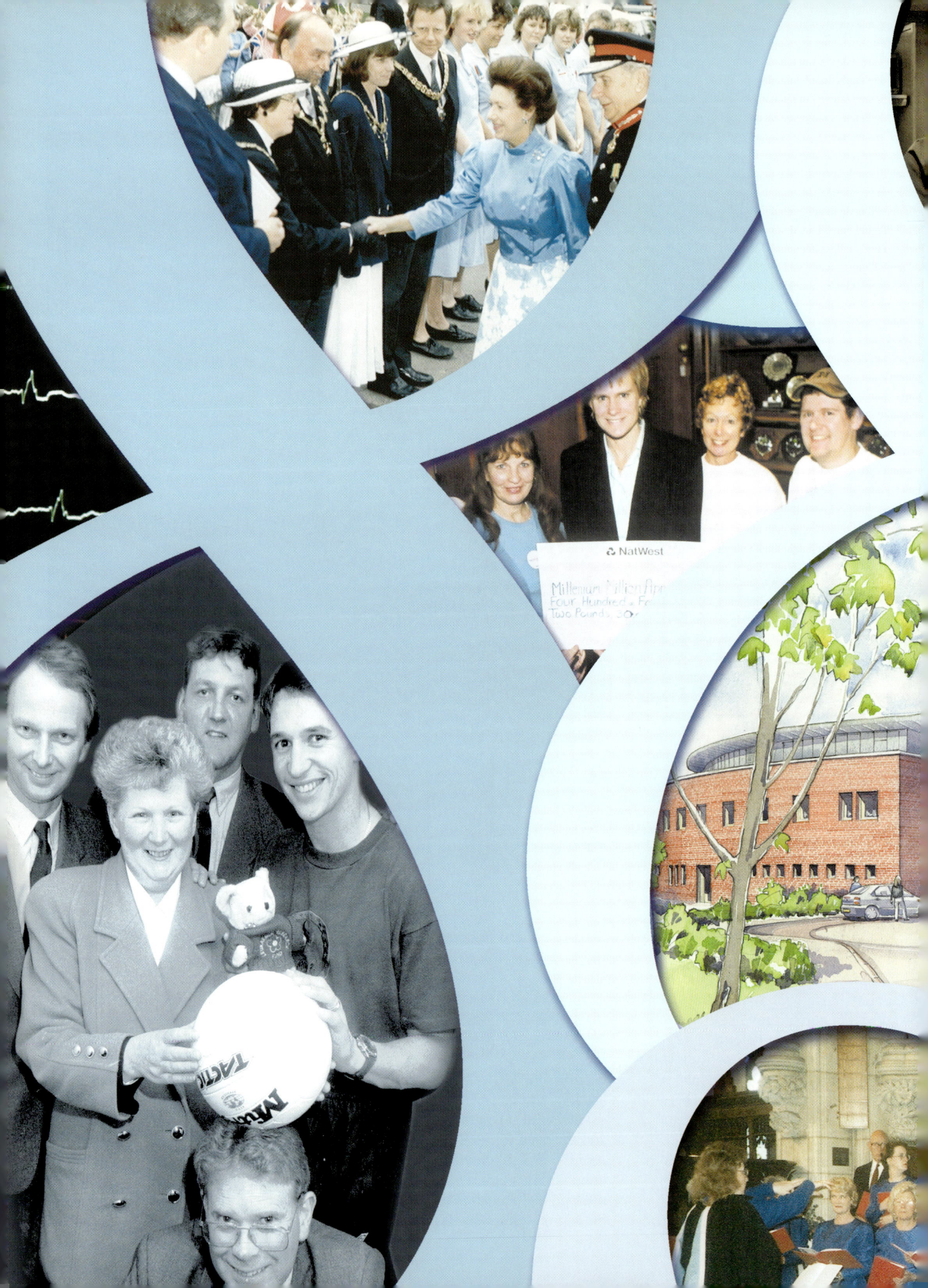

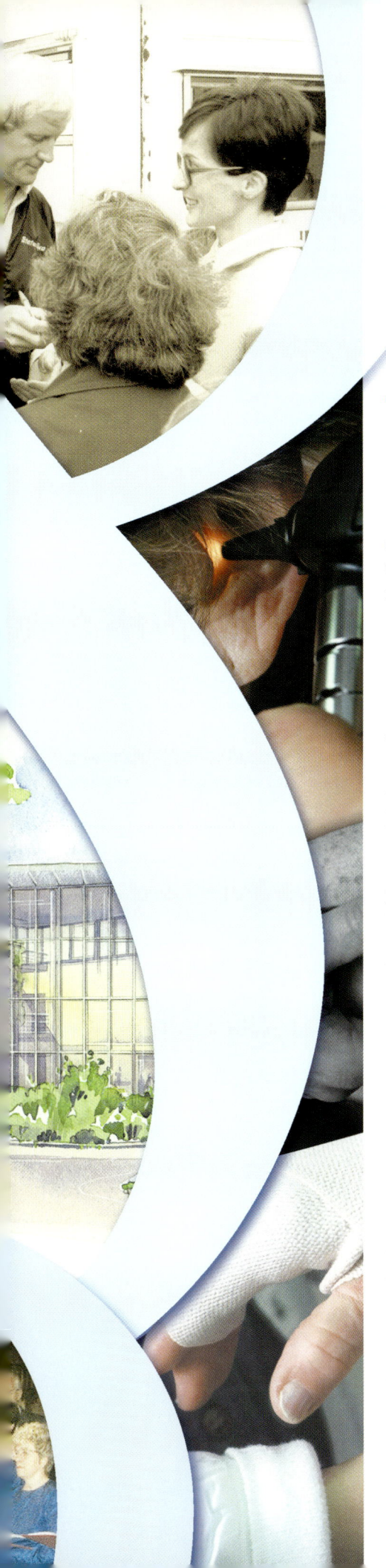

Community involvement

Tremendous team effort boosts hospital

DURING a century of dedicated service, thousands of staff, patients and members of the general public have given invaluable support on behalf of the Nottingham City Hospital. This chapter is a tribute to that continuing work, in which we outline the wonderful team effort behind some of the fundraising appeals and community involvement projects set up since the inception of the NHS in 1948.

The CARE Appeal

THE Medical Research Centre is an excellent example of Nottingham City Hospital and the local community working together for the benefit of patients. In 1977 the hospital received a bequest of £50,000 - at that time its biggest single donation - for research. A working party concluded that the greatest need was for purpose-built laboratories but at a time of worsening recession there was little prospect of the NHS or the University Grants Committee financing such a building.

Dr Richard Burden suggested a research centre on similar lines to the one developed in Stoke. David Evans, a former banker and Chairman of the Area Health Authority, who had been closely involved with the Nottingham hospitals for many years, became the energetic Chairman of the appeal committee formed in 1981. A real breakthrough came when the Nottingham Building Society became a partner in what became known as The CARE Appeal, which quickly caught the imagination of the Nottingham public. Three sponsored Robin Hood marathons raised more than £200,000 and there were numerous other fundraising events, including hospital open days when many people had their blood pressure taken in payment for an appeal donation. City Hospital staff performed at a memorable Christmas concert in aid of the appeal. Dewi Davis read *A Child's Christmas in Wales* and a selection of songs were sung by Chris Howell, Tony Woolfson, Mike Bishop and Brian Houldsworth. An amusing homage to Beatrix Potter was performed by Louise Alderman (flute), Penny Browne (oboe), Charlie Tomson (clarinet), Elizabeth Horne (horn), Tim Dornan (bassoon), Geoff Gilbert (slide projector) and William Jeffcoate (voice).

The £1million appeal target was reached in just four years and by the end of 1983 building work began. The university agreed to furnish a seminar room and the Regional Health Authority paid the architect's fees. The Medical Research Centre was built next to the department of therapeutics (the old Fleming wards) to encourage interaction between staff in the two buildings. It was officially opened by the Duchess of Gloucester in 1986 and during the ceremony Sir Michael Carlisle, Chairman of Trent Regional Health Authority said the local community had "responded magnificently" in raising cash for the development. David White, Chairman of Nottingham Health Authority, paid tribute to the tremendous public support and praised David Evans for chairing the appeal which made the project possible. District General Manager Dr David Banks later presented David Evans with a portrait to remind him of the memorable day. Mr Evans died in November 1996 and the trustees decided it would be appropriate to rename the building in his honour. A ceremony was held in July 1997 with his son Brian unveiling a commemorative plaque. The David Evans Research Centre, providing extensive laboratory and other facilities that were sadly lacking on the campus, has become a focus for many important research projects. It continues to be used by NHS staff interested in bone disease, diabetes, haematology, infectious diseases, renal medicine and gastroenterology.

Scores of papers and presentations have taken place and helped promote the City Hospital's world-wide reputation for the quality of its research. The two vice chairmen of the CARE Appeal were Dr Stephen Jones and Dr Richard Burden, who is still associated with the centre and is the current Chairman of Trustees. For the future, discussions are taking place to integrate the David Evans Research Centre more closely with the research and development plans of the hospital. There is no doubt that the centre will continue to be a major asset of Nottingham City Hospital for many years to come.

Nottingham Forest manager Brian Clough (front right) presents a cheque to David Evans (second right) for the Scanner Appeal

The Nottingham and Nottinghamshire Kidney Fund

THE appeal was launched in 1966 with a target of £35,000 to provide dialysis equipment. Two of the original trustees were the then Lord Mayor Alderman Percy Holland and former Nottinghamshire County Council Chairman Alderman Sir Frank Small. Secretary of the fund was Tony Higgins. By 1972 more than £75,000 had been raised. It was announced that a special unit to investigate and treat kidney disease and a 10-bed unit for patients learning to use artificial kidney machines would be set up at Nottingham City Hospital.

The fund continues to raise money - thanks to dedicated people like Marks & Spencer worker Ian Hill.

He needed a kidney transplant in 1993 and has since led countless charity events.

Hayward House

HAYWARD House is Nottingham's only specialist 'hospice within a hospital.' This palliative care unit is dedicated to relieving the suffering of progressive cancer, suffering which can be physical, emotional, social and spiritual and which involves both the patient and the family. Such care and support are also given to patients with advancing motor neurone disease and to their families.

Built within the grounds of the City

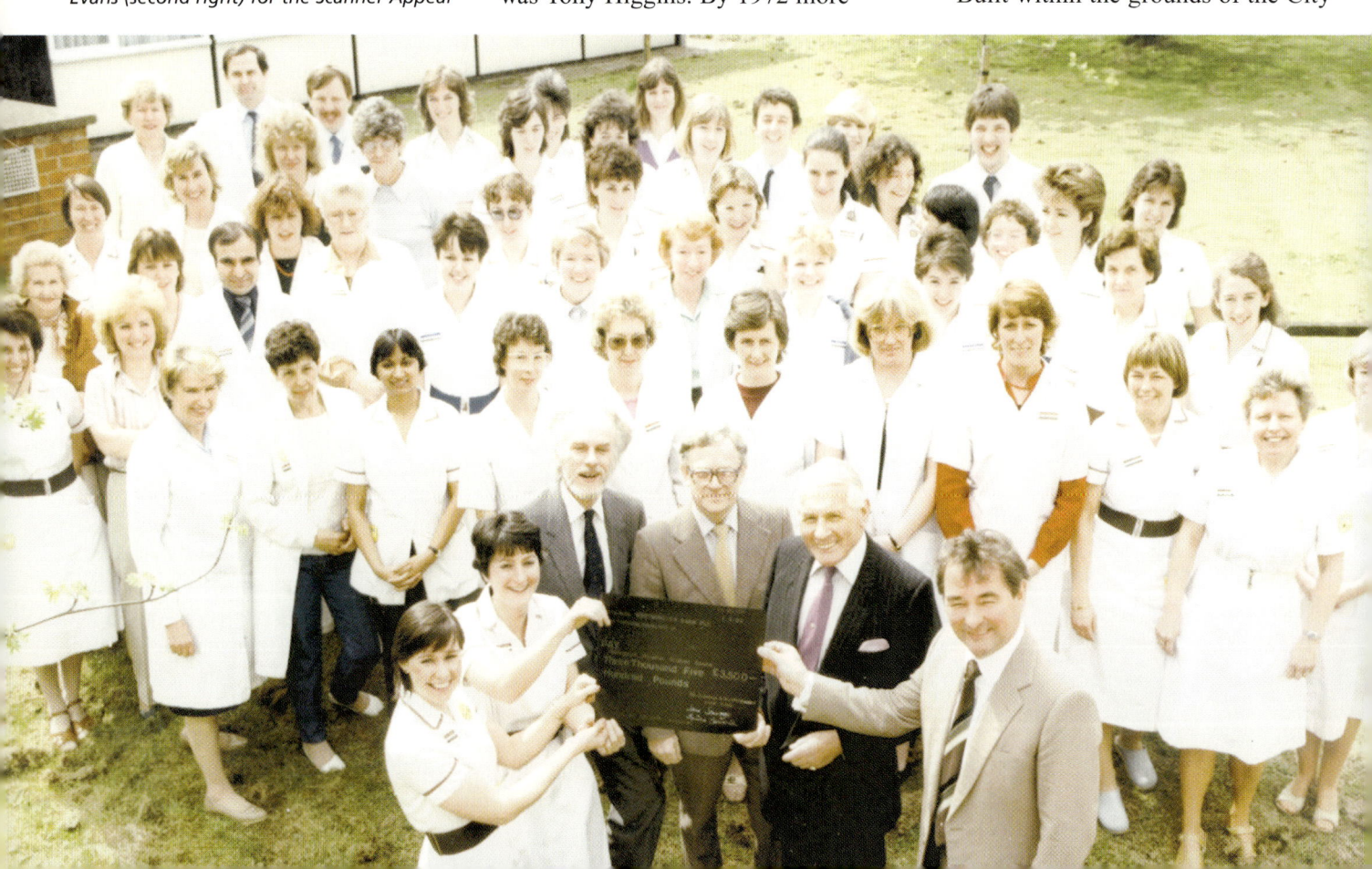

The People's Hospital

Hospital by Cancer Relief Macmillan Fund, aided by generous contributions from the people of Nottingham and a number of business leaders, Hayward House was opened in 1979. Since then the running costs have been maintained by the NHS but a significant element of support from charitable funds has continued to be needed with constant generous help from friends, the general public and voluntary and business organisations. Valuable core finance is obtained from the unit's two volunteer-staffed cancer charity shops.

The building of a new extension in 1990 (again funded by Cancer Relief Macmillan Fund) provided an extensive day care facility and a new education and training unit and this, linked to the appointment of a senior lecturer in palliative medicine (also funded by Cancer Relief) between Hayward House and the University of Nottingham, was the springboard for a succession of significant developments over the year. Hayward House is now a centre of considerable repute and experience.

From an initial inpatient unit, a small day care service and a community Macmillan nurse team, Hayward House today comprises an extensive matrix of specialist services. Its 'total care' is provided now through an inpatient unit (of 17 beds; soon to be increased to 20), a substantial day care/outpatient unit, a seven member community Macmillan nurse home care team, a hospital palliative care support team (led by four hospital Macmillan nurses), a comprehensive counselling service, a highly structured bereavement service, a volunteer home sitter service and a purpose-built complementary therapy unit. Hayward House is respected nationally and internationally for its extensive contribution to education and training in palliative care and for the calibre of its highly motivated research department. Hayward House also acts as a significant general resource for advice, knowledge and support for patients, families and caring professionals on all aspects of palliative care.

Scanner appeal

PRINCESS Margaret visited the hospital on May 24, 1988 to officially open a £1m scanner suite and put the crowning glory on four years of intensive fundraising. She also visited the new occupational therapy department which had opened that year. Princess Margaret talked to Consultant Radiologist Dr Donald Rose and Superintendent Radiographer Jeff Summerlin about the scanner and its role in the future. It has proved invaluable to many patients.

One of the many enjoyable fundraising events in aid of the appeal was the hospital's open day and carnival on June 1, 1985, opened by Hucknall-born actor Robin Bailey, famous for his Uncle Mort character in the hit TV series *I Didn't Know You Cared*. Another successful fundraising event was a Pro-Am golf tournament at Radcliffe-on-Trent Golf Club. Appeal organiser Mrs Cynthia Gaythorpe said Princess Margaret's visit had been a wonderful end to the appeal and paid tribute to the tremendous support it had received from a wide cross-section of people.

Leukaemia appeal

THE Nottinghamshire Leukaemia Appeal was launched in February 1994 as a result of discussions between the Leukaemia Research Fund (LRF) and Nottingham City Hospital medical staff. The intention was to give fundraising for research a local focus by linking it to the development of bone marrow transplantation at the hospital. This was, and still is, a unique co-operation between the national LRF and a major local teaching hospital.

The result has been a huge success with more than £1.5 million raised in 8½ years. This has come about in two ways. Firstly, the continuing activities

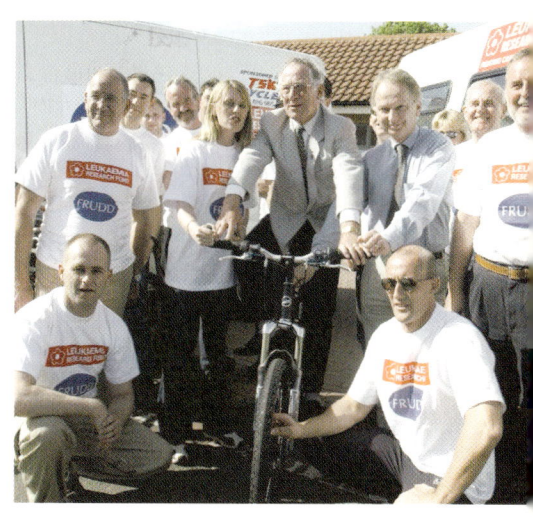

A bike ride from Nottingham City Hospital in 2002 raised money for the Leukaemia Research Fund. Pictured on the bike is Peter Menhennet, Chairman of the Gedling Borough Branch of the fund. Next to him is Professor Nigel Russell

of the local network of LRF branches were given a new impetus and they have raised approximately half of the money. This has been sent directly to the LRF in London but comes back to Nottingham in the form of research grants for projects approved by the LRF scientific committee.

The other half of the money has been raised by the Appeal committee with the help of local organisations, trusts and many generous individuals who have given their time and enthusiasm. This money has been used to buy state-of-the-art equipment, including a gene scanner and flow cytometer, and to fund key research staff.

The appeal has complemented developments both in the university and NHS. In 1999 the research and stem cell laboratories moved into the new university Clinical Sciences Building on the Nottingham City Hospital campus where they enjoy excellent modern facilities. Now there is to be an even more important development with the reconfiguration of Nottingham's clinical services.

A new leukaemia/transplant unit is to be built at Nottingham City Hospital so that all adult patients with leukaemia, myeloma, lymphoma and related conditions will be treated on

The People's Hospital

one site. This is scheduled for completion in 2005 and will bring together clinical and research staff in a way which has not been possible before and no doubt will result in improved treatment for more patients, a boost to the transplant programme and new opportunities for both clinical and laboratory research.

Heart research unit appeal

AN appeal was launched in 1997 towards establishing a £100,000 research unit at Nottingham City Hospital. The National Heart Research Fund had already given £50,000 towards the cost of the project. Plans were drawn up to convert a former infirmary building on the site where research and staff training is carried out, backed by a library and an office. The project will work in tandem with the hospital's cardiac unit, set up in September 1995 after years of campaigning from heart patients for Nottingham to have its own facilities.

Donations

OVER the years the hospital has benefited from bequests and donations, varying from a few pounds to substantial amounts. This generous support from individuals, companies and community organisations, is valuable in assisting the hospital's work.

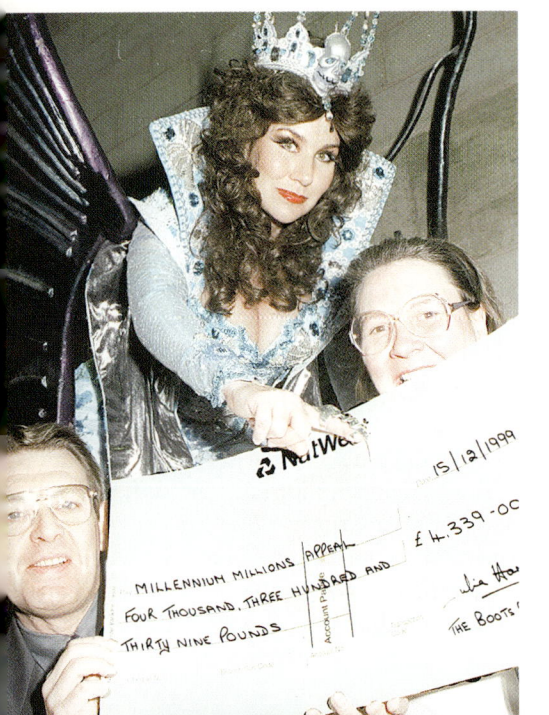

Often a gift is an expression of gratitude for the care a loved one has received. For example in 1998 Suzannah Evans-Farley gave the maternity unit £105,000 for vital equipment - to say thank you for her 'miracle' baby. She was left £160,000 to give to charity by her late father Peter Evans.

She had no hesitation in deciding what to do with a huge chunk of the money after the birth of her son Oliver at Nottingham City Hospital.

Her gift is the largest single donation the maternity unit has ever received and has enabled managers to get new equipment they would not otherwise have been able to afford.

Suzannah, from Arnold, thought she couldn't have children because she suffered from endometriosis, a condition which usually leads to infertility.

But soon after her father died in November, 1996, she learned she had become pregnant.

Suzannah said: "The staff at Nottingham City Hospital who looked after me were absolutely brilliant when Oliver was born.

"I was in labour for 49 hours and Oliver was born with the umbilical cord wrapped twice around his neck. He is my miracle baby."

Suzannah's money has bought an ultrasound scanner and several foetal heart monitors for the hospital.

She said: "This equipment is helping babies' lives, and giving the money towards new life is one of the most satisfying feelings I have ever had."

Suzannah also gave money to Marie Curie Cancer Care and another charity.

Left: *Linda Lusardi, who played the wicked Queen Lucretia in Snow White at the Theatre Royal in 1999, received a "wicked" cheque for £4,339 from the Boots Association on behalf of the Millennium Millions Appeal.*

The Nottingham Breast Institute

WORK has started on the £5.3million Nottingham Breast Institute at the City Hospital. It has taken four years to raise £1.3million, the remainder coming from hospital and national NHS funds. Scheduled to open late summer 2003, the purpose-built centre will bring together all outpatient diagnosis, treatment and follow-up clinics, teaching, research and education for the 35,000 patients who will use it each year. It will replace the Helen Garrod unit, which has been in temporary buildings since 1979 when it was established in memory of a patient, and will bring together other outpatient breast care services under one roof.

The appeal to raise the money for the new institute began in 1998 with the launch of the Millennium Millions Appeal, chaired by Marilyn Harrison.

Hospital Chairman Christine Bowering said: "We have had tremendous support from the local community in helping us to reach this stage . . .I would like to thank everyone who has been involved with this project, from the people who have made major cash donations to those who have been contributed just a few pounds."

Medical Research Fund

IN addition to successful fundraising appeals and donations to the hospital there are other clear cases of helping others. When a cremation form is signed the second part attracts a fee. This can be signed by any suitably qualified doctor but is usually signed by the pathologists.

In the 1980s they agreed to forgo their fees and put the money into a central fund to help others. This is called the Medical Research Fund. It is used to help pay the cost of producing scientific theses written by junior doctors and to help send junior

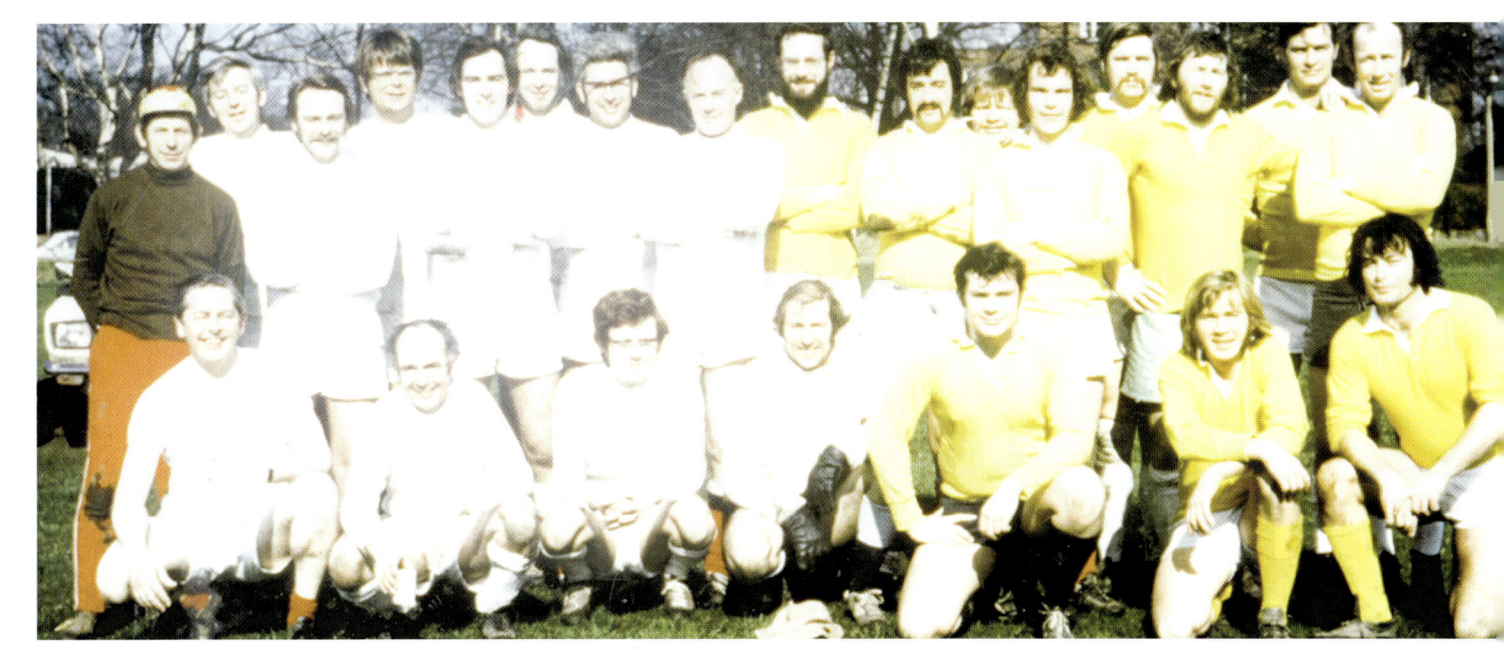

The People's Hospital

Some familiar faces can be seen in the senior and junior staff football teams in the 1970s

and senior colleagues to conferences so they can keep up to date. It also allows them to present their data to doctors in other parts of the country or world and thereby promote Nottingham City Hospital.

Nottingham Hospitals' Choir

THE Nottingham Hospitals' Choir was set up by Vic Bradley from the Medical School in 1970 with David Evans as President. When David died he was replaced by Dr Peter Toghill. The choir holds two major concerts a year - one in the Concert Hall at Christmas, which is always a sell-out, and a smaller one in the summer months. They go from strength-to-strength under Jacky Smith who took over from Vic when he retired. The choir has raised £200,000 for the Malcolm Sergeant Cancer Fund for Children. Anyone with an association with any of the hospitals can join this mixed choir if they meet the standard.

Hospital sport

WHEN the Medical School was being planned, part of the process was to bring to Nottingham a large group of young doctors. These proved to be fit, energetic people and it was not uncommon for the senior staff to take on the junior staff at some sport or other. Soccer was played, either five-a-side or, less often, 11-a-side. Cricket featured outside what is now the hospital headquarters. This activity depended on the agreement of John Gilby, the hospital's former Principal Pharmacist and Director of Service Development, who was, and is the protector of the pitch. Later, golf became one of the most popular sports and matches are held between the University Hospital and the City Hospital at Hollinwell.

There is a thriving Hospitals Golf Society. Founded in 1982, the society meets on different courses every month during the summer and has proved a good social way of Nottingham hospitals' staff working together.

Hospital staff often lend a hand in the community. A good example came in 1981 and 1982 when many staff took part in the first and second Robin Hood marathons to raise funds for the CARE Appeal. The medical care and feeding stations were also manned by hospital staff. Some staff continue to be involved with the marathon today.

The Rotary Club of Sherwood Sunrisers

THIS club started in 1994 with Pauline Johnston (then Head of Occupational Therapy) one of the key individuals responsible for its formation. It is a club with an almost equal membership of men and women and it is unusual in being a breakfast club, meeting every Tuesday morning at 7am.

In the early days the club tried a number of venues for meetings but soon settled at the City Hospital, using the facilities provided by the City Side Restaurant, which opens specially to accommodate the club and sets aside a separate area for the meetings. Visitors to Sherwood Sunrisers are pleasantly surprised at the range of hot and cold breakfasts available to them - perhaps compensating for the early start!

Membership is drawn from a wide variety of backgrounds, occupations and professions, as required by Rotary International regulation, and so the club has only a handful of members drawn from the hospital staff. In spite of that three of those have been elected to the office of president in the first eight years since formation.

SUPPORT GROUPS

The League of Friends of the City Hospital

THE League of Friends of the City Hospital has raised hundreds of thousands of pounds since it was founded in 1954. The first president was the Duchess of Portland.

The League's early aims were to supply extra comforts and benefits for patients and staff which were outside the range of the NHS and it began in a small way, providing chocolates, tobacco and flowers for patients.

The League's first major project was providing substantial kitchen equipment for the training of disabled patients in the occupational therapy unit, and later they funded a playroom and schoolroom for long-stay younger patients.

During the League's first 20 or 30 years they bought many televisions for wards and the nurses' homes. It also initiated a self-supporting telephone trolley service. One of the League's major achievements was providing, in association with the local authority, a creche to enable mothers to come and work in the hospital. The League also equipped a hairdressing salon for nursing staff with a service to patients on the wards. Day rooms were provided on the orthopaedic wards and a visitors' waiting room on the intensive care unit. The League helped promote fundraising for the Leisure Centre which opened in 1974 and played a significant part in raising funds for the CARE Appeal.

Basford Hospital League of Friends continued until the hospital closed in 1993 and in 1995 Linden Lodge League of Friends amalgamated with the City Hospital League.

Members of the Hospital League of Friends of Sherwood and St Francis Hospitals continued their work until 1996 when they decided to disband. They had been active for more than 30 years and raised large sums of money for the comfort of elderly patients. The City Hospital League took over the Sherwood wards, now South Corridor and the management of St Francis Hospital transferred to the mental health services.

In 1999 the National Association of Hospital and Community League of Friends celebrated its 50th anniversary. During that year the City Hospital League hosted a special concert by the Nottingham Hospitals' Choir and opened a gallery in the entrance to the outpatients department. Local artists and art groups display their paintings for two weeks and the League receives a percentage from any sales. The project has proved very popular and given added interest to the outpatients entrance. The League also provided a £15,000 minibus to help improve the award-winning park-and-ride service.

In the last 10 years the League has raised and donated more than half a million pounds.

Christine Bowering, Chairman of the City Hospital, said: "The League of Friends has done a superb amount of work at the hospital for many years and we are indebted to it for its practical help and its fundraising efforts."

The Women's Royal Voluntary Service

A TROLLEY service operated by the WVS (now Women's Royal Voluntary Service) was available as early as 1949. The WRVS, which has more than 200 volunteers on the campus, runs five canteens, plus a trolley service in the oncology department. It operates a creche two hours a day in the maternity unit, where mothers can leave their children while they are having scans.

The WRVS is also a friendly 'first port of call' in the outpatients department, where escorts and hostesses direct patients to appointments and perform other valuable roles. Over the years the WRVS has presented many TV sets to

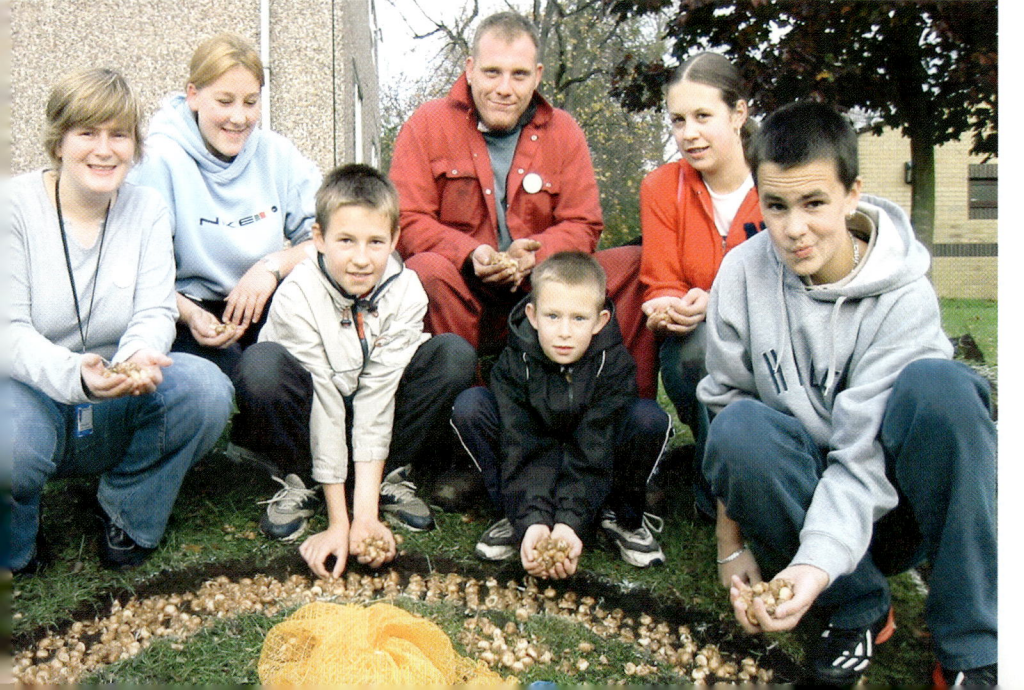

Left: A warming cuppa from WRVS volunteer Eileen Kenton for Lynn Palmer, a visitor to the hospital
Below: Hospital Youth Worker Donna Hilton (left) and NHS gardener Chris Gray (centre) help some of the children with their bulb planting project in the hospital grounds

The People's Hospital

wards and donated medical equipment from canteen profits.

Radio City

RADIO City - Nottingham City Hospital's own radio station - went on air on April 2, 1974. On that evening 5,000 listeners, staff and patients at the City, Heathfield, Sherwood and St Francis Hospitals, were able to tune into 'The Voice that Cares' for requests, music, news and views around the hospital.

An old store room connected to the social club was converted to house the station equipment, provided by the hospital. Eventually the project was moved to the new Leisure Centre. The original team of volunteers comprised Station Manager Peter Wagstaff, Programme Controller Tony Monoghan, Publicity and Promotion Manager Barrie Pierpoint (who presented 'BJ's World' under his station name of Barrie James), Tony Davis (who was in control of 'Wardwaves') and Disc Jockey Jeff Widdowson (who used the name Jeff Hunt to present the programme 'Sounds Contemporary'). Consultant John Cochrane became President of the project and a 100lb iced fruit cake was cut to celebrate the station's birthday in 1977. In the same year a £10,000 appeal was launched to equip three new studios. The service was eventually amalgamated into Nottingham Hospitals' Radio.

SELF HELP GROUPS

THE City Hospital has close and long standing links with Self Help Nottingham. The Cardiac Support Group (Nottingham) and BUSH are two examples of support groups benefiting patients, their families and carers.

BUSH

DURING the 1980s the hospital became a catalyst for several self help groups. BUSH (Burns Unit Self Help), formed in 1982, was the first of its kind in the country, set up to provide counselling, friendship, mutual support and after-care for patients and relatives coming to terms with the trauma of burns injuries.

It was the idea of a consultant surgeon, who said: "They can talk about it better than anyone. They can listen too and that's something staff on a busy ward, however caring, don't always have time to do." Chairman Ray James had himself suffered severe burns when he was a fireman. BUSH won a county council award in 1987 in recognition of its "outstanding contribution to the lives of local disabled people."

The Cardiac Support Group (Nottingham)

THE group started in February 1991. Tracey Riley, a staff nurse in the coronary care unit, supported by Occupational Therapy Manager Judy Briggs, invited four patients on the cardiac rehabilitation programme and members of Self Help Nottingham to an initial meeting. It was agreed that a self help group would be beneficial to patients recovering from heart problems.

From small beginnings it has grown into the largest cardiac support group in the country with more than 300 members. This includes carers, who are considered every bit as important as patients.

The group aims to boost the morale of both patients and their families by providing support, guidance and advice so that together they can face the future with confidence. Meetings are held in the hospital's Sherwood Hall on the last Thursday of every month from 7pm to 9pm.

Seeing a roomful of vibrant people helps newcomers realise that a useful and productive life can, and does, continue after heart problems. Outings, socials and pub lunches are organised and an exercise club, Fitness for Life, is run for the benefit of members.

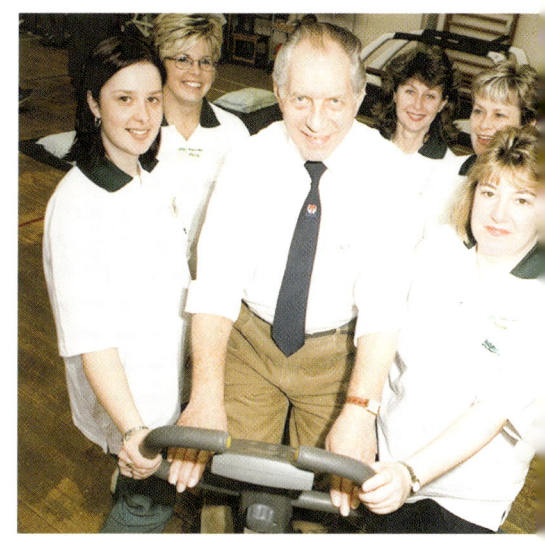

ASDA staff joined the cardiac rehabilitation patients in an exercise class at the hospital's physiotherapy gym in 1999. They donated £250 towards the Cardiac Support Group. Pictured is George Christian (centre) from the hospital Cardiac Support Group and ASDA staff, from left to right, Carla Goodman, Penny Taylor, Veronica Stuart, Maureen O'Donnell and Tracey Little

The group supports cardiac rehabilitation and raises funds to provide items of equipment for the cardiac rehabilation units at both the City Hospital and Queen's Medical Centre.

INTERNATIONAL LINKS

THE City Hospital has forged many significant overseas links. For example Dr Dewi Davies, in association with the Royal College of Physicians, started sending used medical journals to Sri Lanka as they were unable to pay for themselves. As a consequence he visited the island to give lectures.

When he retired the system was taken over by Dr David Banks who continued the link until he retired. In recognition of this work he was made an honorary member of the Ceylon College of Physicians in 1996. The link work is now carried on by Professor John Britton, who has also been involved in setting up an exchange programme with a medical school in Ethiopia at a place called Jimma. The project has been visited by various people including the

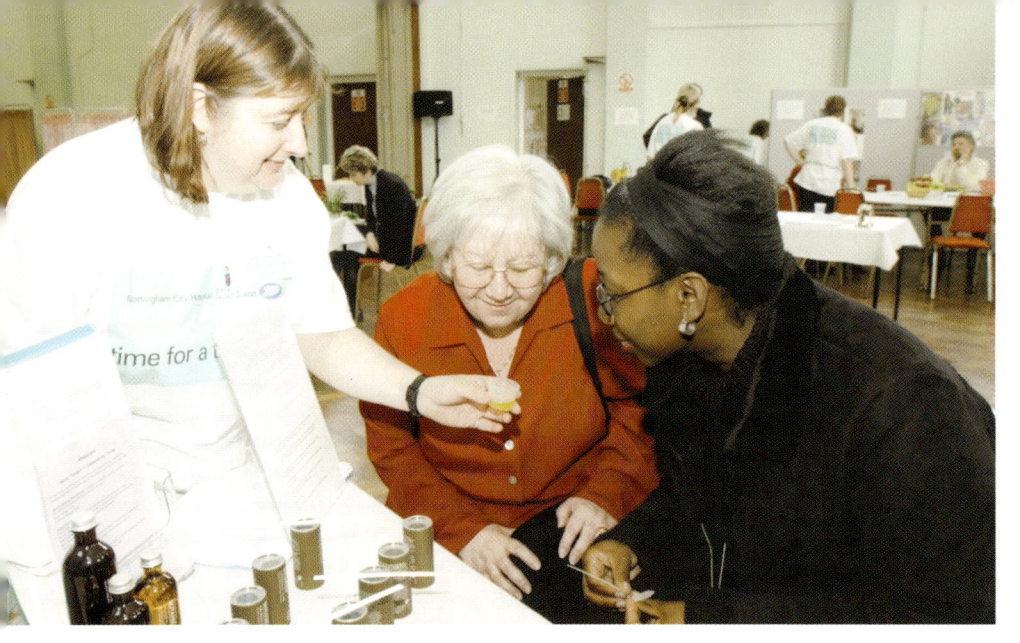

The People's Hospital

Hospital staff flocked to the Sherwood Hall which had been transformed into a 'health spa' for a day. Beauty treatments and complementary therapies were on offer in a partnership between the hospital, New College Nottingham and Boots. Sandra Cox from Boots demonstrates some aromatherapy products to hospital canteen waitress Maria Green and Audra Castor

hospital's former Chief Executive Thelma Holland.

The hospital has been able to help with advice, teaching and their examinations system. In turn, many people from Jimma have visited the City Hospital on fact-finding visits. Research programmes have also been set up so that they are able to apply to other bodies for funds to develop the service in the hospital. The Ethiopians face overwhelming problems. For example, they see rheumatic heart disease so severe that there is a major problem for patients in their late teens. They know what to do but there are not the facilities to tackle the problem. There is only one cardiothoracic surgeon in the whole of Ethiopia and yet in a clinic in Jimma, there are 30 or so patients who would benefit from an operation.

VOLUNTEERS

FOR many years local people have visited patients at the hospital, bringing comforts and contact with the 'outside world.' As patient numbers increased post-war, it was recognised that no matter how efficient treatment may be, there was still room for voluntary effort, which today involves more than 800 people.

The development of specialised services for elderly patients resulted in the creation of a paid post to co-ordinate volunteers in 1967. Services grew from this beginning at Sherwood Hospital. The patients' request programme became Nottingham Hospitals' Radio; a Sunday escort service was introduced by the chaplain and a worker to administer a volunteer programme at the outlying Basford Hospital was appointed in 1972.

Further programmes were developed during the 1970s and 80s including a library trolley service to most of the adult wards.

The Sandfield unit for special needs, now the Children's Centre, opened its doors in 1976. Volunteers were a new and welcome addition to the team of dedicated workers based there.

Opened in 1980, Hayward House, a purpose-built hospice offering specialist palliative care, began to introduce a comprehensive range of services provided by volunteers, co-ordinated by a paid organiser.

Linden Lodge, a care unit for younger disabled adults opened in 1981. The services of volunteers, so successful at its sister unit, Ellerslie House, were introduced to this new unit.

A volunteer, specially trained by the Red Cross in skin camouflage, began advising plastic surgery patients in the use of make up techniques in 1986, following a request from hospital consultants.

In 1990, at the suggestion of Professor Roger Blamey, the Nottingham Breast Cancer Support Group was initiated.

Experience in the value of mutual support from those experiencing similar health problems led to the appointment of a Self Help Co-ordinator in November, 1994.

In 1995 a scheme involving volunteers to support older patients at home, on discharge from hospital, was established. Age Concern was commissioned to run the scheme on behalf of the Trust.

The development of volunteering in children's services took a significant step forward with the appointment of a part-time co-ordinator in 1999, to support volunteers working alongside ward and clinic staff, play leaders and hospital-based teachers.

A volunteer 'meet and greet' service was introduced to complement the hospital's Patient Advice and Liaison Service (PALS). Recruitment of volunteers began in the autumn of 2001, and following a development programme, including accredited customer service modules, the service was officially launched, in association with a parallel scheme at the University Hospital, on April 1, 2002. A further voluntary scheme, jointly funded by the Department of Health, is being developed to enhance patient services in surgery, cancer services and children's services.

'Time For a Treat', a collaborative, ground-breaking project sponsored by Boots, New College Nottingham and Nottingham City Hospital, was launched in January 2002, enabling patients from a wide cross-section of hospital wards and community groups, referred by Nottingham City Primary Care Trust, to benefit from beauty and therapy-based 'treats.' In addition to the skills of beauticians and students from New College Nottingham, a number of the hospital's own volunteers have gained accreditation to deliver a programme of therapeutic massage to patients.

The People's Hospital

The future vision

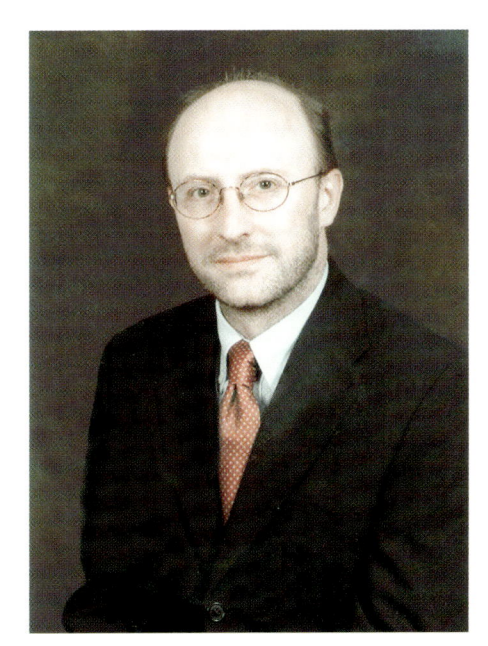

Gerry McSorley has been the Chief Executive at Nottingham City Hospital since 2000

THE previous chapters have illustrated the significant changes on the hospital campus over the last 100 years. They have also emphasised the emotional relationship the hospitals have had with the people of Nottingham, Nottinghamshire, and further afield as the years have passed. From the founding citizens of the original Board of Guardians with their foresight to create a vision for hospital services at the end of the 19th century, through the years of war, to the creation of the National Health Service in 1948, the hospital has developed through the drive and imagination of individuals who have cared for the health and well-being of so many.

As we look forward to the second hundred years of the hospital we can be sure of further improvements being made. In 2003 the hospital will see the opening of the Nottingham Breast Institute, paid for by a determined combination of the people of the county along with financial support from the NHS and the Nottingham City Hospital, the start of construction of the new centre for clinical haematology and a new centre for urology. Final plans are also in hand to create a new centre for patients with coronary heart disease to open in 2005.

But most importantly of all 2003 will see agreement on the need for a complete redevelopment of many of the older facilities, especially so for those original Edwardian wards. Whilst this redevelopment may mark the most dramatic break with our past, none doubt the significance of carrying on the drive to create a hospital fit for the 21st century. The new hospital that will replace much of which exists today will be at the forefront of technology and facilities. The needs of patients will, as in 1903, be at the heart of its design. The campus is much loved as a place of trees and green and it is our aim to preserve such characteristics, which sets us apart from so many hospitals. As well as placing the needs of patients at the very centre of this redevelopment, the importance of the hospital continuing, and expanding as a major partner in the training and development of undergraduates and post graduates in medicine and other health care professions is set fair. As well as our commitment to developing our staff for the next century we are also determined to enhance our reputation in clinical research for which we have a large number of staff of national and international reputation.

We could not achieve these aims alone however. It has never been truer that for the hospital to really care for its patients it must do so in collaboration with others. Our historical roots are found in this tradition, from the large number of voluntary groups, to other health care staff that work in the local community, to those who work in social care, and to those who work in other hospitals, most notably at our neighbouring hospital the Queen's Medical Centre.

The Nottingham City Hospital faces the future with hope and excitement, able to look back at a proud history. I am especially proud to be its Chief Executive at this important point in time and to be able to record my personal appreciation of the work done by my predecessors over the last 100 years.

Gerry McSorley
Chief Executive

Glossary

THE co-authors hope this glossary of medical terms will be useful for readers who are unfamiliar with medical terminology.

Angiogram - special X-ray to show arteries
Angioplasty - dilation of narrowed arteries with a balloon
Autoclave - equipment for sterilising surgical instruments
Biochemistry - the science of chemical processes in the living organism
Cardiac catheterisation - a tube put into the heart to take samples and pictures and to measure pressures
Cardiology - the study of the heart and its disorders
Cardiothoracic - relating to the heart and chest
Chemotherapy - treatment with drugs, usually for cancer
CT scanner - equipment which produces cross-sectional images of a selected part of the body
Cytology - the study of tissues and their cells
Cytotoxic - drugs used in the treatment of cancer to suppress the division of cells
Defibrillator - equipment which delivers a controlled electric shock to restore a regular heart beat
Dialysis - a technique for purifying the blood as a substitute for the normal function of the kidney
ECG (electrocardiograph) - machine to measure the small, varying, electrical impulses which occur in heart muscle at each beat
Endoscopy - direct visual internal examination using a flexible optical instrument (endoscope)
Enzyme - complex proteins produced by the body to trigger biochemical changes essential to life
Gastro-enterology - the study of the function and diseases of the stomach and intestines
Genito-urinary medicine - relating to the reproductive and urinary organs
Genetics - the study of genes and heredity
Gynaecology - specialty dealing with diseases of women
Haematology - the science of blood and blood disorders
Histology - study of the microscopic structure of tissues
HIV - Human Immunodeficiency Virus which can cause AIDS
Hydrotherapy - use of water in treatment
Immunology - study of the body's mechanism for recognising and responding to foreign materials such as bacteria
Keyhole surgery - minimally invasive surgery carried out through a very small incision
Laminar airflow - a special form of ventilation system used in operating theatres
Lithotriptor - equipment to shatter kidney stones
Mammography - an X-ray technique for diagnosing and locating abnormalities of the breast
Maxillo-facial surgery - specialty dealing with disease or injury of the face and mouth
Microbiology - study of micro organisms
Microsurgery - intricate surgery performed using microscopes
Mitral valve surgery - repair/replacement of the heart valves
MRI - Magnetic Resonance Imaging, using scanners to show cross-sections of the body
Neonatal - relating to the first month of life
Nephrology - specialty concerned with the treatment of kidney disease
Neurology - the study of the nervous system and its disorders
Obstetrics - care of women during pregnancy, childbirth and the weeks immediately after
Oncology - the study of the causes and treatment of cancer
Paediatrics - specialty concerned with childhood development and disease
Palliative care - treatment to alleviate symptoms
Pathology - the study of the causes and effects of disease
Pharmacology - the study of drugs, their uses and effectiveness
Radiology - specialty which uses X-rays and other diagnostic tools such as scanners
Radiotherapy - treatment of disease by means of radioactivity
Respiratory medicine - specialty concerned with breathing problems
Rheumatology - the study of rheumatic diseases such as arthritis
Therapeutic - contributing to the treatment or cure of disease
Ultrasound - use of inaudible sound waves to show internal structures
Urology - specialty dealing with the function and disease of the kidneys and urinary tract

HOW THE HOSPITAL LAUNCHED ITS CENTENARY CELEBRATIONS

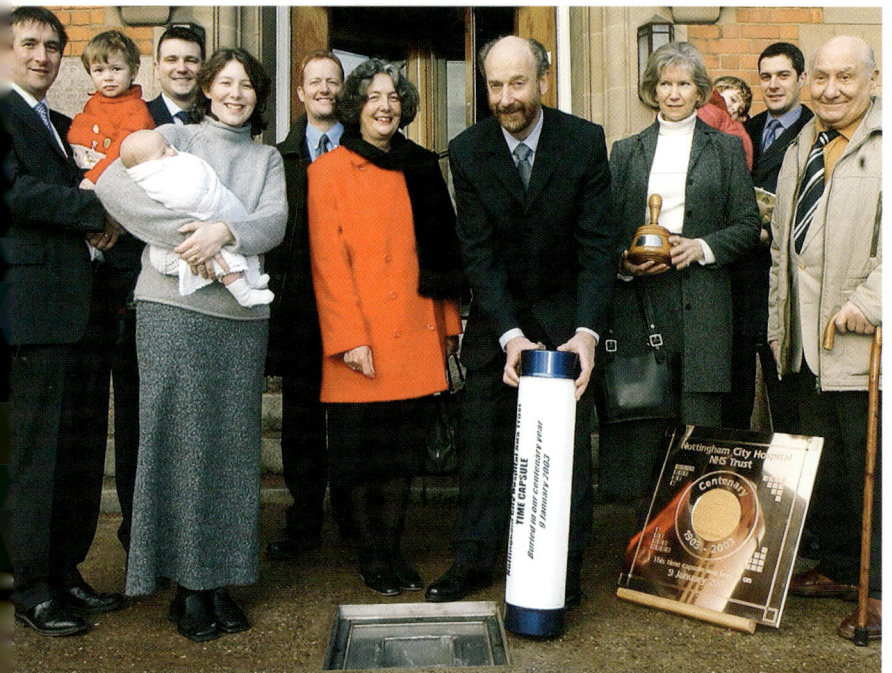

Nottingham City Hospital began its centenary celebrations in January 2003 — by burying a time capsule.

It was a particularly proud occasion for John Palmer, of Wilford, and his family. His grandfather, Councillor Thomas Palmer, Chairman of the Board of Guardians, received a gold key when he opened the workhouse and infirmary in 1903.

A century later 11 members of the Palmer family, ranging in age from 88-year-old John to baby Toby Lloyd, who was born at Nottingham City Hospital in October 2002, were invited to bury the time capsule to give future generations an idea of what the hospital was like in the early 21st century.

The capsule was buried in the pavement at the foot of the steps leading into the hospital's headquarters building — just beneath the foundation stone which was put in place in 1897 as construction began.

Among the items buried in the capsule were a copy of the Nottingham Evening Post for January 9, 2003, minutes from recent hospital board meetings, statistics on the hospital and a CD of the hospital website.

Also in the cylinder are aerial pictures of the hospital site, early proofs of this book, a surgical instrument and letters from the hospital's Chairman Christine Bowering, Chief Executive Gerry McSorley and Secretary of State for Health Alan Milburn.

Mr John Palmer (far right) is pictured with members of his family at the ceremony to bury the time capsule.

Picture credits and bibliography

PHOTOGRAPHS and illustrations used in this book were from many sources. Every endeavour has been made to obtain permission to reproduce copyright material but apology is offered to any whose rights may have been inadvertently infringed.

Grateful thanks are expressed to the following:

Front and back cover: Kenneth Adams of Derby; Nottingham City Hospital; John Birdsall Social Issues Photo Library (www.JohnBirdsall.co.uk) and Nottingham Evening Post
 i www.JohnBirdsall.co.uk
iii City Hospital
 v City Hospital
 1 *Montage* Paul Swift and City Hospital
2 Paul Swift
3 City Hospital
4 & 5 *Montage* Paul Swift and City Hospital
6 Paul Swift and City Hospital
7 Paul Swift
8 Paul Swift
9 Paul Swift
10 Paul Swift
11 Paul Swift
12 Paul Swift
13 Paul Swift
14 Paul Swift
15 Evening Post
16 & 17 *Montage* Paul Swift, City Hospital and Evening Post
18 Kenneth Adams, Paul Swift and Mrs Joan Tomlinson
19 Mrs Joan Tomlinson
20 Paul Swift and Mrs Mavis Astill
21 Paul Swift and Miss Lesley Baker
22 City Hospital
23 Paul Swift
24 Paul Swift
25 Mrs Margaret Lander, Beeston
26 Paul Swift
27 Evening Post
28 Evening Post and City Hospital
29 Evening Post
30 Evening Post
32 & 33 *Montage* Evening Post, www.JohnBirdsall.co.uk, Paul Swift and City Hospital
34 Paul Swift
35 Paul Swift
36 Judith Scott
37 Paul Swift
38 Sister Audrey Wade, Paul Swift and City Hospital
39 City Hospital
40 City Hospital and Mrs McDermott of Chilwell
41 Mrs McDermott, Mrs Joy Browne of Old Clipstone, Mansfield
42 Evening Post and Paul Swift
43 F W Loasby of Mapperley, Paul Swift and Evening Post
44 www.JohnBirdsall.co.uk, City Hospital
45 www.JohnBirdsall.co.uk and City Hospital
46 and **47** *Montage* Evening Post, www.JohnBirdsall.co.uk and City Hospital
48 Evening Post
49 www.JohnBirdsall.co.uk
50 City Hospital and Evening Post
51 City Hospital
52 David Banks
53 City Hospital
54 Evening Post
55 Evening Post
56 www.JohnBirdsall.co.uk and Evening Post
57 Evening Post
58 Evening Post
59 Evening Post
60 Evening Post
61 Evening Post
62 Evening Post
63 www.JohnBirdsall.co.uk
64 Evening Post
65 Evening Post and City Hospital
66 Neil Culm
67 Evening Post
68 and **69** *Montage* Evening Post and www.JohnBirdsall.co.uk
70 City Hospital and www.JohnBirdsall.co.uk
71 Evening Post
72 www.JohnBirdsall.co.uk
73 Evening Post
74 City Hospital and www.JohnBirdsall.co.uk
75 Evening Post
76 Evening Post and www.JohnBirdsall.co.uk
77 www.JohnBirdsall.co.uk and City Hospital
78 www.JohnBirdsall.co.uk
79 www.JohnBirdsall.co.uk
80 and **81** Paul Swift and City Hospital
82 City Hospital
83 City Hospital
84 Paul Swift
85 City Hospital
86 City Hospital
87 Paul Swift and Evening Post
88 and **89** Evening Post and Department of Manuscripts and Special Collections, the University of Nottingham
90 Paul Swift
91 Evening Post
92 City Hospital
93 City Hospital and Evening Post
94 and **95** *Montage* Evening Post and City Hospital
96 Paul Swift
97 Evening Post
98 Evening Post
99 David Banks
100 Evening Post
101 Evening Post
102 Evening Post
103 City Hospital
104 Evening Post

Many references have been used by David Lowe and Paul Swift in compiling this book. The authors gratefully acknowledge the following sources:

Bagthorpe to the City, Story of a Nottingham Hospital by James Macfie, published by Nottingham Health Authority.

Nottingham General Hospital: Personal Reflections by John Bittiner and David Lowe, published by Special Trustees for Nottingham University Hospitals.

A Nurse in Time by Evelyn Prentis, published by Hutchinson. Reprinted by permission of The Random House Group Ltd.

Archive material held by the Nottingham Evening Post, the University of Nottingham and Nottingham City Council Leisure and Community Services (Angel Row Library).

Index

NB: Page numbers in *italics* indicate illustrations or photographs

Administration/management 82-3
Airie, Tom 53, 90
Aitken, Sir Robert 23
Alexandra ward 14
Ambulance service 81
Annakin, Miss 38, 39
Ashwell, H G 2, 9, 14
Astill, Mavis 20

Bader, Douglas 3, 23, *26*, 64
Bagthorpe to the City: A Story of a Nottingham Hospital 13, 25
Bagthorpe Workhouse and Infirmary 1, 2, 5-6, *6*, 7, *7*, 8-13, 31, *34*, 36-7, 50
Bain, Mr 64
Baker, Lesley, 64-5
Balfour, Tom 53
Banks, David 26, 50, 52, 53-4, 61, 91, 96, 101
Barclay, Robert 48-9, 75
Barer, D 53
Bark, Chris *56*
Barkla, Paul 64
Barnett, Minnie 36, *36*
Basford Hospital 100
Bates, Patrick 27, 54-5
Bath, Philip 51
Batterbury, Roy 29, 31, 82
Battersby, Tom 61
Beckingham, Ian 56
Beers, Mary 17, 19
Bell, Duncan 53
Benton, Myles 55
Bessell, Eric 73
Beveridge, Sir William 2
Birkett, Noel 14, 63
Bishop, Michael 54-5, *95*
Black, Douglas 71
Blamey, Roger 26, 27, 55-6, *56*, 90, 102
Bone marrow transplantation 59
Boobbyer, Philip, 7-8, *8*
Booth, Ann 71
Boots Company 29, 53, 102
Bossingham, David 91, 92
Boswell, Tim 61
Bowering, Christine iii, *iii*, 77, 98, 100
Bowman, Christine 91, 92
Braddock, Alderman E A *38*
Bramall, Alan 53
Breast care/Helen Garrod screening unit 3, 48, *54*, 55, 71, 75, 98
Briddon, Margaret *41*
Briggs, Judy 101
Britton, John 101
Brock, Sir Russell 49
Bromige, Mike 49
Brook, David 67
Brooksbank, Judy 42, 49, 50
Bruce, John 64
Buckley, William 48, 49
Bullen, Margaret (née Haugh) 38
Burden, Richard 55, 95, 96

Burns Unit 3, 28, 50, 61, 62, *64*, 71, 101
BUSH (Burns Unit Self-Help) 101
Butchery service 86
Butterfield, Lord 26, 91
Byrne, Jenny 59

Campbell, J P 63
Cancer/cancer care 3, 57-8, 60, 73, 79, 83
Cancer Relief Macmillan Fund 97
Cancer Research Campaign 57, 73
Cardiac intensive care 3, *74*
Cardiac support group 101
Cardiac surgery/cardiology 3, 48-9, 51-2
Cardiology 51-2, *52*
CARE Appeal 3, 95-6, 99
Carlisle, Sir Michael 95
Carmichael, Jim 57, 73
Car parking/bus services 75-6
Catering department 85, *85*, 86
Cayley, Mrs 92
Chambers, John 86-7
Chaplaincy/church services 87, *87*
Charity ward 11
Charnley, Sir John 9, 63
Charnley Suite 9, 14
Chest diseases 50-1
Children and Young People's Clinic 66
Children's education 22-3
Children's outpatients 3, 71
Children's wards 9
Christmas shows 29, 95
City Hospital School of Nursing 2
City Infirmary/City Hospital 2, 9, *10*, 11, *11*, 28, 38, 39-41
City Side Restaurant 86
Clark, Rebecca *78*
Clayton, Sir Stanley 26, *28*
Cleaning services 84
Cleft lip/palate surgery 15, 62
Clinical genetics 3, 28, 67
Clinical nurse managers 45
Clinical radiology 3
Clinical Sciences Building 3, 59, 64, 73, 90, *92*, 97
Cochrane, J B 2, *11*, 12, *24*, 24-25, *25*, 28, 38, 39, 64, 101
Cocor, Cristina 60, *61*, 79
Community involvement 95-102
Cooke, Pat 67
Cooksey, Graeme 56
Cooper, Irene *41*
Corcoran, Ray 96
Coronary care 3, 27, 28
Cotton, Roger 23, 31, 57, *59*, 71, 91
Coultas, Robert 49
Cove-Smith, Rodney 28-9
Cox, Don 11
Crocker, Cheryl 77
Cross, Gareth 67
Crowe, Crawford 13, 24, *24*
Crowther, Leslie 29
Curnock, David *61*, 66, 75
Cystic fibrosis 51, 65, 90
Cystic Fibrosis Trust 65

Dale, Lynne 52
David Evans Research Centre 14, 59, 96
Davies, Dewi 50, 95, 101
Daykin triplets *21*
Day surgery 3, 75
Deakin, Norman *61*, 77

Dennis, Dr 56
Dialysis 3, 28, 55-6, 61, 73, 90
Dinners/parties 29
Diphtheria 5, 9, 17
Disablement services centre 3
Don, Dr 65
Donald, Fiona 61
Donaldson, Sir Liam 3
Donations/fundraising 30, *54*, 55, 87, *96*, 97, 98, *98*
Dorrell, Stephen 75
Duff, Robert 30, 52
Dunn, Mike 54
Dwight, Miss *34*
Dyson, Jenny 57

Edward ward 35
Edward One ward 37, 64
Edward Two ward 64
Elderly, health care of the 52-3
Electricity supplies 86-7
Ellerslie House 102
Ellis, Ian 28
Elston, Christopher 55, 57
Elston, Doreen *38*
Emergency admissions 79
Emsley, Ken 64
Endoscopy 3, 75, 77
Ethiopia 101-2
Evans, Christine 56
Evans, David 14, *14*, 59, 95, 96, *96*, 99
Evans, J M *43*
Evans-Farley, Suzannah 98

Fell, Kim 79
Fentem, Peter 51
Finance department 83
Finch, Roger 60-61
Firs Maternity Hospital 24, 35, 37, 39, 49, 50
First World War 2, 8, 35, 82
Fitzsimmons, John 65-6, 67, 73
Fleming, Sir Alexander 14
Fleming ward 30
Fletcher, John 14, 30-1, 58, 59, 71, 91
Fletcher ward, 14
Foote, J B 22
Forest Dean 50, 51
Foster, Alderman Eric 37
Foster, Dr 56
Fox, Jenny 52
Frankton, Anne *58*
Fraser ward 57
Fraser, William 14, 57
French, Shelagh, 59
Frostick, Simon 63
Future vision 103

Gastro-enterology 53
Gaythorpe, Cynthia 97
Gedling ward 27, 71
Genetics 67, 83
Genito-urinary 3, 71
Geriatric medicine 3, 13, 31, 52-3
Gerrard, Miss 39
Gervis Pearson, Noel 15, 58
Gervis Pearson ward 57-8
Gilby, John 69, *71*, 77, 99
Giles, Martin 52
Gill, Ivy 35-6
Gloucester, HRH the Duchess of 2, *2*, 3, 19, 31, 57, 71, 95
Gordon, K 27
Gould, Geoffrey *2*
Graham, Robert 90
Gray, Matt 27 54
Green, Alderman W 9

Greenfield, David 25
Guardians, Nottingham Board of 2, 5-7, 8, *8*, 9
Guilbert, Penny 67

Haematology 28, 58-9, *79*, 90, 103
Hale, Paula 66
Hall, Leslie 22, 47
Hamilton, Lady 3, 25
Hampton, John 30
Harlow Wood Orthopaedic Hospital 63
Haynes, Andrew 59
Hayre, Greta 39
Hayward House - palliative care 3, 28, *28*, 96-7, 102
H Block 3, 21, 28, 31, 55, 61, 65, 67, 73
Heart research unit appeal 98
Heathfield 9, 28, 40, 51, 65, 84, 100
Heathfield wards 17
Henry, David 53
Higgins, Tony 96
Higginson, Marie *64*
Hill, Ian 96
Hiller, Joan 65, 66
Hilton, Donna *67*, 77, *100*
Histopathology *27*, 56, 57, *57*, 78
Hodges, Janet 43
Hodson, Sue 92
Hogarth, Roger 58
Hogarth ward 58, 59
Holland, Alderman Percy 96
Holland, Thelma 72-3, 77-8, 102
Holmes-Sellors, Sir Thomas 26
Hooley, Mary M 24, *24*, *34*, 37
Hopkins, Harold 54
Horan, Dr 53
Hospital Information Support System (HISS) 83-4
Hospital name changes 2, 3, 8, 9, 11, 33, 75
Hospital sport 99
Hospitals' choir 99
Hounsfield, Sir Godfrey 48
HRH Princess Margaret 3, 62, 97
HRH Queen Elizabeth 23, 51
Hucknall Orthopaedic Clinic 63
Hughes, John *85*, 86
Hull, Sir David 66
Hurley, Mr 28

Ilkeston Community Hospital 62
Infection control service 60, 61
Infectious diseases 3, 60-1, *61*
Influenza epidemic 36-7
Information and communication technology (ICT) 83-4
Institute of Genetics 67
Intensive care 48-9, 70
International links 101-2
Isolation Hospital 5-7, 9, 17

Jackson, Peter 90
Jagger, Chris 73
James, Ray 101
James, Sam 9, 15, 62
James ward, 9, 49
Jarvis, Chris 65
Jeffcoate, William 91, 92, 95
Jeffier, J V 27
Jelley, Alderman John 6-7
Jenkins, Gladys *41*
Jenner ward 22
Jequier, Miss 64
Jew, Sister *18*, *40*